WORLD HEALTH ORGANIZATION

CORRIGENDA

ENVIRONMENTAL HEALTH CRITERIA
NO. 216

DISINFECTANTS AND DISINFECTANT BYPRODUCTS

Section 4.5.1, page 237, 2nd paragraph: The last four lines should read

[Rats] tolerated doses of 200 mg/kg of body weight administered by gavage but displayed severe symptoms including dyspnoea, laborious breathing, depressed motor activity and cyanosis at higher doses (Komulainen et al., 1994). At necropsy, gastrointestinal inflammation was observed, and oedema was noted in the lungs and kidneys. An LD_{50} of 230 kg/kg in 48 hours was identified in this study

Sections 3.1.4, 3.2.4, 4.1.2.5, 4.1.3.5, and 4.1.4.5

After the printing of the document, Dr James Huff kindly brought to the attention of the Secretariat that a study on the carcinogenicity of sodium hypochlorite, and another on the carcinogenicity of bromodichloromethane, chlorodibromomethane, bromoform, chlorine, and chloramine, were not cited in the document. The authors' abstracts of these studies are given below.

*Soffritti M, Belpoggi F, Lenzi A, Maltoni C (1997) Results of long-term carcinogenicity studies of chlorine in rats. **Ann NY Acad Sci**, 837: 189-208.*

Four groups, each of 50 male and 50 female Sprague-Dawley rats, of the colony used in the Cancer Research Center of Bentivoglio of the Ramazzini Foundation, 12 weeks old at the start of the study, received drinking water containing sodium hypochlorite, resulting in concentrations of active chlorine of 750, 500, and 100 mg/l (treated groups), and tap water (active chlorine < 0.2 mg/l) (control group), respectively, for 104 weeks. Among the female rats of the treated groups, an increased incidence of lymphomas and leukemias has been observed, although this is not clearly dose related. Moreover, sporadic cases of some tumors, the occurrence of which is extremely unusual among the untreated rats of the colony used (historical controls), were detected in chlorine-exposed animals. The results of this study confirm the results of the experiment of the United States National Toxicology Program (1991), which showed an increase of leukemia among female Fischer 344/N rats following the administration of chlorine (in the form of sodium hypochlorite and chloramine) in their drinking water. The data here presented call for further research aimed at quantifying the oncogenic risks related to the chlorination of drinking water, to be used as a basis for consequent public health measures.

Dunnick JK, Melnick RL (1993) Assessment of the carcinogenic potential of chlorinated water: experimental studies of chlorine, chloramine, and trihalomethanes. **J Natl Cancer Inst**, 85: 817-822

BACKGROUND: Water chlorination has been one of the major disease prevention treatments of this century. While epidemiologic studies suggest an association between cancer in humans and consumption of chlorination byproducts in drinking water, these studies have not been adequate to draw definite conclusions about the carcinogenic potential of the individual byproducts.

PURPOSE: The purpose of this study was to investigate the carcinogenic potential of chlorinated or chloraminated drinking water and of four organic trihalomethane byproducts of chlorination (chloroform, bromodichloromethane, chlorodibromomethane, and bromoform) in rats and mice.

METHODS: Bromodichloromethane, chlorodibromomethane, bromoform, chlorine, or chloramine was administered to both sexes of F344/N rats and (C57BL/6 x C3H)F1 mice (hereafter called B6C3F1 mice). Chloroform was given to both sexes of Osborne-Mendel rats and B6C3F1 mice. Chlorine or chloramine was administered daily in the drinking water for 2 years at doses ranging from 0.05 to 0.3 mmol/kg per day. The trihalomethanes were administered by gavage in corn oil at doses ranging from 0.15 to 4.0 mmol/kg per day for 2 years, with the exception of chloroform, which was given for 78 weeks.

RESULTS: The trihalomethanes were carcinogenic in the liver, kidney, and/or intestine of rodents. There was equivocal evidence for carcinogenicity in female rats that received chlorinated or chloraminated drinking water: this evidence was based on a marginal increase in the incidence of mononuclear cell leukemia. Rodents were generally exposed to lower doses of chlorine and chloramine than to the trihalomethanes, but the doses in these studies were the maximum that the animals would consume in the drinking water. The highest doses used in the chlorine and chloramine studies were equivalent to a daily gavage dose of bromodichloromethane that induced neoplasms of the large intestine in rats. In contrast to the results with the trihalomethanes, administration of chlorine or chloramine did not cause a clear carcinogenic response in rats or mice after long-term exposure.

CONCLUSION: These results suggest that organic byproducts of chlorination are the chemicals of greatest concern in assessment of the carcinogenic potential of chlorinated drinking water.

Environmental Health Criteria 216

DISINFECTANTS AND DISINFECTANT BY-PRODUCTS

First draft prepared by G. Amy, University of Colorado, Boulder, Colorado, USA; R. Bull, Battelle Pacific Northwest Laboratory, Richland, Washington, USA; G.F. Craun, Gunther F. Craun and Associates, Staunton, Virginia, USA; R.A. Pegram, US Environmental Protection Agency, Research Triangle Park, North Carolina, USA; and M. Siddiqui, University of Colorado, Boulder, Colorado, USA

Published under the joint sponsorship of the United Nations Environment Programme, the International Labour Organisation and the World Health Organization, and produced within the framework of the Inter-Organization Programme for the Sound Management of Chemicals.

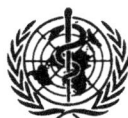

World Health Organization
Geneva, 2000

The **International Programme on Chemical Safety (IPCS)**, established in 1980, is a joint venture of the United Nations Environment Programme (UNEP), the International Labour Organisation (ILO) and the World Health Organization (WHO). The overall objectives of the IPCS are to establish the scientific basis for assessment of the risk to human health and the environment from exposure to chemicals, through international peer review processes, as a prerequisite for the promotion of chemical safety, and to provide technical assistance in strengthening national capacities for the sound management of chemicals.

The **Inter-Organization Programme for the Sound Management of Chemicals (IOMC)** was established in 1995 by UNEP, ILO, the Food and Agriculture Organization of the United Nations, WHO, the United Nations Industrial Development Organization and the Organisation for Economic Co-operation and Development (Participating Organizations), following recommendations made by the 1992 UN Conference on Environment and Development to strengthen cooperation and increase coordination in the field of chemical safety. The purpose of the IOMC is to promote coordination of the policies and activities pursued by the Participating Organizations, jointly or separately, to achieve the sound management of chemicals in relation to human health and the environment.

WHO Library Cataloguing-in-Publication Data

Disinfectants and disinfectant by-products.

(Environmental health criteria ; 216)

1.Disinfectants - chemistry 2.Disinfectants - toxicity 3.Drinking water
4.Risk assessment 5.Epidemiologic studies I.Series

ISBN 92 4 157216 7 (NLM Classification: QV 220)
ISSN 0250-863X

CONTENTS

ENVIRONMENTAL HEALTH CRITERIA FOR DISINFECTANTS AND DISINFECTANT BY-PRODUCTS

NOTE TO READERS OF THE CRITERIA MONOGRAPHS

Every effort has been made to present information in the criteria monographs as accurately as possible without unduly delaying their publication. In the interest of all users of the Environmental Health Criteria monographs, readers are requested to communicate any errors that may have occurred to the Director of the International Programme on Chemical Safety, World Health Organization, Geneva, Switzerland, in order that they may be included in corrigenda.

* * *

A detailed data profile and a legal file can be obtained from the International Register of Potentially Toxic Chemicals, Case postale 356, 1219 Châtelaine, Geneva, Switzerland (telephone no. + 41 22 – 9799111, fax no. + 41 22 – 7973460, E-mail irptc@unep.ch).

Environmental Health Criteria

PREAMBLE

Objectives

In 1973, the WHO Environmental Health Criteria Programme was initiated with the following objectives:

(i) to assess information on the relationship between exposure to environmental pollutants and human health, and to provide guidelines for setting exposure limits;

(ii) to identify new or potential pollutants;

(iii) to identify gaps in knowledge concerning the health effects of pollutants;

(iv) to promote the harmonization of toxicological and epidemiological methods in order to have internationally comparable results.

The first Environmental Health Criteria (EHC) monograph, on mercury, was published in 1976, and since that time an ever-increasing number of assessments of chemicals and of physical effects have been produced. In addition, many EHC monographs have been devoted to evaluating toxicological methodology, e.g., for genetic, neurotoxic, teratogenic and nephrotoxic effects. Other publications have been concerned with epidemiological guidelines, evaluation of short-term tests for carcinogens, biomarkers, effects on the elderly and so forth.

Since its inauguration, the EHC Programme has widened its scope, and the importance of environmental effects, in addition to health effects, has been increasingly emphasized in the total evaluation of chemicals.

The original impetus for the Programme came from World Health Assembly resolutions and the recommendations of the 1972 UN Conference on the Human Environment. Subsequently, the work became an integral part of the International Programme on Chemical

Safety (IPCS), a cooperative programme of UNEP, ILO and WHO. In this manner, with the strong support of the new partners, the importance of occupational health and environmental effects was fully recognized. The EHC monographs have become widely established, used and recognized throughout the world.

The recommendations of the 1992 UN Conference on Environment and Development and the subsequent establishment of the Intergovernmental Forum on Chemical Safety with the priorities for action in the six programme areas of Chapter 19, Agenda 21, all lend further weight to the need for EHC assessments of the risks of chemicals.

Scope

The criteria monographs are intended to provide critical reviews on the effects on human health and the environment of chemicals and of combinations of chemicals and physical and biological agents. As such, they include and review studies that are of direct relevance for the evaluation. However, they do not describe *every* study carried out. Worldwide data are used and are quoted from original studies, not from abstracts or reviews. Both published and unpublished reports are considered, and it is incumbent on the authors to assess all the articles cited in the references. Preference is always given to published data. Unpublished data are used only when relevant published data are absent or when they are pivotal to the risk assessment. A detailed policy statement is available that describes the procedures used for unpublished proprietary data so that this information can be used in the evaluation without compromising its confidential nature (WHO (1990) Revised Guidelines for the Preparation of Environmental Health Criteria Monographs. PCS/90.69, Geneva, World Health Organization).

In the evaluation of human health risks, sound human data, whenever available, are preferred to animal data. Animal and *in vitro* studies provide support and are used mainly to supply evidence missing from human studies. It is mandatory that research on human subjects is conducted in full accord with ethical principles, including the provisions of the Helsinki Declaration.

The EHC monographs are intended to assist national and international authorities in making risk assessments and subsequent risk management decisions. They represent a thorough evaluation of risks and are not, in any sense, recommendations for regulation or standard setting. These latter are the exclusive purview of national and regional governments.

Content

The layout of EHC monographs for chemicals is outlined below.

- Summary — a review of the salient facts and the risk evaluation of the chemical
- Identity — physical and chemical properties, analytical methods
- Sources of exposure
- Environmental transport, distribution and transformation
- Environmental levels and human exposure
- Kinetics and metabolism in laboratory animals and humans
- Effects on laboratory mammals and *in vitro* test systems
- Effects on humans
- Effects on other organisms in the laboratory and field
- Evaluation of human health risks and effects on the environment
- Conclusions and recommendations for protection of human health and the environment
- Further research
- Previous evaluations by international bodies, e.g., IARC, JECFA, JMPR

Selection of chemicals

Since the inception of the EHC Programme, the IPCS has organized meetings of scientists to establish lists of priority chemicals for subsequent evaluation. Such meetings have been held in: Ispra, Italy, 1980; Oxford, United Kingdom, 1984; Berlin, Germany, 1987; and North Carolina, USA, 1995. The selection of chemicals has been based on the following criteria: the existence of scientific evidence that the substance presents a hazard to human health and/or the environment; the possible use, persistence, accumulation or degradation of the substance shows that there may be significant human or environmental exposure; the size and nature of populations at risk (both human and other species) and risks for the environment; international concern, i.e., the substance is of major interest to several countries; adequate data on the hazards are available.

If an EHC monograph is proposed for a chemical not on the priority list, the IPCS Secretariat consults with the cooperating organizations and all the Participating Institutions before embarking on the preparation of the monograph.

Procedures

The order of procedures that result in the publication of an EHC monograph is shown in the flow chart. A designated staff member of IPCS, responsible for the scientific quality of the document, serves as Responsible Officer (RO). The IPCS Editor is responsible for layout and language. The first draft, prepared by consultants or, more usually, staff from an IPCS Participating Institution, is based initially on data provided from the International Register of Potentially Toxic Chemicals and from reference databases such as Medline and Toxline.

The draft document, when received by the RO, may require an initial review by a small panel of experts to determine its scientific quality and objectivity. Once the RO finds the document acceptable as a first draft, it is distributed, in its unedited form, to well over 150 EHC contact points throughout the world who are asked to comment on its completeness and accuracy and, where necessary, provide additional material. The contact points, usually designated by governments, may be Participating Institutions, IPCS Focal Points or individual scientists known for their particular expertise. Generally, some four months are allowed before the comments are considered by the RO and author(s). A second draft incorporating comments received and approved by the Director, IPCS, is then distributed to Task Group members, who carry out the peer review, at least six weeks before their meeting.

The Task Group members serve as individual scientists, not as representatives of any organization, government or industry. Their function is to evaluate the accuracy, significance and relevance of the

EHC PREPARATION FLOW CHART

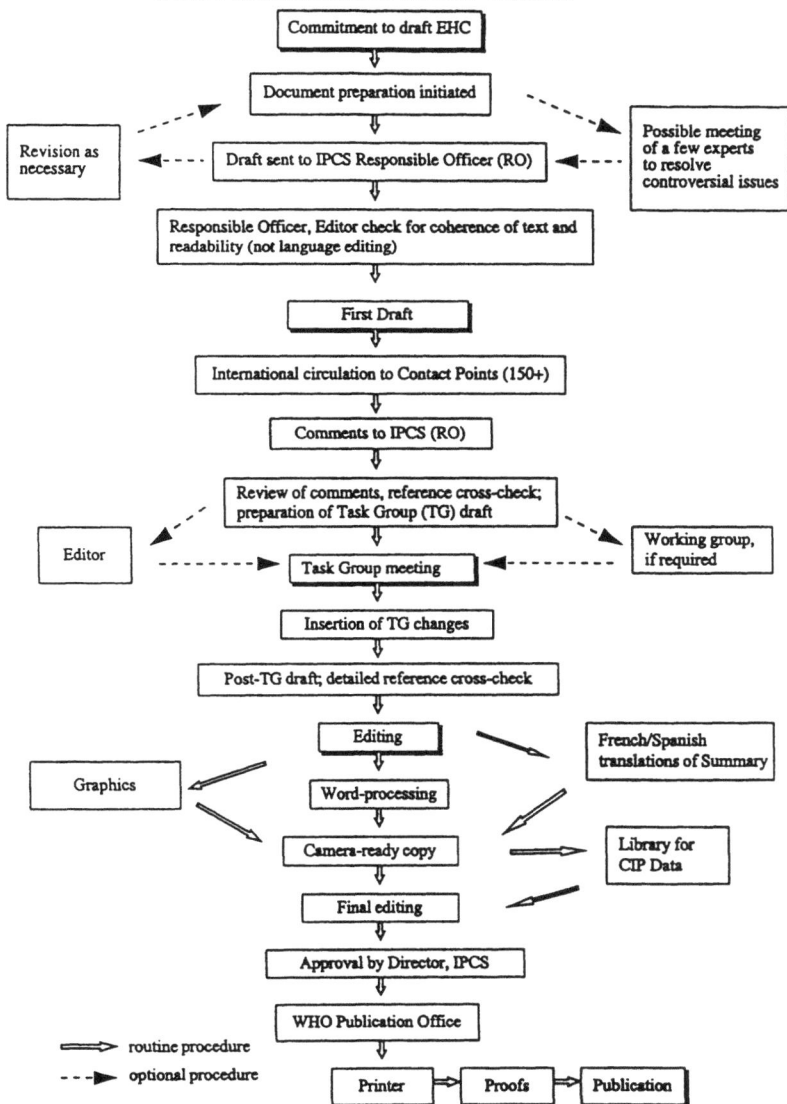

```
                    ┌─────────────────────────┐
                    │  Commitment to draft EHC │
                    └─────────────────────────┘
                                 ⇓
                    ┌─────────────────────────────┐
                    │ Document preparation initiated │
                    └─────────────────────────────┘
```

Commitment to draft EHC

Document preparation initiated

┌──────────────┐
│ Revision as │
│ necessary   │
└──────────────┘

Draft sent to IPCS Responsible Officer (RO)

┌─────────────────────┐
│ Possible meeting   │
│ of a few experts   │
│ to resolve   │
│ controversial issues │
└─────────────────────┘

Responsible Officer, Editor check for coherence of text and readability (not language editing)

First Draft

International circulation to Contact Points (150+)

Comments to IPCS (RO)

Review of comments, reference cross-check; preparation of Task Group (TG) draft

Editor

Task Group meeting

Working group, if required

Insertion of TG changes

Post-TG draft; detailed reference cross-check

Editing

French/Spanish translations of Summary

Graphics

Word-processing

Camera-ready copy

Library for CIP Data

Final editing

Approval by Director, IPCS

WHO Publication Office

⇒ routine procedure

- - ▶ optional procedure

Printer ⇨ Proofs ⇨ Publication

information in the document and to assess the health and environmental risks from exposure to the chemical. A summary and recommendations for further research and improved safety aspects are also required. The composition of the Task Group is dictated by the range of expertise required for the subject of the meeting and by the need for a balanced geographical distribution.

The three cooperating organizations of the IPCS recognize the important role played by nongovernmental organizations. Representatives from relevant national and international associations may be invited to join the Task Group as observers. While observers may provide a valuable contribution to the process, they can speak only at the invitation of the Chairperson. Observers do not participate in the final evaluation of the chemical; this is the sole responsibility of the Task Group members. When the Task Group considers it to be appropriate, it may meet *in camera*.

All individuals who as authors, consultants or advisers participate in the preparation of the EHC monograph must, in addition to serving in their personal capacity as scientists, inform the RO if at any time a conflict of interest, whether actual or potential, could be perceived in their work. They are required to sign a conflict of interest statement. Such a procedure ensures the transparency and probity of the process.

When the Task Group has completed its review and the RO is satisfied as to the scientific correctness and completeness of the document, the document then goes for language editing, reference checking and preparation of camera-ready copy. After approval by the Director, IPCS, the monograph is submitted to the WHO Office of Publications for printing. At this time, a copy of the final draft is sent to the Chairperson and Rapporteur of the Task Group to check for any errors.

It is accepted that the following criteria should initiate the updating of an EHC monograph: new data are available that would substantially change the evaluation; there is public concern for health or environmental effects of the agent because of greater exposure; an appreciable time period has elapsed since the last evaluation.

All Participating Institutions are informed, through the EHC progress report, of the authors and institutions proposed for the drafting of the documents. A comprehensive file of all comments received on drafts of each EHC monograph is maintained and is available on request. The Chairpersons of Task Groups are briefed before each meeting on their role and responsibility in ensuring that these rules are followed.

WHO TASK GROUP ON ENVIRONMENTAL HEALTH CRITERIA FOR DISINFECTANTS AND DISINFECTANT BY-PRODUCTS

Members

Dr G. Amy, Department of Civil, Environmental, and Architectural Engineering, University of Colorado, Boulder, Colorado, USA

Mr J. Fawell, Water Research Centre, Marlow, Buckinghamshire, United Kingdom (*Co-Rapporteur*)

Dr B. Havlik, Ministry of Health, National Institute of Public Health, Prague, Czech Republic

Dr C. Nokes, Water Group, Institute of Environmental Science and Research, Christchurch, New Zealand (*Co-Rapporteur*)

Dr E. Ohanian, Office of Water/Office of Science and Technology, United States Environmental Protection Agency, Washington, DC, USA (*Chairman*)

Dr E. Soderlund, Department of Environmental Medicine, National Institute of Public Health, Torshov, Oslo

Secretariat

Dr J. Bartram, Water, Sanitation and Health Unit, Division of Operational Support in Environment Health, World Health Organization, Geneva, Switzerland

Dr R. Bull, Battelle Pacific Northwest Laboratory, Richland, Washington, USA

Mr G.F. Craun, Gunther F. Craun and Associates, Staunton, Virginia, USA

Dr H. Galal-Gorchev, Chevy Chase, Maryland, USA (*Secretary*)

Mr N. Nakashima, Assessment of Risk and Methodologies, International Programme on Chemical Safety, World Health Organization, Geneva, Switzerland

Dr R.A. Pegram, United States Environmental Protection Agency, Research Triangle Park, North Carolina, USA

Mr S.T. Yamamura, Water, Sanitation and Health Unit, Division of Operational Support in Environment Health, World Health Organization, Geneva, Switzerland

Representatives/Observers

Dr N. Drouot, Dept Toxicologie Industrielle, Paris, France (representing European Centre for Ecotoxicology and Toxicology of Chemicals)

Mr O. Hydes, Drinking Water Inspectorate, London, United Kingdom

Dr B.B. Sandel, Olin Corporation, Norwalk, Connecticut, USA (representing American Industrial Health Council/International Life Sciences Institute)

IPCS TASK GROUP ON ENVIRONMENTAL HEALTH CRITERIA FOR DISINFECTANTS AND DISINFECTANT BY-PRODUCTS

A WHO Task Group on Environmental Health Criteria for Disinfectants and Disinfectant By-products met in Geneva from 17 to 21 August 1998. Dr Peter Toft, Associate Director, IPCS, welcomed the participants on behalf of the three IPCS cooperating organizations (UNEP/ILO/WHO). The Task Group reviewed and revised the draft document and made an evaluation of risks for human health from exposure to certain disinfectants and disinfectant by-products.

The first draft of the chemistry section was prepared by G. Amy and M. Siddiqui, University of Colorado, Boulder, Colorado, USA; the toxicology section was prepared by R. Bull, Battelle Pacific Northwest Laboratory, Richland, Washington, USA, and R.A. Pegram, US Environmental Protection Agency, Research Triangle Park, North Carolina, USA; and the epidemiology section was prepared by G.F. Craun, Gunther F. Craun and Associates, Staunton, Virginia, USA.

The efforts of all who helped in the preparation and finalization of the monograph are gratefully acknowledged.

* * *

The preparation of the first draft of this Environmental Health Criteria monograph was made possible by the financial support afforded to IPCS by the International Life Sciences Institute.

A financial contribution from the United States Environmental Protection Agency for the convening of the Task Group is gratefully acknowledged.

ACRONYMS AND ABBREVIATIONS

ALAT	alanine aminotransferase
AP	alkaline phosphatase
ARB	atypical residual bodies
ASAT	aspartate aminotransferase
AWWA	American Water Works Association
BAN	bromoacetonitrile
BCA	bromochloroacetic acid/bromochloroacetate
BCAN	bromochloroacetonitrile
BDCA	bromodichloroacetic acid/bromodichloroacetate
BDCM	bromodichloromethane
BUN	blood urea nitrogen
bw	body weight
CAN	chloroacetonitrile
CHO	Chinese hamster ovary
CI	confidence interval
CoA	coenzyme A
C_{max}	maximum concentration
CMCF	3-chloro-4-(chloromethyl)-5-hydroxy-2(5H)-furanone
2-CP	2-chloropropionate
CPN	chloropropanone
CT	computerized tomography
CYP	cytochrome P450
DBA	dibromoacetic acid/dibromoacetate
DBAC	dibromoacetone
DBAN	dibromoacetonitrile
DBCM	dibromochloromethane
DBP	disinfectant by-product
DCA	dichloroacetic acid/dichloroacetate
DCAN	dichloroacetonitrile
DCPN	dichloropropanone
DHAN	dihaloacetonitrile
DOC	dissolved organic carbon
ECD	electron capture detector
ECG	electrocardiogram
EEG	electroencephalogram
EHEN	*N*-ethyl-*N*-hydroxyethylnitrosamine
EPA	Environmental Protection Agency (USA)

ESR	electron spin resonance
FAO	Food and Agriculture Organization of the United Nations
GAC	granular activated carbon
GC	gas chromatography
GGT	γ-glutamyl transpeptidase
GOT	glutamate–oxalate transaminase
GPT	glutamate–pyruvate transaminase
GSH	glutathione-SH
GST	glutathione-*S*-transferase
HAA	haloacetic acid
HAN	haloacetonitrile
HDL	high-density lipoprotein
HPLC	high-performance liquid chromatography
hprt	hypoxanthine phosphoribosyl transferase
IARC	International Agency for Research on Cancer
IC	ion chromatography
i.p.	intraperitoneal
IPCS	International Programme on Chemical Safety
JECFA	Joint FAO/WHO Expert Committee on Food Additives
LD_{50}	median lethal dose
LDH	lactate dehydrogenase
LDL	low-density lipoprotein
LOAEL	lowest-observed-adverse-effect level
MA	3,4-(dichloro)-5-hydroxy-2(5H)-furanone
MBA	monobromoacetic acid/monobromoacetate
MCA	monochloroacetic acid/monochloroacetate
MNU	methylnitrosourea
MOR	mortality odds ratio
MRI	magnetic resonance imaging
MTBE	methyl *tert*-butyl ether
MX	3-chloro-4-(dichloromethyl)-5-hydroxy-2(5H)-furanone
NADP	nicotinamide adenine dinucleotide phosphate
NOAEL	no-observed-adverse-effect level
NOEL	no-observed-effect level
NOM	natural organic matter
NTP	National Toxicology Program (USA)
8-OH-dG	8-hydroxy-2-deoxyguanosine
OR	odds ratio

PAS	periodic acid/Schiff's reagent
PBPK	physiologically based pharmacokinetic model
PFBHA	O-(2,3,4,5,6-pentafluorobenzyl)-hydroxylamine
pK_a	log acid dissociation constant
PPAR	peroxisome proliferator activated receptor
PPRE	peroxisome proliferator responsive element
RR	relative risk
SCE	sister chromatid exchange
SD	standard deviation
SDH	sorbitol dehydrogenase
SE	standard error
SGOT	serum glutamate–oxaloacetate transaminase
SGPT	serum glutamate–pyruvate transaminase
SMR	standardized mortality ratio
SSB	single strand breaks
TBA	tribromoacetic acid/tribromoacetate
TBARS	thiobarbituric acid reactive substances
TCA	trichloroacetic acid/trichloroacetate
TCAN	trichloroacetonitrile
TCPN	trichloropropanone
TDI	tolerable daily intake
TGF	transforming growth factor
THM	trihalomethane
TOC	total organic carbon
TOX	total organic halogen
TPA	12-O-tetradecanoylphorbol-13-acetate
UDS	unscheduled DNA synthesis
UV	ultraviolet
UVA_{254}	UV absorbance at 254 nm
V_{max}	maximum rate of metabolism
WHO	World Health Organization

1. SUMMARY AND EVALUATION

Chlorine (Cl_2) has been widely used throughout the world as a chemical disinfectant, serving as the principal barrier to microbial contaminants in drinking-water. The noteworthy biocidal attributes of chlorine have been somewhat offset by the formation of disinfectant by-products (DBPs) of public health concern during the chlorination process. As a consequence, alternative chemical disinfectants, such as ozone (O_3), chlorine dioxide (ClO_2) and chloramines (NH_2Cl, mono-chloramine), are increasingly being used; however, each has been shown to form its own set of DBPs. Although the microbiological quality of drinking-water cannot be compromised, there is a need to better understand the chemistry, toxicology and epidemiology of chemical disinfectants and their associated DBPs in order to develop a better understanding of the health risks (microbial and chemical) associated with drinking-water and to seek a balance between micro-bial and chemical risks. It is possible to decrease the chemical risk due to DBPs without compromising microbiological quality.

1.1 Chemistry of disinfectants and disinfectant by-products

The most widely used chemical disinfectants are chlorine, ozone, chlorine dioxide and chloramine. The physical and chemical properties of disinfectants and DBPs can affect their behaviour in drinking-water, as well as their toxicology and epidemiology. The chemical disinfec-tants discussed here are all water-soluble oxidants, which are produced either on-site (e.g., ozone) or off-site (e.g., chlorine). They are adminis-tered as a gas (e.g., ozone) or liquid (e.g., hypochlorite) at typical doses of several milligrams per litre, either alone or in combination. The DBPs discussed here are measurable by gas or liquid chromatography and can be classified as organic or inorganic, halogenated (chlorinated or brominated) or non-halogenated, and volatile or non-volatile. Upon their formation, DBPs can be stable or unstable (e.g., decomposition by hydrolysis).

DBPs are formed upon the reaction of chemical disinfectants with DBP precursors. Natural organic matter (NOM), commonly measured by total organic carbon (TOC), serves as the organic precursor, whereas bromide ion (Br⁻) serves as the inorganic precursor. DBP formation is influenced by water quality (e.g., TOC, bromide, pH, temperature, ammonia, carbonate alkalinity) and treatment conditions (e.g., disinfectant dose, contact time, removal of NOM before the point of disinfectant application, prior addition of disinfectant).

Chlorine in the form of hypochlorous acid/hypochlorite ion (HOCl/OCl⁻) reacts with bromide ion, oxidizing it to hypobromous acid/hypobromite ion (HOBr/OBr⁻). Hypochlorous acid (a more powerful oxidant) and hypobromous acid (a more effective halogenating agent) react collectively with NOM to form chlorine DBPs, including trihalomethanes (THMs), haloacetic acids (HAAs), haloacetonitriles (HANs), haloketones, chloral hydrate and chloropicrin. The dominance of chlorine DBP groups generally decreases in the order of THMs, HAAs and HANs. The relative amounts of TOC, bromide and chlorine will affect the species distribution of THMs (four species: chloroform, bromoform, bromodichloromethane [BDCM] and dibromochloromethane [DBCM]), HAAs (up to nine chlorinated/brominated species) and HANs (several chlorinated/brominated species). Generally, chlorinated THM, HAA and HAN species dominate over brominated species, although the opposite may be true in high-bromide waters. Although many specific chlorine DBPs have been identified, a significant percentage of the total organic halogens still remain unaccounted for. Another reaction that occurs with chlorine is the formation of chlorate (ClO_3^-) in concentrated hypochlorite solutions.

Ozone can directly or indirectly react with bromide to form brominated ozone DBPs, including bromate ion (BrO_3^-). In the presence of NOM, non-halogenated organic DBPs, such as aldehydes, ketoacids and carboxylic acids, are formed during ozonation, with aldehydes (e.g., formaldehyde) being dominant. If both NOM and bromide are present, ozonation forms hypobromous acid, which, in turn, leads to the formation of brominated organohalogen compounds (e.g., bromoform).

The major chlorine dioxide DBPs include chlorite (ClO_2^-) and chlorate ions, with no direct formation of organohalogen DBPs. Unlike the other disinfectants, the major chlorine dioxide DBPs are derived from decomposition of the disinfectant as opposed to reaction with precursors.

2

Use of chloramine as a secondary disinfectant generally leads to the formation of cyanogen chloride (CNCl), a nitrogenous compound, and significantly reduced levels of chlorine DBPs. A related issue is the presence of nitrite (NO_2^-) in chloraminated distribution systems.

From the present knowledge of occurrence and health effects, the DBPs of most interest are THMs, HAAs, bromate and chlorite.

The predominant chlorine DBP group has been shown to be THMs, with chloroform and BDCM as the first and second most dominant THM species. HAAs are the second predominant group, with dichloroacetic acid (DCA) and trichloroacetic acid (TCA) being the first and second most dominant species.

Conversion of bromide to bromate upon ozonation is affected by NOM, pH and temperature, among other factors. Levels may range from below detection (2 μg/litre) to several tens of milligrams per litre. Chlorite levels are generally very predictable, ranging from about 50% to 70% of the chlorine dioxide dose administered.

DBPs occur in complex mixtures that are a function of the chemical disinfectant used, water quality conditions and treatment conditions; other factors include the combination/sequential use of multiple disinfectants/oxidants. Moreover, the composition of these mixtures may change seasonally. Clearly, potential chemically related health effects will be a function of exposure to DBP mixtures.

Other than chlorine DBPs (in particular THMs), there are very few data on the occurrence of DBPs in finished water and distribution systems. Based on laboratory databases, empirical models have been developed to predict concentrations of THMs (total THMs and THM species), HAAs (total HAAs and HAA species) and bromate. These models can be used in performance assessment to predict the impact of treatment changes and in exposure assessment to simulate missing or past data (e.g., to predict concentrations of HAAs from THM data).

DBPs can be controlled through DBP precursor control and removal or modified disinfection practice. Coagulation, granular activated carbon, membrane filtration and ozone biofiltration can remove NOM. Other than through the use of membranes, there is little opportunity to effectively remove bromide. Source water protection and control represent non-treatment alternatives to precursor control. Removal of DBPs after formation is not viable for organic DBPs, whereas bromate and chlorite can be removed by activated carbon or reducing agents. It is expected that the optimized use of combinations of disinfectants, functioning as primary and secondary disinfectants, can further control DBPs. There is a trend towards combination/ sequential use of disinfectants; ozone is used exclusively as a primary disinfectant, chloramines exclusively as a secondary disinfectant, and both chlorine and chlorine dioxide in either role.

1.2 Kinetics and metabolism in laboratory animals and humans

1.2.1 Disinfectants

Residual disinfectants are reactive chemicals that will react with organic compounds found in saliva and stomach content, resulting in the formation of by-products. There are significant differences in the pharmacokinetics of ^{36}Cl depending on whether it is obtained from chlorine, chloramine or chlorine dioxide.

1.2.2 Trihalomethanes

The THMs are absorbed, metabolized and eliminated rapidly by mammals after oral or inhalation exposure. Following absorption, the highest tissue concentrations are attained in the fat, liver and kidneys. Half-lives generally range from 0.5 to 3 h, and the primary route of elimination is via metabolism to carbon dioxide. Metabolic activation to reactive intermediates is required for THM toxicity, and the three brominated species are all metabolized more rapidly and to a greater extent than chloroform. The predominant route of metabolism for all the THMs is oxidation via cytochrome P450 (CYP) 2E1, leading to the formation of dihalocarbonyls (i.e., phosgene and brominated congeners), which can be hydrolysed to carbon dioxide or bind to tissue macromolecules. Secondary metabolic pathways are reductive dehalogenation via CYP2B1/2/2E1 (leading to free radical generation) and glutathione (GSH) conjugation via glutathione-*S*-transferase (GST) T1-1, which generates mutagenic intermediates. The brominated THMs are much more likely than chloroform to proceed through the secondary pathways, and GST-mediated conjugation of chloroform to GSH can occur only at extremely high chloroform concentrations or doses.

1.2.3   Haloacetic acids

The kinetics and metabolism of the dihaloacetic and trihaloacetic acids differ significantly. To the extent they are metabolized, the principal reactions of the trihaloacetic acids occur in the microsomal fraction, whereas more than 90% of the dihaloacetic acid metabolism, principally by glutathione transferases, is observed in the cytosol. TCA has a biological half-life in humans of 50 h. The half-lives of the other trihaloacetic acids decrease significantly with bromine substitution, and measurable amounts of the dihaloacetic acids can be detected as products with brominated trihaloacetic acids. The half-lives of the dihaloacetic acids are very short at low doses but can be drastically increased as dose rates are increased.

1.2.4   Haloaldehydes and haloketones

Limited kinetic data are available for chloral hydrate. The two major metabolites of chloral hydrate are trichloroethanol and TCA. Trichloroethanol undergoes rapid glucuronidation, enterohepatic circulation, hydrolysis and oxidation to TCA. Dechlorination of trichloroethanol or chloral hydrate would lead to the formation of DCA. DCA may then be further transformed to monochloroacetate (MCA), glyoxalate, glycolate and oxalate, probably through a reactive intermediate. No information was found on the other haloaldehydes and haloketones.

1.2.5   Haloacetonitriles

The metabolism and kinetics of HANs have not been studied. Qualitative data indicate that the products of metabolism include cyanide, formaldehyde, formyl cyanide and formyl halides.

1.2.6   Halogenated hydroxyfuranone derivatives

3-Chloro-4-(dichloromethyl)-5-hydroxy-2(5H)-furanone (MX) is the member of the hydroxyfuranone class that has been most extensively studied. From animal studies, it appears that the ^{14}C label of MX is rapidly absorbed from the gastrointestinal tract and reaches systemic circulation. MX itself has not been measured in blood. The MX label is largely excreted in urine and faeces, urine being the major route of excretion. Very little of the initial radiolabel is retained in the body after 5 days.

1.2.7 Chlorite

The ^{36}Cl from chlorite is rapidly absorbed. Less than half the dose is found in the urine as chloride, and a small proportion as chlorite. A significant proportion probably enters the chloride pool of the body, but a lack of analytical methods to characterize chlorite in biological samples means that no detailed information is available.

1.2.8 Chlorate

Chlorate behaves similarly to chlorite. The same analytical constraints apply.

1.2.9 Bromate

Bromate is rapidly absorbed and excreted, primarily in urine, as bromide. Bromate is detected in urine at doses of 5 mg/kg of body weight and above. Bromate concentrations in urine peak at about 1 h, and bromate is not detectable in plasma after 2 h.

1.3 Toxicology of disinfectants and disinfectant by-products

1.3.1 Disinfectants

Chlorine gas, chloramine and chlorine dioxide are strong respiratory irritants. Sodium hypochlorite (NaOCl) is also used as bleach and is frequently involved in human poisoning. These exposures, however, are not relevant to exposures in drinking-water. There have been relatively few evaluations of the toxic effects of these disinfectants in drinking-water in experimental animals or humans. Evidence from these animal and human studies suggests that chlorine, hypochlorite solutions, chloramine and chlorine dioxide themselves probably do not contribute to the development of cancer or any toxic effects. Attention has focused on the wide variety of by-products that result from reactions of chlorine and other disinfectants with NOM, which is found in virtually all water sources.

1.3.2 Trihalomethanes

THMs induce cytotoxicity in the liver and kidneys of rodents exposed to doses of about 0.5 mmol/kg of body weight. The vehicle of administration significantly affects the toxicity of the THMs. The THMs have little reproductive and developmental toxicity, but BDCM has been shown to reduce sperm motility in rats consuming 39 mg/kg of body weight per day in drinking-water. Like chloroform, BDCM, when administered in corn oil, induces cancer in the liver and kidneys after lifetime exposures to high doses. Unlike chloroform and DBCM, BDCM and bromoform induce tumours of the large intestine in rats exposed by corn oil gavage. BDCM induces tumours at all three target sites and at lower doses than the other THMs. Since the publication of the 1994 WHO Environmental Health Criteria monograph on chloroform, additional studies have added to the weight of evidence indicating that chloroform is not a direct DNA-reactive mutagenic carcinogen. In contrast, the brominated THMs appear to be weak mutagens, probably as a result of GSH conjugation.

1.3.3 Haloacetic acids

The HAAs have diverse toxicological effects in laboratory animals. Those HAAs of most concern have carcinogenic, reproductive and developmental effects. Neurotoxic effects are significant at the high doses of DCA that are used therapeutically. Carcinogenic effects appear to be limited to the liver and to high doses. The bulk of the evidence indicates that the tumorigenic effects of DCA and TCA depend on modifying processes of cell division and cell death rather than their very weak mutagenic activities. Oxidative stress is also a feature of the toxicity of the brominated analogues within this class. Both DCA and TCA cause cardiac malformations in rats at high doses.

1.3.4   Haloaldehydes and haloketones

Chloral hydrate induces hepatic necrosis in rats at doses equal to or greater than 120 mg/kg of body weight per day. Its depressant effect on the central nervous system in humans is probably related to its metabolite trichloroethanol. Limited toxicity data are available for the other halogenated aldehydes and ketones. Chloroacetaldehyde exposure causes haematological effects in rats. Exposure of mice to 1,1-dichloropropanone (1,1-DCPN), but not 1,3-dichloropropanone (1,3-DCPN), results in liver toxicity.

Chloral hydrate was negative in most but not all bacterial tests for point mutations and in *in vivo* studies on chromosomal damage. However, it has been shown that chloral hydrate may induce structural chromosomal aberrations *in vitro* and *in vivo*. Chloral hydrate has been reported to cause hepatic tumours in mice. It is not clear if it is the parent compound or its metabolites that are involved in the carcinogenic effect. The two chloral hydrate metabolites, TCA and DCA, have induced hepatic tumours in mice.

Some halogenated aldehydes and ketones are potent inducers of mutations in bacteria. Clastogenic effects have been reported for chlorinated propanones. Liver tumours were noted in a lifetime drinking-water study with chloroacetaldehyde. Other halogenated aldehydes, e.g., 2-chloropropenal, have been identified as tumour initiators in the skin of mice. The haloketones have not been tested for carcinogenicity in drinking-water. However, 1,3-DCPN acted as a tumour initiator in a skin carcinogenicity study in mice.

1.3.5   Haloacetonitriles

Testing of these compounds for toxicological effects has been limited to date. Some of the groups are mutagenic, but these effects do not relate well to the activity of the chemicals as tumour initiators in the skin. There are only very limited studies on the carcinogenicity of this class of substances. Early indications of developmental toxicity of members of this class appear to be largely attributable to the vehicle used in treatment.

1.3.6 Halogenated hydroxyfuranone derivatives

Based on experimental studies, the critical effects of MX appear to be its mutagenicity and carcinogenicity. Several *in vitro* studies have revealed that MX is mutagenic in bacterial and mammalian test systems. MX caused chromosomal aberrations and induced DNA damage in isolated liver and testicular cells and sister chromatid exchanges in peripheral lymphocytes from rats exposed *in vivo*. An overall evaluation of the mutagenicity data shows that MX is mutagenic *in vitro* and *in vivo*. A carcinogenicity study in rats showed increased tumour frequencies in several organs.

1.3.7 Chlorite

The toxic action of chlorite is primarily in the form of oxidative damage to red blood cells at doses as low as 10 mg/kg of body weight. There are indications of mild neurobehavioural effects in rat pups at 5.6 mg/kg of body weight per day. There are conflicting data on the genotoxicity of chlorite. Chlorite does not increase tumours in laboratory animals in chronic exposure studies.

1.3.8 Chlorate

The toxicity of chlorate is similar to that of chlorite, but chlorate is less effective at inducing oxidative damage. It does not appear to be teratogenic or genotoxic *in vivo*. There are no data from long-term carcinogenicity studies.

1.3.9 Bromate

Bromate causes renal tubular damage in rats at high doses. It induces tumours of the kidney, peritoneum and thyroid in rats at doses of 6 mg/kg of body weight and above in chronic studies. Hamsters are less sensitive, and mice are considerably less sensitive. Bromate is also genotoxic *in vivo* in rats at high doses. Carcinogenicity appears to be secondary to oxidative stress in the cell.

1.4 Epidemiological studies

1.4.1 Cardiovascular disease

Epidemiological studies have not identified an increased risk of cardiovascular disease associated with chlorinated or chloraminated drinking-water. Studies of other disinfectants have not been conducted.

1.4.2 Cancer

The epidemiological evidence is insufficient to support a causal relationship between bladder cancer and long-term exposure to chlorinated drinking-water, THMs, chloroform or other THM species. The epidemiological evidence is inconclusive and equivocal for an association between colon cancer and long-term exposure to chlorinated drinking-water, THMs, chloroform or other THM species. The information is insufficient to allow an evaluation of the observed risks for rectal cancer and risks for other cancers observed in single analytical studies.

Various types of epidemiological studies have attempted to assess the cancer risks that may be associated with exposure to chlorinated drinking-water. Chloraminated drinking-water was considered in two studies. Several studies have attempted to estimate exposures to total THMs or chloroform and the other THM species, but the studies did not consider exposures to other DBPs or other water contaminants, which may differ for surface water and groundwater sources. One study considered the mutagenicity of drinking-water as measured by the *Salmonella typhimurium* assay. Assessments of possible cancer risks that may be associated with drinking-water disinfected with ozone or chlorine dioxide have not been performed.

Ecological and death certificate-based case–control studies have provided hypotheses for further evaluation by analytical studies that consider an individual's exposure to drinking-water and possible confounding factors.

Analytical studies have reported weak to moderate increased relative risks of bladder, colon, rectal, pancreatic, breast, brain or lung cancer associated with long-term exposure to chlorinated drinking-water. Single studies reported associations for pancreatic, breast or brain cancer; however, the evaluation of a possible causal relationship for epidemiological associations requires evidence from more than a single study. In one study, a small increased relative risk of lung cancer was associated with the use of surface water sources, but the magnitude of risk was too small to rule out residual confounding.

A case–control study reported a moderately large association between rectal cancer and long-term exposure to chlorinated drinking-water or cumulative THM exposure, but cohort studies have found either no increased risk or a risk too weak to rule out residual confounding.

Decreased bladder cancer risk was associated with increased duration of exposure to chloraminated drinking-water, but there is no biological basis for assuming a protective effect of chloraminated water.

Although several studies found increased risks of bladder cancer associated with long-term exposure to chlorinated drinking-water and cumulative exposure to THMs, inconsistent results were reported among the studies for bladder cancer risks between smokers and non-smokers and between men and women. Estimated exposure to THMs was considered in three of these studies. In one study, no association was found between estimated cumulative exposure to THMs. In another study, a moderately strong increased relative risk was associated with increased cumulative exposure to THMs in men but not in women. The third study reported a weak increased relative risk associated with an estimated cumulative exposure of 1957–6425 μg of THMs per litre-year; weak to moderate associations were also reported for exposure to THM concentrations greater than 24, greater than 49 and greater than 74 μg/litre. No increased relative risk of bladder cancer was associated with exposure to chlorinated municipal surface water supplies, chloroform or other THM species in a cohort of women, but the follow-up period of 8 years was very short, resulting in few cases for study.

Because inadequate attention has been paid to assessing exposure to water contaminants in epidemiological studies, it is not possible to properly evaluate the increased relative risks that were reported.

Specific risks may be due to other DBPs, mixtures of by-products or other water contaminants, or they may be due to other factors for which chlorinated drinking-water or THMs may serve as a surrogate.

1.4.3 Adverse pregnancy outcomes

Studies have considered exposures to chlorinated drinking-water, THMs or THM species and various adverse outcomes of pregnancy. A scientific panel recently convened by the US Environmental Protection Agency reviewed the epidemiological studies and concluded that the results of currently published studies do not provide convincing evidence that chlorinated water or THMs cause adverse pregnancy outcomes.

Results of early studies are difficult to interpret because of methodological limitations or suspected bias.

A recently completed but not yet published case–control study has reported moderate increased relative risks for neural tube defects in children whose mothers' residence in early pregnancy was in an area where THM levels were greater than 40 µg/litre. Replication of the results in another area is required before this association can be properly evaluated. A previously conducted study in the same geographic area reported a similar association, but the study suffered from methodological limitations.

A recently reported cohort study found an increased risk of early miscarriage associated with heavy consumption of water (five or more glasses of cold tapwater per day) containing high levels (≥ 75 µg/litre) of THMs. When specific THMs were considered, only heavy consumption of water containing BDCM (≥ 18 µg/litre) was associated with a risk of miscarriage. As this is the first study to suggest an adverse reproductive effect associated with a brominated by-product, a scientific panel recommended that another study be conducted in a different geographic area to attempt to replicate these results and that additional efforts be made to evaluate exposures of the cohort to other water contaminants.

1.5 Risk characterization

It should be noted that the use of chemical disinfectants in water treatment usually results in the formation of chemical by-products, some of which are potentially hazardous. However, the risks to health from these by-products at the levels at which they occur in drinking-water are extremely small in comparison with the risks associated with inadequate disinfection. Thus, it is important that disinfection not be compromised in attempting to control such by-products.

1.5.1 Characterization of hazard and dose–response

1.5.1.1 Toxicological studies

1) Chlorine

A WHO Working Group for the 1993 *Guidelines for drinking-water quality* considered chlorine. This Working Group determined a tolerable daily intake (TDI) of 150 µg/kg of body weight for free chlorine based on a no-observed-adverse-effect level (NOAEL) of approximately 15 mg/kg of body weight per day in 2-year studies in rats and mice and incorporating an uncertainty factor of 100 (10 each for intra- and interspecies variation). There are no new data that indicate that this TDI should be changed.

2) Monochloramine

A WHO Working Group for the 1993 *Guidelines for drinking-water quality* considered monochloramine. This Working Group determined a TDI of 94 µg/kg of body weight based on a NOAEL of approximately 9.4 mg/kg of body weight per day, the highest dose tested, in a 2-year bioassay in rats and incorporating an uncertainty factor of 100 (10 each for intra- and interspecies variation). There are no new data that indicate that this TDI should be changed.

3) Chlorine dioxide

The chemistry of chlorine dioxide in drinking-water is complex, but the major breakdown product is chlorite. In establishing a specific TDI for chlorine dioxide, data on both chlorine dioxide and chlorite can be considered, given the rapid hydrolysis to chlorite. Therefore, an oral TDI for chlorine dioxide is 30 µg/kg of body weight, based on the NOAEL of 2.9 mg/kg of body weight per day for neurodevelopmental effects of chlorite in rats.

4)   Trihalomethanes

Cancer following chronic exposure is the primary hazard of concern for this class of DBPs. Because of the weight of evidence indicating that chloroform can induce cancer in animals only after chronic exposure to cytotoxic doses, it is clear that exposures to low concentrations of chloroform in drinking-water do not pose carcinogenic risks. The NOAEL for cytolethality and regenerative hyperplasia in mice was 10 mg/kg of body weight per day after administration of chloroform in corn oil for 3 weeks. Based on the mode of action evidence for chloroform carcinogenicity, a TDI of 10 µg/kg of body weight was derived using the NOAEL for cytotoxicity in mice and applying an uncertainty factor of 1000 (10 each for inter- and intraspecies variation and 10 for the short duration of the study). This approach is supported by a number of additional studies. This TDI is similar to the TDI derived in the 1998 WHO *Guidelines for drinking-water quality*, which was based on a 1979 study in which dogs were exposed for 7.5 years.

Among the brominated THMs, BDCM is of particular interest because it produces tumours in rats and mice and at several sites (liver, kidneys, large intestine) after corn oil gavage. The induction of colon tumours in rats by BDCM (and by bromoform) is also interesting because of the epidemiological associations with colo-rectal cancer. BDCM and the other brominated THMs are also weak mutagens. It is generally assumed that mutagenic carcinogens will produce linear dose–response relationships at low doses, as mutagenesis is generally considered to be an irreversible and cumulative effect.

In a 2-year bioassay, BDCM given by corn oil gavage induced tumours (in conjunction with cytotoxicity and increased proliferation) in the kidneys of mice and rats at doses of 50 and 100 mg/kg of body weight per day, respectively. The tumours in the large intestine of the rat occurred after exposure to both 50 and 100 mg/kg of body weight per day. Using the incidence of kidney tumours in male mice from this study, quantitative risk estimates have been calculated, yielding a slope factor of 4.8×10^{-3} [mg/kg of body weight per day]$^{-1}$ and a calculated dose of 2.1 μg/kg of body weight per day for a risk level of 10^{-5}. A slope factor of 4.2×10^{-3} [mg/kg of body weight per day]$^{-1}$ (2.4 μg/kg of body weight per day for a 10^{-5} risk) was derived based on the incidence of large intestine carcinomas in the male rat. The International Agency for Research on Cancer (IARC) has classified BDCM in Group 2B (possibly carcinogenic to humans).

DBCM and bromoform were studied in long-term bioassays. In a 2-year corn oil gavage study, DBCM induced hepatic tumours in female mice, but not in rats, at a dose of 100 mg/kg of body weight per day. In previous evaluations, it had been suggested that the corn oil vehicle may play a role in the induction of tumours in female mice. A small increase in tumours of the large intestine in rats was observed in the bromoform study at a dose of 200 mg/kg of body weight per day. The slope factors based on these tumours are 6.5×10^{-3} [mg/kg of body weight per day]$^{-1}$ for DBCM, or 1.5 μg/kg of body weight per day for a 10^{-5} risk, and 1.3×10^{-3} [mg/kg of body weight per day]$^{-1}$ or 7.7 μg/kg of body weight per day for a 10^{-5} risk for bromoform.

These two brominated THMs are weakly mutagenic in a number of assays, and they were by far the most mutagenic DBPs of the class in the GST-mediated assay system. Because they are the most lipophilic THMs, additional concerns about whether corn oil may have affected their bioavailability in the long-term studies should be considered. A NOAEL for DBCM of 30 mg/kg of body weight per day has been established based on the absence of histopathological effects in the liver of rats after 13 weeks of exposure by corn oil gavage. IARC has classified DBCM in Group 3 (not classifiable as to its carcinogenicity to humans). A TDI for DBCM of 30 μg/kg of body weight was derived based on the NOAEL for liver toxicity of 30 mg/kg of body weight per day and an uncertainty factor of 1000 (10 each for inter- and intraspecies variation and 10 for the short duration of the study and possible carcinogenicity).

Similarly, a NOAEL for bromoform of 25 mg/kg of body weight per day can be derived on the basis of the absence of liver lesions in rats after 13 weeks of dosing by corn oil gavage. A TDI for bromoform of 25 μg/kg of body weight was derived based on this NOAEL for liver toxicity and an uncertainty factor of 1000 (10 each for inter- and intraspecies variation and 10 for the short duration of the study and possible carcinogenicity). IARC has classified bromoform in Group 3 (not classifiable as to its carcinogenicity to humans).

5)   Haloacetic acids

The induction of mutations by DCA is very improbable at the low doses that would be encountered in chlorinated drinking-water. The available data indicate that DCA differentially affects the replication rates of normal hepatocytes and hepatocytes that have been initiated. The dose–response relationships are complex, with DCA initially stimulating division of normal hepatocytes. However, at the lower chronic doses used in animal studies (but still very high relative to those that would be derived from drinking-water), the replication rate of normal hepatocytes is eventually sharply inhibited. This indicates that normal hepatocytes eventually down-regulate those pathways that are sensitive to stimulation by DCA. However, the effects in altered cells, particularly those that express high amounts of a protein that is immunoreactive to a c-Jun antibody, do not seem to be able to down-regulate this response. Thus, the rates of replication in the pre-neoplastic lesions with this phenotype are very high at the doses that cause DCA tumours to develop with a very low latency. Preliminary data would suggest that this continued alteration in cell birth and death rates is also necessary for the tumours to progress to malignancy. This interpretation is supported by studies that employ initiation/promotion designs as well.

On the basis of the above considerations, it is suggested that the currently available cancer risk estimates for DCA be modified by incorporation of newly developing information on its comparative metabolism and modes of action to formulate a biologically based dose–response model. These data are not available at this time, but they should become available within the next 2–3 years.

The effects of DCA appear to be closely associated with doses that induce hepatomegaly and glycogen accumulation in mice. The lowest-observed-adverse-effect level (LOAEL) for these effects in an 8-week study in mice was 0.5 g/litre, corresponding to approxi-mately 100 mg/kg of body weight per day, and the NOAEL was

0.2 g/litre, or approximately 40 mg/kg of body weight per day. A TDI of 40 μg/kg of body weight has been calculated by applying an uncertainty factor of 1000 to this NOAEL (10 each for inter- and intraspecies variation and 10 for the short duration of the study and possible carcinogenicity). IARC has classified DCA in Group 3 (not classifiable as to its carcinogenicity to humans).

TCA is one of the weakest activators of the peroxisome proliferator activated receptor (PPAR) known. It appears to be only marginally active as a peroxisome proliferator, even in rats. Furthermore, treatment of rats with high levels of TCA in drinking-water does not induce liver tumours. These data strongly suggest that TCA presents little carcinogenic hazard to humans at the low concentrations found in drinking-water.

From a broader toxicological perspective, the developmental effects of TCA are the end-point of concern. Animals appear to tolerate concentrations of TCA in drinking-water of 0.5 g/litre (approximately 50 mg/kg of body weight per day) with little or no signs of adverse effect. At 2 g/litre, the only sign of adverse effect appears to be hepatomegaly. Hepatomegaly is not observed in mice at doses of 0.35 g of TCA per litre in drinking-water, estimated to be equivalent to 40 mg/kg of body weight per day.

In another study, soft tissue anomalies were observed at approximately 3 times the control rate at the lowest dose administered, 330 mg/kg of body weight per day. At this dose, the anomalies were mild and would clearly be in the range where hepatomegaly (and carcinogenic effects) would occur. Considering the fact that the PPAR interacts with cell signalling mechanisms that can affect normal developmental processes, a common mechanism underlying hepato-megaly and the carcinogenic effects and developmental effects of this compound should be considered.

The TDI for TCA is based on a NOAEL estimated to be 40 mg/kg of body weight per day for hepatic toxicity in a long-term study in mice. Application of an uncertainty factor of 1000 (10 each for inter- and intraspecies variation and 10 for possible carcinogenicity) to the estimated NOAEL gives a TDI of 40 μg/kg of body weight. IARC has classified TCA in Group 3 (not classifiable as to its carcinogenicity to humans).

Data on the carcinogenicity of brominated acetic acids are too preliminary to be useful in risk characterization. Data available in abstract form suggest, however, that the doses required to induce hepatocarcinogenic responses in mice are not dissimilar to those of the chlorinated acetic acids. In addition to the mechanisms involved in the induction of cancer by DCA and TCA, it is possible that increased oxidative stress secondary to their metabolism might contribute to their effects.

There are a significant number of data on the effects of dibromo-acetic acid (DBA) on male reproduction. No effects were observed in rats at doses of 2 mg/kg of body weight per day for 79 days, whereas an increased retention of step 19 spermatids was observed at 10 mg/kg of body weight per day. Higher doses led to progressively more severe effects, including marked atrophy of the seminiferous tubules with 250 mg/kg of body weight per day, which was not reversed 6 months after treatment was suspended. A TDI of 20 μg/kg of body weight was determined by allocating an uncertainty factor of 100 (10 each for inter- and intraspecies variation) to the NOAEL of 2 mg/kg of body weight per day.

6)   Chloral hydrate

Chloral hydrate at 1 g/litre of drinking-water (166 mg/kg of body weight per day) induced liver tumours in mice exposed for 104 weeks. Lower doses have not been evaluated. Chloral hydrate has been shown to induce chromosomal anomalies in several *in vitro* tests but has been largely negative when evaluated *in vivo*. It is probable that the liver tumours induced by chloral hydrate involve its metabolism to TCA and/or DCA. As discussed above, these compounds are considered to act as tumour promoters. IARC has classified chloral hydrate in Group 3 (not classifiable as to its carcinogenicity to humans).

Chloral hydrate administered to rats for 90 days in drinking-water induced hepatocellular necrosis at concentrations of 1200 mg/litre and above, with no effect being observed at 600 mg/litre (approximately 60 mg/kg of body weight per day). Hepatomegaly was observed in mice at doses of 144 mg/kg of body weight per day administered by gavage for 14 days. No effect was observed at 14.4 mg/kg of body weight per day in the 14-day study, but mild hepatomegaly was observed when chloral hydrate was administered in drinking-water at 70 mg/litre (16 mg/kg of body weight per day) in a 90-day follow-up study. The application of an uncertainty factor of 1000 (10 each for inter- and intraspecies variation and 10 for the use of a LOAEL instead of a NOAEL) to this value gives a TDI of 16 µg/kg of body weight.

7)   Haloacetonitriles

Without appropriate human data or an animal study that involves a substantial portion of an experimental animal's lifetime, there is no generally accepted basis for estimating carcinogenic risk from the HANs.

Data developed in subchronic studies provide some indication of NOAELs for the general toxicity of dichloroacetonitrile (DCAN) and dibromoacetonitrile (DBAN). NOAELs of 8 and 23 mg/kg of body weight per day were identified in 90-day studies in rats for DCAN and DBAN, respectively, based on decreased body weights at the next higher doses of 33 and 45 mg/kg of body weight per day, respectively.

A WHO Working Group for the 1993 *Guidelines for drinking-water quality* considered DCAN and DBAN. This Working Group determined a TDI of 15 µg/kg of body weight for DCAN based on a NOAEL of 15 mg/kg of body weight per day in a reproductive toxicity study in rats and incorporating an uncertainty factor of 1000 (10 each for intra- and interspecies variation and 10 for the severity of effects). Reproductive and developmental effects were observed with DBAN only at doses that exceeded those established for general toxicity (about 45 mg/kg of body weight per day). A TDI of 23 µg/kg of body weight was calculated for DBAN based on the NOAEL of 23 mg/kg of body weight per day in the 90-day study in rats and incorporating an uncertainty factor of 1000 (10 each for intra- and interspecies variation and 10 for the short duration of the study). There are no new data indicating that these TDIs should be changed.

LOAELs for trichloroacetonitrile (TCAN) of 7.5 mg/kg of body weight per day for embryotoxicity and 15 mg/kg of body weight per day for developmental effects were identified. However, later studies suggest that these responses were dependent upon the vehicle used. No TDI can be established for TCAN.

There are no data useful for risk characterization purposes for other members of the HANs.

8) MX

The mutagen MX has recently been studied in a long-term study in rats in which some carcinogenic responses were observed. These data indicate that MX induces thyroid and bile duct tumours. An increased incidence of thyroid tumours was seen at the lowest dose of MX administered (0.4 mg/kg of body weight per day). The induction of thyroid tumours with high-dose chemicals has long been associated with halogenated compounds. The induction of thyroid follicular tumours could involve modifications in thyroid function or a mutagenic mode of action. A dose-related increase in the incidence of cholangiomas and cholangiocarcinomas was also observed, beginning at the low dose in female rats, with a more modest response in male rats. The increase in cholangiomas and cholangiocarcinomas in female rats was utilized to derive a slope factor for cancer. The 95% upper confidence limit for a 10^{-5} lifetime risk based on the linearized multi-stage model was calculated to be 0.06 μg/kg of body weight per day.

9) Chlorite

The primary and most consistent finding arising from exposure to chlorite is oxidative stress resulting in changes in the red blood cells. This end-point is seen in laboratory animals and, by analogy with chlorate, in humans exposed to high doses in poisoning incidents. There are sufficient data available with which to estimate a TDI for humans exposed to chlorite, including chronic toxicity studies and a two-generation reproductive toxicity study. Studies in human volunteers for up to 12 weeks did not identify any effect on blood parameters at the highest dose tested, 36 μg/kg of body weight per day. Because these studies do not identify an effect level, they are not informative for establishing a margin of safety.

In a two-generation study in rats, a NOAEL of 2.9 mg/kg of body weight per day was identified based on lower auditory startle amplitude, decreased absolute brain weight in the F_1 and F_2 generations, and altered liver weights in two generations. Application of an uncertainty factor of 100 (10 each for inter- and intraspecies variation) to this NOAEL gives a TDI of 30 μg/kg of body weight. This TDI is supported by the human volunteer studies.

10) Chlorate

Like chlorite, the primary concern with chlorate is oxidative damage to red blood cells. Also like chlorite, 0.036 mg of chlorate per kg of body weight per day for 12 weeks did not result in any adverse effect in human volunteers. Although the database for chlorate is less extensive than that for chlorite, a recent well conducted 90-day study in rats identified a NOAEL of 30 mg/kg of body weight per day based on thyroid gland colloid depletion at the next higher dose of 100 mg/kg of body weight per day. A TDI is not derived because a long-term study is in progress, which should provide more information on chronic exposure to chlorate.

11) Bromate

Bromate is an active oxidant in biological systems and has been shown to cause an increase in renal tumours, peritoneal mesotheliomas and thyroid follicular cell tumours in rats and, to a lesser extent, hamsters, and only a small increase in kidney tumours in mice. The lowest dose at which an increased incidence of renal tumours was observed in rats was 6 mg/kg of body weight per day.

Bromate has also been shown to give positive results for chromosomal aberrations in mammalian cells *in vitro* and *in vivo* but not in bacterial assays for point mutation. An increasing body of evidence, supported by the genotoxicity data, suggests that bromate acts by generating oxygen radicals in the cell.

In the 1993 WHO *Guidelines for drinking-water quality*, the linearized multistage model was applied to the incidence of renal tumours in a 2-year carcinogenicity study in rats, although it was noted that if the mechanism of tumour induction is oxidative damage in the kidney, application of the low-dose cancer model may not be appropriate. The calculated upper 95% confidence interval for a 10^{-5} risk was 0.1 µg/kg of body weight per day.

The no-effect level for the formation of renal cell tumours in rats is 1.3 mg/kg of body weight per day. If this is used as a point of departure from linearity and if an uncertainty factor of 1000 (10 each for inter- and intraspecies variation and 10 for possible carcinogenicity) is applied, a TDI of 1 µg/kg of body weight can be calculated. This compares with the value of 0.1 µg/kg of body weight per day associated with an excess lifetime cancer risk of 10^{-5}.

At present, there are insufficient data to permit a decision on whether bromate-induced tumours are a result of cytotoxicity and reparative hyperplasia or a genotoxic effect.

IARC has assigned potassium bromate to Group 2B (possibly carcinogenic to humans).

5.1.2   *Epidemiological studies*

Epidemiological studies must be carefully evaluated to ensure that observed associations are not due to bias and that the design is appropriate for an assessment of a possible causal relationship. Causality can be evaluated when there is sufficient evidence from several well designed and well conducted studies in different geographic areas. Supporting toxicological and pharmacological data are also important. It is especially difficult to interpret epidemiological data from ecological studies of disinfected drinking-water, and these results are used primarily to help develop hypotheses for further study.

Results of analytical epidemiological studies are insufficient to support a causal relationship for any of the observed associations. It is especially difficult to interpret the results of currently published analytical studies because of incomplete information about exposures to specific water contaminants that might confound or modify the risk. Because inadequate attention has been paid to assessing exposures to water contaminants in epidemiological studies, it is not possible to properly evaluate the increased relative risks that were reported. Risks may be due to other water contaminants or to other factors for which chlorinated drinking-water or THMs may serve as a surrogate.

1.5.2 Characterization of exposure

1.5.2.1 Occurrence of disinfectants and disinfectant by-products

Disinfectant doses of several milligrams per litre are typically employed, corresponding to doses necessary to inactivate micro-organisms (primary disinfection) or doses necessary to maintain a residual in the distribution system (secondary disinfection).

A necessary ingredient for an exposure assessment is DBP occurrence data. Unfortunately, there are few published international studies that go beyond case-study or regional data.

Occurrence data suggest, on average, exposure to about 35–50 µg of total THMs per litre in chlorinated drinking-water, with chloroform and BDCM being the first and second most dominant species. Exposure to total HAAs can be approximated by a total HAA concentration (sum of five species) corresponding to about one-half of the total THM concentration (although this ratio can vary significantly); DCA and TCA are the first and second most dominant species. In waters with a high bromide to TOC ratio or a high bromide to chlorine ratio, greater formation of brominated THMs and HAAs can be expected. When a hypochlorite solution (versus chlorine gas) is used, chlorate may also occur during chlorination.

DBP exposure in chloraminated water is a function of the mode of chloramination, with the sequence of chlorine followed by ammonia leading to the formation of (lower levels of) chlorine DBPs (i.e., THMs and HAAs) during the free-chlorine period; however, the suppression of chloroform and TCA formation is not paralleled by a proportional reduction in DCA formation.

All factors being equal, bromide concentration and ozone dose are the best predictors of bromate formation during ozonation, with about a 50% conversion of bromide to bromate. A study of different European water utilities showed bromate levels in water leaving operating water treatment plants ranging from less than the detection limit (2 μg/litre) up to 16 μg/L. The brominated organic DBPs formed upon ozonation generally occur at low levels. The formation of chlorite can be estimated by a simple percentage (50–70%) of the applied chlorine dioxide dose.

5.2.2   Uncertainties of water quality data

A toxicological study attempts to extrapolate a laboratory (controlled) animal response to a potential human response; one possible outcome is the estimation of cancer risk factors. An epidemiological study attempts to link human health effects (e.g., cancer) to a causative agent or agents (e.g., a DBP) and requires an exposure assessment.

The chemical risks associated with disinfected drinking-water are potentially based on several routes of exposure: (i) ingestion of DBPs in drinking-water; (ii) ingestion of chemical disinfectants in drinking-water and the concomitant formation of DBPs in the stomach; and (iii) inhalation of volatile DBPs during showering. Although the *in vivo* formation of DBPs and the inhalation of volatile DBPs may be of potential health concern, the following discussion is based on the premise that the ingestion of DBPs present in drinking-water is the most significant route of exposure.

Human exposure is a function of both DBP concentration and exposure time. More specifically, human health effects are a function of exposure to complex mixtures of DBPs (e.g., THMs versus HAAs, chlorinated versus brominated species) that can change seasonally/temporally (e.g., as a function of temperature, nature and concentration of NOM) and spatially (i.e., throughout a distribution system). Each individual chemical disinfectant can form a mixture of DBPs; combinations of chemical disinfectants can form even more complex mixtures. Upon their formation, most DBPs are stable, but some may undergo transformation by, for example, hydrolysis. In the absence of DBP data, surrogates such as chlorine dose (or chlorine demand), TOC (or ultraviolet absorbance at 254 nm [UVA_{254}]) or bromide can be used to indirectly estimate exposure. While TOC serves as a good surrogate for organic DBP precursors, UVA_{254} provides additional insight into NOM characteristics, which can vary geographically. Two key water quality variables, pH and bromide, have been identified as significantly affecting the type and concentrations of DBPs that are produced.

An exposure assessment should first attempt to define the individual types of DBPs and resultant mixtures likely to form, as well as their time-dependent concentrations, as affected by their stability and transport through a distribution system. For epidemiological studies, some historical databases exist for disinfectant (e.g., chlorine) doses, possibly DBP precursor (e.g., TOC) concentrations and possibly total THM (and, in some cases, THM species) concentrations. In contrast to THMs, which have been monitored over longer time frames because of regulatory scrutiny, monitoring data for HAAs (and HAA species), bromate and chlorite are much more recent and hence sparse. However, DBP models can be used to simulate missing or past data. Another important consideration is documentation of past changes in water treatment practice.

1.5.2.3 Uncertainties of epidemiological data

Even in well designed and well conducted analytical studies, relatively poor exposure assessments were conducted. In most studies, duration of exposure to disinfected drinking-water and the water source were considered. These exposures were estimated from residential histories and water utility or government records. In only a few studies was an attempt made to estimate a study participant's water consumption and exposure to either total THMs or individual species of THMs. In only one study was an attempt made to estimate exposures to other DBPs. In evaluating some potential risks, i.e., adverse outcomes of pregnancy, that may be associated with relatively short term exposures to volatile by-products, it may be important to consider the inhalation as well as the ingestion route of exposure from drinking-water. In some studies, an effort was made to estimate both by-product levels in drinking-water for etiologically relevant time periods and cumulative exposures. Appropriate models and sensitivity analysis such as Monte Carlo simulation can be used to help estimate these exposures for relevant periods.

A major uncertainty surrounds the interpretation of the observed associations, as exposures to a relatively few water contaminants have been considered. With the current data, it is difficult to evaluate how unmeasured DBPs or other water contaminants may have affected the observed relative risk estimates.

More studies have considered bladder cancer than any other cancer. The authors of the most recently reported results for bladder cancer risks caution against a simple interpretation of the observed associations. The epidemiological evidence for an increased relative risk of bladder cancer is not consistent — different risks are reported for smokers and non-smokers, for men and women, and for high and low water consumption. Risks may differ among various geographic areas because the DBP mix may be different or because other water contaminants are also present. More comprehensive water quality data must be collected or simulated to improve exposure assessments for epidemiological studies.

2. CHEMISTRY OF DISINFECTANTS AND DISINFECTANT BY-PRODUCTS

2.1 Background

The use of chlorine (Cl_2) as a water disinfectant has come under scrutiny because of its potential to react with natural organic matter (NOM) and form chlorinated disinfectant by-products (DBPs). Within this context, NOM serves as the organic DBP precursor, whereas bromide ion (Br^-) serves as the inorganic precursor. Treatment strategies generally available to water systems exceeding drinking-water standards include removing DBP precursors and using alternative disinfectants for primary and/or secondary (distribution system) disinfection. Alternative disinfectant options that show promise are chloramines (NH_2Cl, monochloramine), chlorine dioxide (ClO_2) and ozone (O_3). While ozone can serve as a primary disinfectant only and chloramines as a secondary disinfectant only, both chlorine and chlorine dioxide can serve as either primary or secondary disinfectants.

Chloramine presents the significant advantage of virtually eliminating the formation of chlorination by-products and, unlike chlorine, does not react with phenols to create taste- and odour-causing compounds. However, the required contact time for inactivation of viruses and *Giardia* cysts is rarely obtainable by chloramine post-disinfection at existing water treatment facilities (monochloramine is significantly less biocidal than free chlorine). More recently, the presence of nitrifying bacteria and nitrite (NO_2^-) and nitrate (NO_3^-) production in chloraminated distribution systems as well as the formation of organic chloramines have raised concern.

The use of chlorine dioxide, like chloramine, can reduce the formation of chlorinated by-products during primary disinfection. However, production of chlorine dioxide, its decomposition and reaction with NOM lead to the formation of by-products such as chlorite (ClO_2^-), a compound that is of health concern.

If used as a primary disinfectant followed by a chloramine residual in the distribution system, ozone can eliminate the need for contact between DBP precursors and chlorine. Ozone is known to react both with NOM to produce organic DBPs such as aldehydes and increase levels of assimilable organic carbon and with bromide ion to form bromate.

A thorough understanding of the mechanisms of DBP formation allows microbial inactivation goals and DBP control goals to be successfully balanced. This chapter examines a range of issues affecting DBP formation and control to provide guidance to utilities considering the use of various disinfecting chemicals to achieve microbial inactivation with DBP control.

2.2 Physical and chemical properties of common disinfectants and inorganic disinfectant by-products

The important physical and chemical properties of commonly used disinfectants and inorganic DBPs are summarized in Table 1.

2.2.1 Chlorine

Chlorine, a gas under normal pressure and temperature, can be compressed to a liquid and stored in cylindrical containers. Because chlorine gas is poisonous, it is dissolved in water under vacuum, and this concentrated solution is applied to the water being treated. For small plants, cylinders of about 70 kg are used; for medium to large plants, tonne containers are common; and for very large plants, chlorine is delivered by railway tank cars or road (truck) tankers. Chlorine is also available in granular or powdered form as calcium hypochlorite ($Ca(OCl)_2$) or in liquid form as sodium hypochlorite (NaOCl; bleach).

Chlorine is used in the form of gaseous chlorine or hypochlorite (OCl^-). In either form, it acts as a potent oxidizing agent and often dissipates in side reactions so rapidly that little disinfection is accomplished until amounts in excess of the chlorine demand have been added. As an oxidizing agent, chlorine reacts with a wide variety of compounds, in particular those that are considered reducing agents (hydrogen sulfide [H_2S], manganese(II), iron(II), sulfite [SO_3^{2-}], Br^-, iodide [I^-], nitrite). From the point of view of DBP formation and

Table 1. Physical and chemical properties of commonly used disinfectants and inorganic disinfectant by-products

Chemical[a]	$E°$ (V)[b]	Oxidation number of Cl or Br	λ_{max} (nm)[c]	e (mol⁻¹ litre⁻¹ cm⁻¹)[d]	$pe°$[e]	pK_a'[f]
HOCl/Cl⁻	+1.49	+1	254 / 292 (OCl⁻)	60 / 419	+25.2	7.5
ClO₂/ClO₂⁻	+0.95	+4	359	1250	+16.1	–
NH₂Cl	–	+1	245	416	–	–
O₃/O₂	+2.07	–	254	3200	+35.0	
HOBr/Br⁻	+1.33	+1	330	50	+22.5	8.7
ClO₂⁻/Cl⁻	+0.76	+3	262	–	+12.8	1.96
ClO₃⁻/Cl⁻	+0.62	+5	360	–	+10.5	1.45
BrO₃⁻/Br⁻	+0.61	+5	195	–	–	0.72

[a] Half-cell reactants/products.

[b] $E°$ = standard electrode potential (redox potential) in water at 25 °C. The oxidation–reduction state of an aqueous environment at equilibrium can be stated in terms of its redox potential. In the chemistry literature, this is generally expressed in volts, E, or as the negative logarithm of the electron activity, pe. When pe is large, the electron activity is low and the system tends to be an oxidizing one: i.e., half-reactions tend to be driven to the right. When pe is small, the system is reducing, and reactions tend to be driven to the left.

[c] λ_{max} = maximum absorbance wavelength of that particular solution in nm.

[d] e = molar absorptivity (molar extinction coefficient), in mol⁻¹ litre⁻¹ cm⁻¹. This can be used for quantitative determination of the various species of chemicals and is the only direct physical measurement. There is often some background absorbance that may interfere with the measurement in natural waters that should be considered.

[e] $pe°$ = – log {e⁻} where {e⁻} = electron activity.

[f] pK_a = negative logarithm of the acid ionization constant (e.g., at pH 7.5, the molar concentration of HOCl is same as that of OCl⁻). As this parameter is dependent upon temperature, the values listed were determined at 25 °C.

disinfection, these reactions may be important because they may be fast and result in the consumption of chlorine.

Chlorine gas hydrolyses in water almost completely to form hypochlorous acid (HOCl):

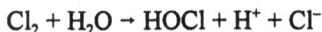

$$Cl_2 + H_2O \rightarrow HOCl + H^+ + Cl^-$$

The hypochlorous acid dissociates into hydrogen ions (H^+) and hypochlorite ions in the reversible reaction:

$$HOCl \leftrightarrow H^+ + OCl^-$$

Hypochlorous acid is a weak acid with a pK_a of approximately 7.5 at 25 °C. Hypochlorous acid, the prime disinfecting agent, is therefore dominant at a pH below 7.5 and is a more effective disinfectant than hypochlorite ion, which dominates above pH 7.5.

The rates of the decomposition reactions of chlorine increase as the solution becomes more alkaline, and these reactions can theoretically produce chlorite and chlorate (ClO_3^-); they occur during the electrolysis of chloride (Cl^-) solutions when the anodic and cathodic compartments are not separated, in which case the chlorine formed at the anode can react with the alkali formed at the cathode. On the other hand, hypochlorous acid/hypochlorite (or hypobromous acid/hypobromite, HOBr/OBr$^-$) can be formed by the action of chlorine (or bromine) in neutral or alkaline solutions. The decomposition of hypohalites (XO^-) is favoured in alkaline solutions ($2XO^- \rightarrow X^- + XO_2^-$) and is such that there is no longer any domain of thermodynamic stability for the hypohalite ions. These oxyhalites are further converted to stable oxyhalates as follows:

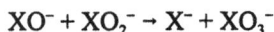

$$XO^- + XO_2^- \rightarrow X^- + XO_3^-$$

Another reaction that occurs in waters containing bromide ion and hypochlorite is the production of hypobromous acid:

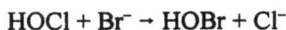

$$HOCl + Br^- \rightarrow HOBr + Cl^-$$

This reaction is irreversible, and the product hypobromous acid is a better halogenating agent than hypochlorous acid and interferes with common analytical procedures for free chlorine. The presence of bromide in hypochlorite solutions can ultimately lead to the formation of bromate (BrO_3^-).

Hypobromous acid is a weak acid ($pK_a = 8.7$); like hypochlorite, hypobromite is metastable. In alkaline solution, it decomposes to give bromate and bromide:

$$3OBr^- \rightarrow BrO_3^- + 2Br^-$$

Bromic acid ($HBrO_3$) is a strong acid ($pK_a = 0.7$). Bromic acid and bromate can be obtained by the electrolytic oxidation of bromide solutions or bromine water using chlorine. Bromic acid and bromate are powerful oxidizing agents, but the speed of their oxidation reactions is generally slow (Mel et al., 1953).

2.2.2 Chlorine dioxide

Chlorine dioxide is one of the few compounds that exists almost entirely as monomeric free radicals. Concentrated chlorine dioxide vapour is potentially explosive, and attempts to compress and store this gas, either alone or in combination with other gases, have been commercially unsuccessful. Because of this, chlorine dioxide, like ozone, must be manufactured at the point of use. Chlorine dioxide in water does not hydrolyse to any appreciable extent. Neutral or acidic dilute aqueous solutions are quite stable if kept cool, well sealed and protected from sunlight.

Chlorine dioxide represents an oxidation state (+4) intermediate between those of chlorite (+3) and chlorate (+5). No acid or ion of the same degree of oxidation is known. Chlorine dioxide is a powerful oxidizing agent that can decompose to chlorite; in the absence of oxidizable substances and in the presence of alkali, it dissolves in water, decomposing with the slow formation of chlorite and chlorate:

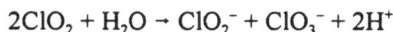

$$2ClO_2 + H_2O \rightarrow ClO_2^- + ClO_3^- + 2H^+$$

Chlorine dioxide has an absorption spectrum with a maximum at 359 nm, with a molar absorptivity of 1250 mol^{-1} $litre^{-1}$ cm^{-1}. This extinction coefficient is independent of temperature, pH, chloride and ionic strength. Chlorine dioxide is readily soluble in water, forming a greenish-yellow solution. It can be involved in a variety of redox reactions, such as oxidation of iodide ion, sulfide ion, iron(II) and manganese(II). When chlorine dioxide reacts with aqueous contaminants, it is usually reduced to chlorite ion. The corresponding electron transfer reactions are comparable to those occurring when singlet oxygen acts as an oxidant (Tratnyek & Hoigne, 1994).

Bromide (in the absence of sunlight) is not oxidized by chlorine dioxide. Therefore, water treatment with chlorine dioxide will not transform bromide ion into hypobromite and will not give rise to the formation of bromoform ($CHBr_3$) or bromate. This is an important difference between the use of chlorine dioxide as an oxidant and the use of chlorine or ozone as an oxidant.

2.2.3 Ozone

Ozone is a strong oxidizing agent ($E° = 2.07$ V). Oxidation reactions initiated by ozone in water are generally rather complex; in water, only part of the ozone reacts directly with dissolved solutes. Another part may decompose before reaction. Such decomposition is catalysed by hydroxide ions (OH^-) and other solutes. Highly reactive secondary oxidants, such as hydroxyl radicals ($OH·$), are thereby formed. These radicals and their reaction products can additionally accelerate the decomposition of ozone. Consequently, radical-type chain reactions may occur, which consume ozone concurrently with the direct reaction of ozone with dissolved organic material.

Many oxidative applications of ozone have been developed, including disinfection, control of algae, removal of tastes and odours, removal of colour, removal of iron and manganese, microflocculation, removal of turbidity by oxidative flocculation, removal of organics by oxidation of phenols, detergents and some pesticides, partial oxidation of dissolved organics and control of halogenated organic compounds. For disinfection and for oxidation of many organic and inorganic contaminants in drinking-water, the kinetics of ozone reactions are favourable; on the other hand, for many difficult-to-oxidize organic compounds, such as chloroform ($CHCl_3$), the kinetics of ozone oxidation are very slow (Hoigne et al., 1985).

2.2.4   Chloramines

Monochloramine has much higher CT values[1] than free chlorine and is therefore a poor primary disinfectant. Additionally, it is a poor oxidant and is not effective for taste and odour control or for oxidation of iron and manganese. However, because of its persistence, it is an attractive secondary disinfectant for the maintenance of a stable distribution system residual. The use of disinfectants such as ozone or chlorine dioxide combined with chloramines as a secondary disinfectant appears to be attractive for minimizing DBP formation (Singer, 1994b).

Monochloramine is the only useful ammonia-chloramine disinfectant. Dichloramine ($NHCl_2$) and nitrogen trichloride (NCl_3) are too unstable to be useful and highly malodorous. Conditions practically employed for chloramination are designed to produce only monochloramine.

2.3   Analytical methods for disinfectant by-products and disinfectants

Analytical methods for various DBPs and their detection limits are summarized in Table 2. Methods for disinfectants are summarized in APHA (1995).

2.3.1   Trihalomethanes, haloacetonitriles, chloral hydrate, chloropicrin and haloacetic acids

Gas chromatographic (GC) techniques are generally employed for organic DBPs. Detection and quantification of haloacetonitriles (HANs) and chloral hydrate in chlorinated natural waters are complicated by (i) hydrolysis of dihaloacetonitriles and chloral hydrate to dihaloacetic acids and chloroform, respectively; (ii) degradation of HANs by dechlorinating agents such as sodium sulfite and sodium thiosulfate; (iii) low purge efficiency for the HANs and chloral hydrate in the purge-and-trap technique; and (iv) low extraction efficiency for

---

[1] The CT value is the product of the disinfectant concentration C in mg/litre and the contact time T in minutes required to inactivate a specified percentage (e.g., 99%) of microorganisms.

Table 2. Summary of analytical methods for various DBPs and their minimum detection limits

DBPs	Analytical method	APHA[a] method	Minimum detection limit (μg/litre)	Major interferences	References
THMs	MTBE extraction Pentane extraction	– 6232B	0.4 0.1	None	AWWARF (1991) AWWARF (1991)
HAAs	Salted MTBE extraction and derivatization with diazomethane	6233B	0.5–1.0	None	AWWARF (1991)
HANs	Pentane extraction	6232B	0.05	None	Koch et al. (1988)
Cyanogen chloride	MTBE extraction	6233A	0.5	None	AWWARF (1991)
Chloramine	Derivatization with 2-mercaptobenzothiazole	–	–	None	Lukasewycz et al. (1989)
Haloketones[b]	Pentane extraction	6232B	0.2	None	Krasner et al. (1995) AWWARF (1991)
Chloral hydrate	MTBE extraction	–	0.5	None	AWWARF (1991)
Aldehydes	Extraction with hexane and derivatization with PFBHA	–	1.0	PFBHA sulfate	Sclimenti et al. (1990)
Bromate	Ion chromatography (H_3BO_3/NaOH)	4500	2.0[c] 0.2	Cl^-	Siddiqui et al. (1996a) Krasner et al. (1993) Weinberg et al. (1998)
Chlorate	Ion chromatography (H_3BO_3/NaOH)	4500	5	Cl^-, acetate	Siddiqui (1996)
Chlorite	Ion chromatography ($NaHCO_3$/Na_2CO_3)	4500	10	Cl^-, acetate	AWWARF (1991)
TOC	UV/persulfate or combustion	5310	200	Metals	APHA (1995)

[a] American Public Health Association.
[b] Sum of 1,1-DCPN and 1,1,1-TCPN.
[c] 1.0 μg/litre with high-capacity column.

chloral hydrate with pentane in the liquid–liquid extraction normally used. Although chloral hydrate is not efficiently extracted from water with pentane, it can be extracted with an efficiency of approximately 36% when the ratio by volume of methyl *tert*-butyl ether (MTBE) to water is 1 : 5 (Amy et al., 1998). MTBE quantitatively extracts HANs, trihalomethanes (THMs), chloral hydrate and chloropicrin, permitting simultaneous analysis for all of these DBPs. Chloral hydrate decomposes on packed columns to trichloroacetaldehyde, resulting in considerable band broadening, although this does not appear to be a significant problem with DB-1 and DB-5 columns.

The extraction of THMs can be accomplished using MTBE (EPA Method 551) or pentane. Method 551 also permits simultaneous extraction and measurement of chloral hydrate, HANs, THMs, chloropicrin and haloketones. The pentane method can be used to extract THMs, HANs, haloketones and chloropicrin but not chloral hydrate in the same run (APHA, 1995).

The haloacetic acid (HAA) analytical method involves using an acidic salted ether or acidic methanol liquid–liquid extraction, requiring esterification with diazomethane prior to analysis on a gas chromatograph equipped with an electron capture detector (ECD). THMs and HANs can be analysed by extraction with pentane prior to analysis on a capillary-column GC equipped with an ECD. The analysis of cyanogen compounds involves extraction with MTBE prior to injection into GC–ECD. Aldehydes require derivatization with O-(2,3,4,5,6-pentafluorobenzyl)-hydroxylamine (PFBHA) (to form an oxime), extraction with hexane and GC–ECD analysis [(C_6F_5)-CH_2ONH_2 + RCHO → (C_6F_5)–$CH_2ON=CHR$ + H_2O]. It should be noted that PFBHA peaks are very large relative to other peaks in the chromatogram from a purge-and-trap system, whereas the peaks are comparable to other peaks in a GC–ECD chromatogram (Trehy et al., 1986).

2.3.2 *Inorganic disinfectant by-products*

An ion chromatography (IC) method (EPA Method 300) has been developed to determine inorganic by-products. The elution order is fluoride, chlorite, bromate, chloride, nitrite, bromide, chlorate, nitrate and sulfate ion. The eluent is a carbonate buffer. Ethylenediamine is used to preserve chlorite samples and to minimize the potential for chlorite ion reaction on the IC separating column. EPA Method 300 involves measurement by an IC system using a separating column (e.g., Ion Pac AS9-SC) fitted with an anion micromembrane suppressor column. An eluent containing 2.0 mmol of sodium carbonate (Na_2CO_3) per litre / 0.75 mmol of sodium bicarbonate ($NaHCO_3$) per litre is used for bromide determination, and an eluent containing 40 mmol of boric acid (H_3BO_3) per litre / 20 mmol of sodium hydroxide (NaOH) per litre is used for bromate and chlorate determination. The analytical mini-mum detection limits for bromate and chlorate using a borate eluent have been reported as 2 µg/litre and 5 µg/litre, respectively (Siddiqui, 1996; Siddiqui et al., 1996a). For samples with high chloride ion content, a silver cartridge can be used to remove chloride prior to IC analysis to minimize its interference with bromate measurement. It should be noted that for natural sources and waters with high total organic carbon (TOC) levels, detection limits will be slightly different because of the masking effect of NOM and high concentrations of carbonate/bicarbonate ions that may interfere with bromate/chlorate measurement.

2.3.3 Total organic carbon and UV absorbance at 254 nm

TOC is the primary surrogate parameter for the measurement of NOM in water supplies. Several investigators have reported that the ultraviolet (UV)/persulfate oxidation method underestimates the TOC concentration in natural waters as compared with the combustion method because of the inability of the persulfate method to oxidize highly polymerized organic matter. It is generally assumed that the calibration of a TOC analyser with a potassium hydrogen phthalate standard is sufficient for the measurement of TOC in natural waters, but potassium hydrogen phthalate has a simple molecular structure and is easy to oxidize. Dissolved organic carbon (DOC) is operationally defined by a (0.45-µm) filtration step. UV absorbance at 254 nm (UVA_{254}) is used to describe the type and character of NOM, whereas TOC describes just the amount of NOM.

2.3.4 Chloramines

Knowledge of the amine content of the water during water treat-ment processes involving chloramination is important to define more adequately the content of a matrix described only as a combined chlorine residual. The presence of organic nitrogen and the instability of many organic chloramines continue to challenge the analyst.

Lukasewycz et al. (1989) developed a technique for the analysis of chloramines and organic chloramines present in water using 2-mercaptobenzothiazole as a derivatizing agent. The resulting sulfanilamides are stable and can be conveniently analysed by high-performance liquid chromatography (HPLC) using UV or electrochemical detection. This method appears to be superior to the use of diazotization or phenylarsine oxide as a method of detection. Organic chloramines are much weaker disinfectants than inorganic monochloramine but are indistinguishable by the common analytical methods.

2.4 Mechanisms involved in the formation of disinfectant by-products

2.4.1 Chlorine reactions

Chlorine reacts with humic substances (dissolved organic matter) present in most water supplies, forming a variety of halogenated DBPs, such as THMs, HAAs, HANs, chloral hydrate and chloropicrin, as follows:

$$HOCl + DOC \rightarrow DBPs$$

It is generally accepted that the reaction between chlorine and humic substances, a major component of NOM, is responsible for the production of organochlorine compounds during drinking-water treatment. Humic and fulvic acids show a high reactivity towards chlorine and constitute 50–90% of the total DOC in river and lake waters (Thurman, 1985). Other fractions of the DOC comprise the hydrophilic acids (up to 30%), carbohydrates (10%), simple carboxylic acids (5%) and proteins/amino acids (5%). The reactivity of carbohydrates and carboxylic acids towards chlorine is low, and they are not expected to contribute to the production of organochlorine compounds. However, hydrophilic acids such as citric acid and amino acids will react with chlorine to produce chloroform and other products and may contribute towards total organochlorine production (Larson & Rockwell, 1979).

Free chlorine reacts with water constituents by three general pathways: oxidation, addition and substitution (Johnson & Jensen, 1986). Chlorine can undergo an addition reaction if the organic compound has a double bond. For many compounds with double bonds, this reaction is too slow to be of importance in water treatment. The oxidation reactions with water constituents such as carbohydrates or fatty acids (e.g., oleic acid) are generally slow.

Most chlorine DBPs are formed through oxidation and substitution reactions. THMs have the general formula CHX_3, where X can be Cl or Br. Chloroform may be produced through a series of reactions with functional groups of humic substances. The major functional groups of humic substances include acetyl, carboxyl, phenol, alcohol, carbonyl and methoxyl. The reactions proceed much more rapidly at high pH than at low pH.

Rook (1977) proposed resorcinol structures to be the major precursor structure in humic material for chloroform formation. In accordance with this hypothesis in the chlorination of terrestrial and aquatic humic substances, a series of intermediates were detected that contained a trichloromethyl group and that could be converted to chloroform by further oxidation or substitution reactions (Stevens et al., 1976).

However, the production of chlorinated compounds such as dichloropropanedoic acid, 2,2-dichlorobutanedoic acid, cyanogen chloride (CNCl), HANs or the cyano-substituted acids cannot be explained on the basis of resorcinol structures, and possible production pathways require protein-type precursors (De Leer et al., 1986). The reaction pathway for amino acids involves initial rapid formation of the monochloramine and dichloramine, which can react further to form aldehyde or HANs, respectively. Trehy et al. (1986) demonstrated the formation of chloral hydrate along with HANs after chlorination of amino acids by substitution reactions, and aldehydes were shown to be the oxidation products. Luknitskii (1975) provided a detailed chemistry of chloral hydrate formation.

Christman et al. (1983) also identified chloroform, chloral hydrate, dichloroacetic acid (DCA), trichloroacetic acid (TCA) and 2,2-dichlorobutanedoic acid as the major products, accounting for 53% of the total organic halogen (TOX). A number of other minor products have been detected, including several chlorinated alkanoic acids and non-chlorinated benzene carboxylic acids. De Leer et al. (1985) extended these studies to incorporate chloroform intermediates, chlorinated aromatic acids and cyano-compounds as potential products in drinking-water. The presence of unhalogenated aldehydes and HANs in chlorinated natural waters can be attributed in part to the presence of amino acids or peptides in natural waters. Humic acids may also contribute to the presence of amino acids in natural waters, as they have amino acids associated with them either in a free or in a combined form. Several studies regarding the chlorination of amino acids have shown that the primary amino group on the amino acids can be converted to either an aldehyde or a nitrile group (Morris et al., 1980; Isaac & Morris, 1983). These studies indicate that with an equimolar amount of halogenating agent, the major product is an aldehyde. However, if an excess of halogenating agent is added, then the corresponding nitrile can also be formed, with the ratio of the aldehyde to nitrile formed increasing with pH.

Many treated waters contain not only chlorinated but also brominated compounds, such as bromoform. These compounds form because aqueous chlorine converts bromide in the water to hypobromous acid. The bromine can then react with the organic matter in the same way as hypochlorous acid to form various bromochlorinated DBPs. However, compared with hypochlorous acid, hypobromous acid is a weaker oxidant and stronger halogenating agent.

Chlorate, an inorganic by-product of chlorine, is formed in concentrated hypochlorite solutions during their production and storage through the following reactions (Gordon et al., 1997):

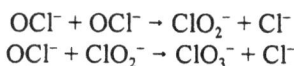

$$OCl^- + OCl^- \rightarrow ClO_2^- + Cl^-$$
$$OCl^- + ClO_2^- \rightarrow ClO_3^- + Cl^-$$

The first reaction proceeds at a much slower rate and is rate limiting, hence the generally observed second-order kinetics. Sodium hypochlorite is stored at pH greater than 12 to prevent rapid decomposition, and most of the sodium hypochlorite is present as hypochlorite ion. The average rate constant for the formation of chlorate is 85×10^{-5} mol^{-1} litre^{-1} d^{-1} (Gordon et al., 1995).

2.4.2 *Chlorine dioxide reactions*

The major chlorine dioxide by-products of concern are chlorite and chlorate. Chlorine dioxide reacts generally as an electron acceptor, and hydrogen atoms present in activated organic C–H or N–H structures are thereby not substituted by chlorine (Hoigne & Bader, 1994). Moreover, in contrast to chlorine, chlorine dioxide's efficiency for disinfection does not vary with pH or in the presence of ammonia, and it does not oxidize bromide. As opposed to chlorine, which reacts via oxidation and electrophilic substitution, chlorine dioxide reacts only by oxidation; this explains why it does not produce organo-chlorine compounds. In addition to this, chlorine dioxide is more selective in typical water treatment applications, as evidenced by its somewhat lower disinfectant demand as compared with chlorine.

Chlorine dioxide is generally produced by reacting aqueous (sodium) chlorite with chlorine (Gordon & Rosenblatt, 1996):

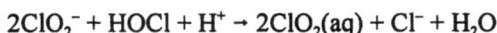

$$2ClO_2^- + HOCl + H^+ \rightarrow 2ClO_2(aq) + Cl^- + H_2O$$

However, under conditions of low initial reactant concentrations or in the presence of excess chlorine, the reactant produces chlorate ion:

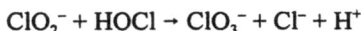

$$ClO_2^- + HOCl \rightarrow ClO_3^- + Cl^- + H^+$$

This reaction scenario is common in generators that overchlorinate to achieve high reaction yields based on chlorite ion consumption.

An alternative approach to chlorine dioxide generation is with hydrochloric acid (HCl), a process that results in less chlorate during production:

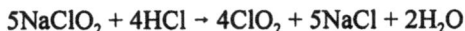

$$5NaClO_2 + 4HCl \rightarrow 4ClO_2 + 5NaCl + 2H_2O$$

Chlorite ion is also produced when chlorine dioxide reacts with organics (Gordon & Rosenblatt, 1996):

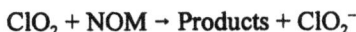

$$ClO_2 + NOM \rightarrow Products + ClO_2^-$$

Chlorine dioxide can also undergo a series of photochemically initiated reactions resulting in the formation of chlorate ion (Gordon et al., 1995).

While bromide is not generally oxidized by chlorine dioxide, bromate can be formed in the presence of sunlight over a wide range of pH values (Gordon & Emmert, 1996). Utilities need to be concerned with bromate ion in the chlorine dioxide treatment of drinking-water if the water contains bromide and is exposed to sunlight. Practically, this means minimizing exposure to sunlight when chlorine dioxide is applied in the presence of bromide ion. There appears to be a problem with chlorine dioxide producing odour-causing compounds at the tap. This has been linked to chlorine dioxide reacting with volatile organic compounds derived from new carpets and office products (Hoehn et al., 1990).

Hoigne & Bader (1994) described the kinetics of reaction between chlorine dioxide and a wide range of organic and inorganic compounds that are of concern in water treatment. Measured rate constants were high for nitrite, hydrogen peroxide, ozone, iodide, iron(II), phenolic compounds, tertiary amines and thiols. Bromide, ammonia, structures containing olefinic double bonds, aromatic hydrocarbons, primary and secondary amines, aldehydes, ketones and carbohydrates are unreactive under the conditions of water treatment. Chlorine dioxide rapidly oxidizes substituted phenoxide anions and many phenols, and second-order rate constants have been measured (Rav-Acha & Choshen, 1987).

2.4.3 Chloramine reactions

Chloramination of drinking-water produces THMs (if chloramine is formed by chlorination followed by ammonia addition), HAAs, chloral hydrate, hydrazine, cyanogen compounds, nitrate, nitrite, organic chloramines and 1,1-dichloropropanone (1,1-DCPN) (Dlyamandoglu & Selleck, 1992; Kirmeyer et al., 1993, 1995).

In the presence of even small quantities of organic nitrogen, it is possible for chloramination to produce organic chloramines. Several researchers have shown that monochloramine readily transfers its chlorine at a comparatively rapid rate to organic amines to form organohalogen amines (Isaac & Morris, 1983; Bercz & Bawa, 1986). Monochloramine was shown to cause binding of radiolabelled halogen to nutrients such as tyrosine and folic acid; the amount of binding varied with pH but was generally less at neutral pH than at higher pH (Bercz & Bawa, 1986). Organic chloramines are much weaker disinfectants than inorganic monochloramine but are indistinguishable by common analytical methods. Organic chloramine formation may necessitate changing chloramination conditions (e.g., ammonia and chlorine addition order, chlorine-to-ammonia ratios and contact time).

HANs and non-halogenated acetonitriles are produced when chloramines are reacted with humic materials and amino acids (Trehy et al., 1986). The reaction pathway for these products is quite complicated and very similar to that for chlorine, with many intermediates and by-products formed. In the case of aspartic acid, De Leer et al. (1986) demonstrated the presence of at least 11 other significant products.

2.4.4 Ozone reactions

Ozone has been shown to oxidize bromide to hypobromite and bromate, and hypochlorite to chlorate (Glaze et al., 1993; Siddiqui et al., 1995; Siddiqui, 1996).

Bromate generally forms through a combination of molecular ozone attack and reaction of bromide with free radical species. The molecular ozone mechanism does not account for hydroxyl radicals always formed as secondary oxidants from decomposed ozone during water treatment. Siddiqui et al. (1995) indicated that there is a radical pathway that is influenced by both pH and alkalinity. The hydroxyl radical and, to a lesser degree, the carbonate radical ($CO_3 \cdot$) pathway may be more important than the molecular ozone pathway. Oxidants such as hydroxyl and carbonate radicals may interact with intermediate bromine species, leading to the formation of hypobromite radicals ($BrO \cdot$), which eventually undergo disproportionation to form hypobromite and bromite (BrO_2^-). Bromate is then formed through oxidation of bromite by ozone. The radical mechanism for the formation of bromate includes two decisive reaction steps still involving molecular ozone: the formation of hypobromite and oxidation of bromite.

Bromate ion formed through reactions with molecular ozone contributes in the range of 30–80% to the overall bromate ion formation in NOM-containing waters (von Gunten and Hoigne, 1994). Siddiqui et al. (1995) reported up to 65% and 100% bromate ion formation through the radical pathway in NOM-free and NOM-containing waters, respectively. Differences in NOM-containing waters can be attributed to differences in the characteristics of the NOM present. A change in mechanism as a function of pH and the competitive roles of the free radical (one electron transfer) mechanism above pH 7 versus oxygen atom (two electron transfer) mechanism help explain both the large variations in bromate ion yield and the sensitivity to reactor design, concentration of organic precursors and ozone/bromide ion concentrations (Gordon, 1993).

The presence of bromide ion in a source water further complicates the reaction of ozone and leads to the formation of additional DBPs, such as bromoform, dibromoacetonitrile (DBAN) and dibromoacetone (DBAC) (Siddiqui, 1992; Amy et al., 1993, 1994).

2.5 Formation of organohalogen disinfectant by-products

Table 3 summarizes the DBPs identified as being formed from the use of chlorine, chlorine dioxide, chloramine and ozone.

The formation of organochlorine and organobromine compounds during drinking-water treatment is a cause of health concern in many countries. These compounds include THMs, HAAs, HANs, chloral hydrate, chloropicrin, acetohalides, halogenated furanones and other compounds.

2.5.1 Chlorine organohalogen by-products

Table 4 summarizes the range of concentrations of chlorinated DBPs formed from the reaction of chlorine with NOM, from various sources.

The major chlorination DBPs identified are THMs, HAAs, HANs, haloketones, chloropicrin and chloral hydrate. HAAs represent a major portion of the non-THM halogenated organic compounds (Miller & Uden, 1983; Reckhow & Singer, 1985). Many researchers have identified HANs and haloketones as other important DBPs (Trehy & Bieber, 1981; Miller & Uden, 1983; Oliver, 1983; Reckhow & Singer, 1985). According to an AWWARF (1991) study, for all eight utilities tested, 1,1,1-trichloropropanone (1,1,1-TCPN) was the more prevalent of the two measured haloketone compounds. In addition, Kronberg et al. (1988) identified the extremely mutagenic compound, MX.

Table 3. Disinfectant by-products present in disinfected waters

Disinfectant	Significant organo-halogen products	Significant inorganic products	Significant non-halogenated products
Chlorine/ hypochlorous acid	THMs, HAAs, HANs, chloral hydrate, chloropicrin, chlorophenols, N-chloramines, halofuranones, bromohydrins	Chlorate (mostly from hypo-chlorite use)	Aldehydes, cyanoalkanoic acids, alkanoic acids, benzene, carboxylic acids
Chlorine dioxide		chlorite, chlorate	unknown
Chloramine	HANs, cyanogen chloride, organic chloramines, chloramino acids, chloral hydrate, haloketones	nitrate, nitrite, chlorate, hydrazine	aldehydes, ketones
Ozone	bromoform, MBA, DBA, DBAC, cyanogen bromide	chlorate, iodate, bromate, hydrogen peroxide, hypobromous acid, epoxides, ozonates	aldehydes, ketoacids, ketones, carboxylic acids

Despite the fact that HAA formation and THM formation have very different pH dependencies, HAA formation correlates strongly with THM formation when treatment conditions are relatively uniform and when the water has a low bromide concentration (Singer, 1993). DBP formation and requisite chlorine dosage for disinfection strongly correspond to the concentration of TOC at the point of chlorine addition, suggesting that optimized or enhanced removal of organic carbon prior to chlorination will decrease the formation of DBPs.

HAA formation can be appreciable when drinking-water is chlorinated under conditions of slightly acidic pH and low bromide concentrations. The concentrations of DCA and TCA are similar to the concentrations of chloroform, and the total HAA concentration can be as much as 50% greater than the THM concentration in the finished water on a weight basis.

Table 4. Concentration range of chlorinated disinfectant by-products in drinking-water[a]

DBPs	Peters et al. (1990); Peters (1991)	Krasner et al. (1989)	Nieminski et al. (1993)	Koch et al. (1991)	Reckhow et al. (1990)
THMs	3.1–49.5	30.0–44.0	17.0–51.0	49.0–81.0	201–1280
HAAs	<0.5–14.7	13.0–21.0	5.0–25.0	22.0–32.0	118–1230
HANs	0.04–1.05	2.5–4.0	0.5–5.0	2.0–2.6	3.0–12.0
Haloketones	–	0.9–1.8	0.2–1.6	1.0–2.0	4.8–25.3
Chlorophenols	–	–	0.5–1.0	–	–
Chloral hydrate	–	1.7–3.0	–	–	–
Chloropicrin	–	0.1–0.16	<0.1–0.6	–	–
TOC	1.7–5.6	2.9–3.2	1.5–6.0	2.5–3.0	4.8–26.6
Bromide	100–500	70–100	–	170–420	–

[a] All values shown in µg/litre, except TOC (mg/litre).

45

McGuire & Meadow (1988) reported that the national average THM concentration in the USA was 42 µg/litre for drinking-water utilities serving more than 100 000 persons, and only 3% of systems were above the US maximum contaminant level of 100 µg/litre. Amy et al. (1993) estimated that the national average THM concentration in the USA was 40 µg/litre, with an average TOC concentration of 3.0 mg/litre. The median annual average THM concentration found for utilities among the American Water Works Association's (AWWA) Water Industry Database was 35 µg/litre, as compared with 50 µg/litre for the non-database utilities (Montgomery Watson, Inc., 1993).

In Germany, 10% of the utilities produced disinfected drinking-water with a THM concentration above 10 µg/litre; the median annual average concentration was between 1 and 4 µg/litre, depending on raw water quality and size of facility (Haberer, 1994).

Total THM levels in treated drinking-water were reported in one survey in the United Kingdom (Water Research Centre, 1980): chlorinated water derived from a lowland river contained a mean level of 89.2 µg/litre, and that from an upland reservoir, 18.7 µg/litre. The study also showed that chlorinated groundwater was contaminated by THMs to a significantly lesser extent than chlorinated surface waters.

In a national survey of the water supplies of 70 communities serving about 38% of the population in Canada, conducted in the winter of 1976–1977, chloroform concentrations in treated water of the distribution system 0.8 km from the treatment plant, determined by the gas sparge technique, averaged 22.7 µg/litre. Levels of the other THMs were considerably lower, averaging 2.9 µg/litre for bromodichloromethane (BDCM), 0.4 µg/litre for dibromochloromethane (DBCM) and 0.1 µg/litre for bromoform. Using direct aqueous injection techniques, average concentrations of most of the THMs were higher (Health Canada, 1993).

Samples collected from the distribution systems of eight major cities in Saudi Arabia showed that THMs occurred in all the water supplies, at concentrations ranging between 0.03 and 41.7 µg/litre. Median total THM concentrations in several cities were higher during the summer than during the winter. In addition, THM concentrations were low in cities that did not mix groundwater and desalinated water.

Brominated THMs dominated (with bromoform the most abundant) and existed at the highest concentration levels, whereas chloroform was the least prevalent compound. This is the opposite of the occurrence pattern found in almost all water distribution systems worldwide (Fayad, 1993).

The concentrations of chloral hydrate in drinking-water in the USA were summarized by IARC (1995) and varied from 0.01 to 28 µg/litre. The highest values were found in drinking-water prepared from surface water.

Chlorination of water as well as the combination of ozonation and chlorination can lead to the formation of chloropicrin (Merlet et al., 1985). In a study conducted for over 25 utilities, very low levels of chloropicrin were observed, and chlorination produced maximum concentrations of less than 2 µg/litre (AWWARF, 1991). The chloropicrin appeared to form slowly during the incubation period, with concentrations tending to level off at approximately 40 h.

Dichloroacetonitrile (DCAN) is by far the most predominant HAN species detected in water sources with bromide levels of 20 µg/litre or less. For sources with higher bromide levels (50–80 µg/litre), bromochloroacetonitrile (BCAN) was the second most prevalent compound. However, none of these sources had a DBAN concentration exceeding 0.5 µg/litre, including one source water that had a much higher bromide level, 170 µg/litre. Thus, it appears that ambient bromide concentration is not the only factor influencing the speciation of HAN compounds.

Chlorine can react with phenols to produce mono-, di- or trichlorophenols, which can impart tastes and odours to waters. The control of chlorophenolic tastes and odours produced when phenol-laden water is treated with chlorine is essential. The sources of phenolic compounds in water supplies are reported to be industrial wastes.

In natural waters, one of the most important sources of organic nitrogen is proteins and their hydrolysis products. The reaction of aqueous chlorine or monochloramine with organic nitrogen may form complex organic chloramines (Feng, 1966; Morris et al., 1980; Snyder

& Margerum, 1982). The formation of *N*-chloramines resulting from the reaction of amines and chlorine has been reported (Weil & Morris, 1949; Gray et al., 1979; Morris et al., 1980). Likewise, the chlorination of amides has been reported (Morris et al., 1980).

Nieminski et al. (1993) reported the occurrence of DBPs for Utah (USA) water treatment plants. All plants used chlorine for primary and secondary disinfection purposes. Overall, THMs and HAAs represented 75% of the total specific DBPs analysed for the survey; however, total DBPs represented only 25–50% of the TOX concentration. THMs constituted 64% of the total DBPs by weight; HAAs were 30% of the total DBPs by weight and approximately one-half of the total THM concentrations. (However, in some waters, HAA concentrations may approach or possibly exceed THM concentrations.) HANs, haloketones, chlorophenols and chloropicrin represented 3%, 1.5%, 1.0% and 0.5%, respectively, of the total surveyed DBPs.

The occurrence of DBPs in drinking-waters in the USA was evaluated at 35 water treatment facilities that had a broad range of source water qualities and treatment processes (Krasner et al., 1989). THMs were the largest class of DBPs, and HAAs were the next most significant class. Aldehydes, by-products of ozonation, were also produced by chlorination. Over four quarterly sampling periods, median total THM concentrations ranged from 30 to 44 µg/litre, with chloroform, BDCM, DBCM and bromoform ranges of 9.6–15, 4.1–10, 2.6–4.5 and 0.33–0.88 µg/litre, respectively. Median total HAA concentrations ranged from 13 to 21 µg/litre, with TCA, DCA, monochloroacetic acid (MCA), dibromoacetic acid (DBA) and monobromoacetic acid (MBA) ranges of 4.0–6.0, 5.0–7.3, <1–1.2, 0.9–1.5 and <0.5 µg/litre, respectively.

Concentrations of DCA and TCA measured in various water sources have been summarized by IARC (1995): in Japan, chlorinated drinking-water contained 4.5 and 7.5 µg of DCA and TCA per litre, respectively; rainwater in Germany contained 1.35 µg of DCA per litre and 0.1–20 µg of TCA per litre, whereas groundwater contained 0.05 µg of TCA per litre; in Australia, a maximum concentration of 200 µg/litre was found for DCA and TCA in chlorinated treated water; and chlorinated water in Switzerland contained 3.0 µg of TCA per litre.

In a survey of 20 drinking-waters prepared from different source waters in the Netherlands, HAAs were found in all drinking-waters prepared from surface water, whereas they could not be detected in drinking-waters prepared from groundwaters. Brominated acetic acids accounted for 65% of the total acid concentration (Peters et al., 1991). In another survey of Dutch drinking waters, the average concentration of dihaloacetonitriles was about 5% of the average THM concentration (Peters, 1990).

2.5.2   Chloramine organohalogen by-products

Chloramine treatment practice involves three potential approaches: free chlorine followed by ammonia addition, ammonia addition followed by chlorine addition (*in situ* production) and pre-formed (off-line formation) chloramines. Generally, the objective is monochloramine formation. Chlorine followed by ammonia is a common approach, and, during the free-chlorine period, DBP formation may mimic that of chlorine. Chloramination results in the production of THMs (predominantly formed by chlorination followed by ammonia addition), HAAs, chloral hydrate, hydrazine, cyanogen compounds, organic chloramines and 1,1-DCPN (Dlyamandoglu & Selleck, 1992; Singer, 1993; Kirmeyer et al., 1993, 1995). Chloramination significantly reduces but does not eliminate THM formation; cyanogen chloride and TOX represent the major DBP issues with respect to chloramines.

Scully et al. (1990) identified chloramino acids such as *N*-chloroglycine, *N*-chloroleucine and *N*-chlorophenylalanine as by-products after chlorination of water containing nitrogen or after chloramination.

2.5.3   Chlorine dioxide organohalogen by-products

Chlorine-free chlorine dioxide does not form THMs (Noack & Doerr, 1978; Symons et al., 1981). Several studies show that the TOX formed with chlorine dioxide is 1–15% of the TOX formed with chlorine under the same reaction conditions (Chow & Roberts, 1981; Symons et al., 1981; Fleischacker & Randtke, 1983).

Treatment of phenol-laden source waters with chlorine dioxide does not produce the typical chlorophenolic taste and odour compounds that are produced when the water is treated using chlorine and is effective in removing existing tastes and odours of this type.

2.5.4 Ozone organohalogen by-products

Ozonation of drinking-water containing bromide ion has been shown to produce hypobromous acid/hypobromite, with hypobromite ion serving as an intermediate to bromate formation. In the presence of NOM, hypobromous acid produces a host of brominated organic compounds, such as bromoform, MBA, DBA, DBAN, cyanogen bromide and DBAC (Glaze et al., 1993; Siddiqui & Amy, 1993). Cavanagh et al. (1992) and Glaze et al. (1993) reported the identification of bromohydrins, a new group of labile brominated organic compounds from the ozonation of a natural water in the presence of enhanced levels of bromide. However, results by Kristiansen et al. (1994) strongly suggest that the bromohydrins, such as 3-bromo-2-methyl-2-butanol, in extracts of unquenched disinfected water are artefacts formed from the reaction of excessive hypobromous acid with traces of olefins in the extraction solvents and not novel DBPs.

Table 5 compares the median concentrations of various DBPs after ozonation and chlorination.

2.6 Formation of inorganic disinfectant by-products

Although organic DBPs have been the subject of study over a longer time frame, the formation of many inorganic by-products is coming under increasing scrutiny.

2.6.1 Chlorine inorganic by-products

Chlorite and chlorate are inorganic by-products formed in some chlorine solutions. This is of interest because many small drinking-water utilities use hypochlorite solutions as a source of free chlorine for disinfection. Bolyard & Fair (1992) examined the occurrence of chlorate in samples of untreated source water, drinking-water and hypochlorite solutions from 14 sites that use hypochlorite solutions. The hypochlorite solutions used were found to contain significant levels of chlorate. Chlorite and bromate were also found in hypochlorite solutions from these same water utilities. Chlorate was present in drinking-water, either as a manufacturing by-product or from

Table 5. Median concentrations of organic disinfectant by-products in drinking-water

DBPs	Median concentration (μg/litre): chlorination[a]	Median concentration (μg/litre): ozonation[b]
THMs	40	<1.0
Chloroform	15	–
BDCM	10	–
DBCM	4.5	–
Bromoform	0.57	<1.0
HANs	2.5	<1.0
TCAN	<0.012	–
DCAN	1.1	–
BCAN	0.58	–
DBAN	0.48	<1.0
Haloketones	0.94	–
DCPN	0.46	–
TCPN	0.35	–
HAAs	20	<5.0
MCA	1.2	–
DCA	6.8	–
TCA	5.8	–
MBA	<0.5	<1.0
DBA	1.5	<5.0
Aldehydes	7.8	45
Formaldehyde	5.1	20
Acetaldehyde	2.7	11
Glyoxal	–	9
Methylglyoxal	–	5
Chloral hydrate	3.0	–
Ketoacids	–	75
Trichlorophenol	<0.4	–

[a] Krasner et al. (1989).
[b] Siddiqui et al. (1993).

decomposition reactions occurring during storage. Approximately 0.2 mg of chlorate per litre was observed in water following the addition of chlorine as sodium hypochlorite at a dose sufficient to maintain a residual of 0.45 mg/litre (Andrews & Ferguson, 1995). The concentration of chlorite in commercial bleach solutions typically ranges from 0.002 to 0.0046 mol/litre; similarly, the chlorate concentration ranges from about 0.02 to 0.08 mol/litre (Gordon et al., 1995).

A detailed study by Bolyard & Fair (1992) demonstrated that hypochlorite solutions used to disinfect drinking-water contain significant levels of chlorite and chlorate. The concentration of chlorite ranged from <2 to 130 mg/litre for free available chlorine concentrations ranging from 3 to 110 g/litre. The concentration of chlorate varied over the range 0.19–50 g/litre, with a median of 12 g/litre. These solutions also contained bromate levels ranging from <2 to 51 mg/litre. The concentrations of chlorate in treated source waters ranged from 11 to 660 µg/litre. In another study involving 25 samples from plants using gaseous chlorine, no chlorate was detected, indicating that the use of gaseous chlorine does not produce chlorate (Bolyard & Fair, 1992). Nieminski et al. (1993) measured chlorate and chlorite for six water treatment plants that use liquid chlorine (i.e., hypochlorite) and found chlorate concentrations ranging from 40 to 700 µg/litre, with no chlorite or bromate detected in finished waters. These chlorate concentrations may be attributed to high concentrations of chlorate, ranging from 1000 to 8000 mg/litre, detected in a bleach used for disinfection and resulting from the decomposition of hypochlorite stock solution. However, no chlorite or chlorate was detected in any of the samples of finished water of the treatment plants that apply gaseous chlorine. Chlorate formation is expected to be minimal in low-strength hypochlorite solutions freshly prepared from calcium hypochlorite, because of the low hypochlorite concentration and only mildly alkaline pH.

2.6.2 Chloramine inorganic by-products

Inorganic by-products of chloramination include nitrate, nitrite, hydrazine and, to some extent, chlorate (Dlyamandoglu & Selleck, 1992; Kirmeyer et al., 1995).

2.6.3 Chlorine dioxide inorganic by-products

The major inorganic by-products of chlorine dioxide disinfection have been identified as chlorite and chlorate. Andrews & Ferguson (1995) measured a chlorate concentration of 0.38 mg/litre when a chlorine dioxide residual of 0.33 mg/litre was maintained. The application of chlorine dioxide produces about 0.5–0.7 mg of chlorite and 0.3 mg of chlorate per mg of chlorine dioxide consumed or applied (Andrews & Ferguson, 1995).

2.6.4 Ozone inorganic by-products

When bromide or iodide ions are present in waters, some of the halogen-containing oxidants that can be produced during ozonation include free bromine, hypobromous acid, hypobromite ion, bromate ion, free iodine, hypoiodous acid and iodate ion.

During the oxidation or chemical disinfection of natural waters containing bromide ion with ozone, bromate ion can be formed at concentrations ranging from 0 to 150 µg/litre under normal water treatment conditions (Siddiqui, 1992). Chlorate formation with an initial total chlorine concentration of 0.6 mg/litre was evaluated at pH levels of 8.0, 7.0 and 6.0, and chlorate concentrations ranging from 10 to 106 µg/litre were formed after ozonation (Siddiqui et al., 1996a).

It has been reported that ozone reacts with many metal ions and with cyanide ion (Hoigne et al., 1985; Yang & Neely, 1986). Bailey (1978) discussed the formation of ozonates, compounds of metal cations having the general formula $M^+O_3^-$. Hydrogen peroxide has been identified as a by-product of ozonation of organic unsaturated compounds (Bailey, 1978).

Table 6 provides the range of bromate concentrations normally encountered in drinking-waters with a variety of source water characteristics after ozonation.

2.7 Formation of non-halogenated organic disinfectant by-products

2.7.1 Chlorine organic by-products

Lykins & Clark (1988) conducted a 1-year pilot plant study of the effects of ozone and chlorine and determined that the concentration of aldehydes increased by 144% upon ozonation. In the chlorinated stream, the concentration of these aldehydes increased by 56%. This study indicates that aldehyde formation, although greater with ozone, is not unique to ozonation, but is associated with chlorination and other oxidants as well.

Table 6. Summary of bromate ion formation potentials in different source waters under different conditions following ozonation

N*	Bromide (µg/litre)	Ozone (mg/litre)	pH	Alkalinity (mg/litre)	DOC (mg/litre)	Bromate (µg/litre)	Reference
18	10–800	1–9.3	5.6–9.4	20–132	2.2–8.2	<5–60	Krasner et al. (1992)
4	60–340	3–12	6.5–8.5	90–230	3–7	<5–40	Siddiqui & Amy (1993)
28	10–100	2–4	6.8–8.8	20–120	0.3–11	<5–100	Amy et al. (1993, 1994)
4	12–37	0–3.97	7.8	N/A	N/A	<7–35	Hautman & Bolyard (1993)
1	500	2.3–9.5	7.2–8.3	N/A	N/A	13–293	Yamada (1993)
23	12–207	0.3–4.3	5.7–8.2	14–246	0.5–6.8	<2–16	Legube et al. (1993)
8	107–237	1–5	6.8–8.0	N/A	2–5	<5–50	Kruithof & Meijers (1993)

* N = number of sources studied.

2.7.2   Chloramine organic by-products

When Suwannee River (USA) fulvic acid was reacted with aqueous solutions of ^{15}N-labelled chloramine and ^{15}N-labelled ammonia, lyophilized products exhibiting nuclear magnetic resonances between 90 and 120 ppm were observed, denoting the formation of amides, enaminones and aminoquinones (Ginwalla & Mikita, 1992). This represents evidence for the formation of nitrogen-containing compounds from the chlorination of NOM in natural waters.

Amino acids, peptides and amino sugars were chlorinated under various chlorine/nitrogen ratios (Bruchet et al., 1992). Six natural amino acids (alanine, methionine, valine, phenylalanine, leucine and isoleucine) were shown to induce tastes and odours at concentrations in the range of 10–20 µg/litre. Detectable odours were consistently induced in a multicomponent mixture containing each of these amino acids after a 2-h contact time with chlorine. Investigation of the by-products indicated that the odours generated were systematically linked to the aliphatic aldehydes formed. The peptides investigated had varying degrees of odour formation potential, while the amino sugars did not impart any odour. Chlorinous odours occasionally detected during these experiments were found to be due to organic chloramines and other oxidation by-products.

2.7.3   Chlorine dioxide organic by-products

Gilli (1990) showed the formation of carbonyl compounds (34 µg/litre) such as *n*-valeraldehyde (7–15 µg/litre), formaldehyde (3.4–9 µg/litre), acetaldehyde (4.5 µg/litre) and acetone (3.2 µg/litre) after using chlorine dioxide.

2.7.4   Ozone organic by-products

Ozone aliphatic oxidation products from organic impurities in water are usually acids, ketones, aldehydes and alcohols. So-called ultimate oxidation products of organic materials are carbon dioxide, water, oxalic acid and acetic acid. However, ozonation conditions generally employed in treating drinking-water are rarely sufficient to form high concentrations of these ultimate products.

When source waters containing NOM and unsaturated organic compounds are ozonated, ozonides, peroxides, diperoxides, triperoxides and peroxy acids, for example, can be produced. The limited research that has been conducted in aqueous solutions indicates that these intermediates decompose readily in water to form products such as aldehydes, ketones, carboxylic acids and ketoacids.

Coleman et al. (1992) identified numerous compounds in addition to the following in ozonated humic samples: monocarboxylic acids up to C-24, dicarboxylic acids up to C-10, ketoacids, furan carboxylic acids, and benzene mono-, di- and tricarboxylic acids. Among the various aldehydes, Paode et al. (1997) found four (formaldehyde, acetaldehyde, glyoxal and methylglyoxal) to be dominant. Table 7 provides a range of concentrations for aldehydes from the ozonation of a variety of source waters.

2.8   Influence of source water characteristics on the amount and type of by-products produced

The extensive literature pertaining to DBP levels in disinfected source waters and control of DBPs by various treatment processes attests to the wide variety of factors influencing DBP formation and the complex interrelationships between these factors. Variables including the concentration and characteristics of precursor material, pH, chlorine concentration, bromide level, presence of chlorine-demanding substances such as ammonia, temperature and contact time all play a role in DBP formation reactions.

2.8.1   Effect of natural organic matter and UV absorbance at 254 nm

NOM consists of a mixture of humic substances (humic and fulvic acids) and non-humic (hydrophilic) material. Both the amount (as indicated by TOC or UVA_{254}) and the character (as described by UVA_{254}) of NOM can affect DBP formation. NOM provides the precursor material from which organic DBPs are formed; consequently, increasing concentrations of NOM lead to increasing concentrations of by-products. This relationship has led to the use of TOC and UVA_{254} measurements as surrogate parameters for estimating the extent of DBP formation.

Table 7. Effect of ozone dose and TOC on non-halogenated organic by-products

Ozone dose (mg/litre)	TOC (mg/litre)	Formal (µg/litre)	Acetal (µg/litre)	Glyoxal (µg/litre)	Methyl-glyoxal (µg/litre)	Reference
1.2–4.4	2.66	8–24	2–4	4–11	4–15	Miltner et al. (1992)
1.0–9.2	1.0–25.9	3–30	7–65	3–15	3–35	Weinberg et al. (1993)
5.5–28.5	5.4–17.4	58–567	6–28	15–166	17–54	Schechter & Singer (1995)

The removal of NOM is strongly influenced by those properties embodying the size, structure and functionality of this heterogeneous mixture. The humic acids are more reactive than fulvic acids with chlorine (Reckhow et al., 1990) and ozone, in terms of both oxidant/ disinfectant demand and DBP formation. Processes such as coagulation, adsorption and membrane filtration are separation processes that remove NOM intact, while ozonation transforms part of the NOM into biodegradable organic matter, potentially removable by biofiltration. Coagulation preferentially removes humic/higher molecular weight NOM; the selectivity of membranes for NOM removal is largely dictated by the molecular weight cutoff of the membrane; the use of granular activated carbon (GAC) requires a significant empty bed contact time; biofiltration can remove only the rapidly biodegradable NOM fraction.

In an investigation of the nature of humic and fulvic acids isolated from a variety of natural waters, Reckhow et al. (1990) found that the fulvic fractions had a lower aromatic content and smaller molecular size than the humic fractions. UV absorbance was correspondingly higher for the humic fractions, owing to the higher aromatic content and larger size. These researchers also found that for all of the organic material investigated, the production of chloroform, TCA, DCA and DCAN was higher upon chlorination of the humic fractions than upon chlorination of the corresponding fulvic fractions. These findings support the findings of other researchers and show that the UV absorbance measurement is an indicator of the nature of the precursor material present in a sample. This measurement, in conjunction with the TOC (or DOC) measurement, can be employed in the evaluation of data to provide an indication of the reactivity of NOM towards forming DBPs.

The reaction of ozone with NOM can occur directly or by radical processes. The disappearance of disinfecting chemical is influenced by the type and concentration of NOM present in natural waters. Direct consumption of these chemicals is greater when the UV absorbance (due to electrophilic and nucleophilic sites of NOM) of the source water is significant, resulting in decreased DBP formation potential.

It appears that the nature of the organic material in a source water may have some impact on the relative concentrations of THMs and HAAs formed upon chlorination. Treatment techniques that lower the levels of DOC without affecting bromide levels have been implicated in a shift from chlorinated to brominated THM compounds. This is of concern because the theoretical risk to humans varies for the individual THMs, with the brominated species generally being of more concern (Bull & Kopfler, 1991).

2.8.2 Effect of pH

The impact of pH on THM concentrations has been reported by a number of researchers since THMs in drinking-water first came to the attention of the water industry (Stevens et al., 1976; Lange & Kawczynski, 1978; Trussell & Umphres, 1978). More recently, the impact of pH on a number of other chlorination by-products has been reported (Miller & Uden, 1983; Reckhow & Singer, 1985). The rate of THM formation increases with the pH (Stevens et al., 1976). Kavanaugh et al. (1980) reported a 3-fold increase in the reaction rate per unit pH.

In general, increasing pH has been associated with increasing concentrations of THMs and decreasing concentrations of HAAs (pH primarily impacting TCA), HANs and haloketones. The concentrations of TCA tend to be higher in waters with pH levels less than 8.0 than in waters with pH levels greater than 8.0; a less marked trend is observed for DCA. Other researchers have reported similar findings with respect to the pH dependency of HAA concentrations. For example, Stevens et al. (1976) found that TCA concentrations were significantly lower at a pH of 9.4 than at pH levels of approximately 5 and 7. TCA was by far the most predominant of the measured HAA species at six of the eight utilities surveyed. Carlson & Hardy (1998) reported that at pH levels greater than 9.0, THM formation decreased with increasing pH. It is possible that the shift in chlorine species from hypochlorous acid to hypochlorite affects THM formation during short reaction times.

AWWARF (1991) observed no relationship between pH and the concentrations of THMs at eight utilities over time, suggesting that although THM concentrations for a particular water are known to be pH dependent, factors other than pH influence THM concentrations over a variety of source waters. Nieminski et al. (1993) reported that treatment plants with a pH of about 5.5 in finished water produced equal amounts of THMs and HAAs, whereas plants with pHs greater than 7.0 in finished water produced higher amounts of THMs as compared with HAAs.

No strong relationship has been observed between HAN concentration and pH over time. Within the approximate pH range 7–8.5, HAN concentrations increased slightly over time. In general, a trend of decreasing HAN concentrations with increasing pH would be expected, since these compounds are known to undergo base-catalysed hydrolysis and have been identified as intermediates in the formation of chloroform (Reckhow & Singer, 1985). Therefore, these compounds may be unstable in the presence of free chlorine or under basic conditions. In general, after an initial formation period, HAN and haloketone concentrations level off or begin to decline over the remainder of the reaction period. This indicates that base-catalysed hydrolysis may not be a significant mechanism of reaction for the relatively low pH sources.

Stevens et al. (1989) evaluated the effects of pH and reaction time (4, 48 and 144 h) on the formation of chloral hydrate. Chloral hydrate formation increased over time at pH 5 and 7, whereas chloral hydrate that had formed within 4 h at pH 9.4 decayed over time at the elevated pH.

The pH of the source water can also affect the formation of by-products after chloramine addition. The disproportionation of mono-chloramine, which is an important reaction leading to an oxidant loss, has been shown by several researchers to be catalysed by hydrogen ion, phosphate, carbonate and silicate (Valentine & Solomon, 1987).

Humic acids have shown reaction rates with chlorine dioxide that increased by a factor of 3 per pH unit (pH 4–8) (Hoigne & Bader, 1994).

In addition to the impact of pH on THM and HAA formation noted above, overall TOX formation decreases with increasing pH. Many of the halogenated DBPs tend to hydrolyse at alkaline pH levels (>8.0) (Singer, 1994a). This has significant implications, for example, for precipitative softening facilities.

pH has a strong effect on aldehyde formation (Schechter & Singer, 1995). Higher ozonation pH values produced lower amounts of aldehydes, supporting the theory that these DBPs are formed primarily through the direct molecular ozone reaction pathway, as opposed to the radical pathway. These results may also reflect greater destruction of aldehydes by hydroxyl radicals at elevated pH levels.

2.8.3 *Effect of bromide*

The presence of bromide ion during water treatment disinfection can lead to the formation of DBPs such as brominated organics and bromate ion. Low but significant levels of bromide, the ultimate precursor to bromate and other brominated compounds, may occur in drinking-water sources as a result of pollution and saltwater intrusion in addition to bromide from natural sources. An understanding of the sources and levels of bromide ion in different source waters is crucial for an understanding of the bromate ion formation potential in drinking-waters. There are no known treatment techniques available for economically removing bromide ion present in source waters during drinking-water treatment.

The impact of bromide on the speciation of DBPs within a class of compounds such as THMs or HAAs has been discussed by Cooper et al. (1983, 1985) and Amy et al. (1998). Rook et al. (1978) reported that bromine is more effective than chlorine in participating in substitution reactions with organic molecules; furthermore, precursor materials may differ in their susceptibility to bromination versus chlorination reactions. Hypobromous acid formed from bromide may also react with ammonia to form bromamines (Galal-Gorchev & Morris, 1965).

2.8.4 *Effect of reaction rates*

After chlorine addition, there is a period of rapid THM formation for the initial few hours (e.g., 4 h), followed by a decline in the rate of THM formation, suggesting fast and slow NOM reactive sites. Many authors have indicated that the concentration of chloroform appears to increase slowly even after 96 h, suggesting that as long as low concentrations of free chlorine are present, chloroform continues to form. Bromochlorinated THM species have been found to form more rapidly than chloroform. Further data from many sources indicate that bromoform formation slows at approximately 7–8 h and levels off almost completely after 20 h (AWWARF, 1991; Koch et al., 1991).

The same general kinetic trend observed for THMs also appears to apply to HAAs. A period of rapid formation occurs during the first 4–8 h, followed by a reduction in the formation rate. In general, for most sources, concentrations of chlorinated HAAs appear to slowly increase even after 96 h, while the formation of DBA levels off after about 18–20 h.

Miller & Uden (1983) observed that nearly 90% of the final concentrations of THMs, TCA and DCA form within the first 24 h of chlorine addition to waters containing NOM. Reckhow et al. (1990) found that although waters containing precursor materials isolated from six different water sources differed in their yields of chlorinated organic by-products, the formation curves for chloroform, TCA and DCA had the same general shapes for all six precursor materials. Some researchers have suggested that DCA may be an intermediate in TCA formation; however, for all eight source waters studied, both DCA and TCA concentrations increased or remained stable throughout the 96-h reaction period, suggesting that DCA was an end-product (AWWARF, 1991). Carlson & Hardy (1998) indicated that HAA formation followed a pattern similar to that of THM formation. As with the THMs, HAA formation rate appeared to be rapid for the first 30 min; after 30 min, HAAs formed at nearly a constant rate in four of the source waters studied.

Different trends were observed in the HAN concentrations of different source waters. For two source waters, HAN levels formed rapidly for the first 8 h and continued to increase slowly or levelled off after 96 h (AWWARF, 1991). DBAN levels remained relatively stable over the 96 h, as did BCAN and DCAN levels. For other sources, levels of HANs consisting mostly of DCAN increased rapidly up to 4–8 h and began to decline by the end of the 96-h period. For these sources, BCAN appeared to be slightly more stable than DCAN.

Very low levels of chloropicrin formation have been observed by many researchers (AWWARF, 1991). The highest concentration observed was 4.0 µg/litre. Chloropicrin appears to form slowly during the incubation period, with concentrations tending to level off at approximately 40 h.

2.8.5 Effect of temperature

The formation rates of THMs, HAAs, bromate ion and HANs have been shown to increase with temperature (AWWARF, 1991; Siddiqui & Amy, 1993). Both haloketone and chloropicrin levels were found to be higher at a lower temperature, while the concentrations of other DBP species were similar or not significantly different. These results suggest that a higher temperature allows for more rapid progression of the transformation of haloketones to other by-products. In studies on the effect of temperature on THMs, Peters et al. (1980) found an Arrhenius dependency between the rate constant and temperature with an activation energy of 10–20 kJ/mol.

The impact of temperature on THMs was strongest at longer contact times (Carlson & Hardy, 1998). On a conceptual basis, it may be that rapidly forming compounds are more reactive and form DBPs regardless of temperature. On the other hand, slowly forming compounds require higher activation energy, and an increase in the temperature supplies the energy. In addition to reaction kinetics, the temperature of a source water can also affect disinfection efficiency. The biocidal effectiveness of monochloramine is significantly less than that of free chlorine and is dependent on temperature, pH and residual concentration.

2.8.6 Effect of alkalinity

Although pH is a very influential variable and alkalinity affects pH, alkalinity itself does not appear to directly affect the formation of THMs and HAAs (by chlorination) and has only a slight effect on aldehydes and other organic by-products following ozonation (Andrews et al., 1996). However, the majority of studies on the effect of alkalinity on the formation of bromate during ozonation indicate that increased alkalinity increases bromate formation (Siddiqui et al., 1995). The quantity of aldehydes produced remains approximately constant for similar changes in alkalinity and pH; however, deviation from equivalent changes in pH and alkalinity results in increased aldehyde concentrations. Therefore, conditions of high alkalinity and low pH or low alkalinity and high pH produce greater quantities of aldehydes than do intermediate values of these parameters (Andrews et al., 1996).

2.9 Influence of water treatment variables on the amount and type of by-products produced

Since DBPs are formed by all of the above chemical disinfectants, the adoption of alternative disinfectants for DBP control often means only a trade-off between one group of DBPs and another. The most effective DBP control strategy is organic precursor (NOM) removal through enhanced coagulation, biofiltration, GAC or membrane filtration. There has been little success with bromide removal. Other DBP control options include water quality modifications — for example, acid or ammonia addition for bromate minimization.

2.9.1 Effect of ammonia

The presence of ammonia in source waters during disinfection can cause chlorine and ozone demand and participation in the formation of by-products such as nitrate, cyanogen chloride and other nitrogenous compounds.

Ammonia also does not consume chlorine dioxide. In contrast to chlorine, chlorine dioxide can therefore be considered as a virucide when ammonia is present. This might be one of the historical reasons why chlorine dioxide has been adopted as a disinfectant by some treatment plants using well oxidized waters but containing changing ammonia concentrations. The addition of ammonia has been shown to reduce the formation of bromate after ozonation (Siddiqui et al., 1995), and the ammonia has been shown to participate in the formation of HANs and cyanogen bromide (CNBr) (Siddiqui & Amy, 1993).

The growth of nitrifying bacteria is a potential problem in chloraminated water supplies or chlorination of sources containing nitrogen. In a study conducted by Cunliffe (1991), nitrifying bacteria were detected in 64% of samples collected from five chloraminated water supplies in South Australia and in 21% of samples that contained more than 5 mg of monochloramine per litre. Increased numbers of the bacteria were associated with monochloramine decay within the distribution systems.

2.9.2   Effect of disinfectant dose

Chlorine dose is a factor affecting the type and concentration of DBPs formed. The THM level rises with increasing chlorine dose (Kavanaugh et al., 1980). However, there is some disagreement regarding the quantitative relations between chlorine concentration and THM levels (or the rate of THM production). Most investigators found a linear relationship between chlorine consumption and THM production, with an order of reaction greater than or equal to unity (Trussell & Umphres, 1978; Kavanaugh et al., 1980). However, it is also possible that the order of reaction changes during the course of the reaction.

Reckhow & Singer (1985) found that the concentration of DBP intermediates such as DCAN and 1,1,1-TCPN formed after 72 h of reaction time was dependent on chlorine dose. DCAN, which was measured at a concentration of approximately 5 µg/litre at a chlorine dose of 10 mg/litre, was not detected in samples dosed with 50 mg of chlorine per litre. The concentration of chloroform was about 150 µg/litre in a sample dosed with 10 mg of chlorine per litre but was approximately 200 µg/litre in a sample dosed with 20 mg of chlorine per litre. Thus, it is imperative to have uniform chlorine doses for performing DBP formation kinetic measurements.

Since chloramine residuals are longer-lasting than free chlorine residuals, the doses for each set of chlorinated and chloraminated samples will be different in order to achieve the prescribed target residual. The disappearance of chloramines can be explained approximately by a second-order reaction. However, as the chlorine dose increased, the observed rate constant was found to decrease, then increased after reaching a minimum value (Dlyamandoglu & Selleck, 1992). Below the chlorine dose at the minimum value of the observed rate constant, the rate constant was proportional to the 1.4 power of the chlorine dose, regardless of the ammonia concentration (Yamamoto et al., 1988).

2.9.3   Effect of advanced oxidation processes

Water utilities can add treatment processes that remove DBP precursors or DBPs. Many utilities will be using both approaches. The hydrogen peroxide/UV process, an advanced oxidation process, offers small water utilities a treatment process with the potential to provide primary disinfection and a method of DBP control (Symons & Worley, 1995). This process has been shown to oxidize dissolved organic halogens and decrease TOC. TOC removal as a function of UV dose has also been demonstrated by Worley (1994), with TOC removals of between 0% and 80%. Andrews et al. (1996) evaluated the effect of the hydrogen peroxide/UV process on THM formation and concluded that this process is only slightly effective in reducing the formation of DBPs. However, using hydrogen peroxide at 1 mg/litre in combination with UV effectively reduced or prevented the formation of aldehydes. Other advanced oxidation processes (e.g., hydrogen peroxide/ozone, ozone/UV) involving hydroxyl (and hydroperoxyl) radical formation may provide similar opportunities.

2.9.4 Effect of chemical coagulation

Enhanced coagulation and softening will remove TOC. Enhanced coagulation is characterized by coagulant doses greater than those required for optimum turbidity removal; as an alternative to higher doses, a combination of acid (pH depression) and coagulant addition can be practised.

All organic DBPs were reduced by the addition of commonly used coagulants. Iron-based coagulants, such as ferric chloride, were consistently more effective than alum in removing NOM (Crozes et al., 1995). Alum coagulation removed all DBP precursors to a significant extent. The percentage removals showed the same trends as, but were not identical to, the percentage removals of TOC and UV absorbance. UV absorbance was removed to a somewhat greater extent than TOC. Hence, TOC and UV absorbance can serve as surrogate parameters for DBP formation potential. A fairly good correlation was observed between the ratio of HAAs to THMs and the ratio of UV absorbance to TOC, indicating that the relative concentrations of HAAs and THMs do to some extent depend on the nature of the precursor material. However, more data from waters of different qualities would be required to evaluate the validity of this relationship.

The effectiveness of coagulants in removing DBP precursors is dependent upon the molecular size of the dissolved organic matter. Normally, higher molecular weight fractions are effectively removed through coagulation. In a study conducted by Teng & Veenstra (1995), water containing dissolved organic matter with molecular weights in the range 1000–10 000 daltons generally produced the largest amounts of THMs and HAAs under conditions of free chlorination. Coagulation and ozonation shift a proportionately greater amount of the THM and HAA formation potential to the smallest molecular weight range (<1000 daltons).

Coagulation and filtration remove NOM but not bromide, hence increasing the ratio of bromide to TOC. As a result, the subsequent use of chlorine generally favours the formation of brominated organic DBPs.

2.9.5   Effect of pre-ozonation

Several studies of ozone oxidation followed by chlorination showed increased, rather than decreased, levels of THMs (Trussell & Umphres, 1978). This is attributed, at least partially, to the formation of aldehydes by ozonation. Another possibility is hydroxylation of aromatic compounds to produce *m*-dihydroxy aromatic derivatives, which are known THM precursors (Lykins & Clark, 1988). Although the aldehydes produced contain polar groupings, they are nevertheless not easily removed during the flocculation step by complexation with aluminium or iron salts. A convenient and more appropriate method for the removal of the aldehydes formed during ozonation is the incorporation of a biological treatment step (biofiltration) in the water treatment process following ozone oxidation.

Pre-ozonation can have both positive and negative effects on DBP formation. Pre-ozonation with typical water treatment dosages and bicarbonate levels has been shown to remove TCA and DCAN precursors. However, such treatment can result in no net change in the DCA precursors and may lead to an increase in 1,1,1-TCPN precursors (Reckhow & Singer, 1985). According to Teng & Veenstra (1995), pre-ozonation resulted in enhanced formation of DCA during chlorination and chloramination in the presence of precursors in the <1000 dalton molecular weight range. They also indicated that pre-ozonation plus chloramination controlled the overall production of THMs and HAAs. However, the use of pre-ozonation coupled with free chlorination increased the yield of DCA for both the hydrophilic and hydrophobic fractions of NOM as compared with free chlorination alone.

With ozone–chlorine treatment, chloral hydrate formation can be enhanced. This behaviour, which has also been observed for DCA, suggests that the reaction that produces chloral hydrate is accelerated under the conditions of ozonation in combination with prechlorination and warm water temperatures (LeBel et al., 1995).

Ozonation in the presence of traces of hypochlorite ion can form inorganic by-products such as chlorate. Siddiqui et al. (1996a) showed that if there is any residual chlorine present, ozone can potentially oxidize hypochlorite ion to chlorate.

Coleman et al. (1992) suggested that brominated MX analogues and other mixed bromochlorinated by-products formed after ozonation and chlorination can possibly increase mutagenic activity.

2.9.6 *Effect of biofiltration*

Biofiltration (ozone–sand filtration or ozone–GAC) can potentially reduce TOC, organic by-products and the formation of halogenated DBPs.

Passage of ozonated water samples through a rapid sand filter reduced the concentration of aldehydes by 62% (Lykins & Clark, 1988). Chlorinated samples experienced a 26% reduction in aldehyde concentrations under the same conditions. These reductions in aldehyde levels are attributable to biological activity in the sand filters. If GAC filtration follows sand filtration, ozone oxidation can be expected to promote more bioactivity in the GAC filter, because a better colonization environment is provided for microorganisms on GAC particles than on sand. Thus, the biological conversion of oxidized water impurities to carbon dioxide and water will be greater during passage through GAC media. Similar aldehyde removals have been observed by several researchers (Van Hoof et al., 1985; Sketchell et al., 1995).

Drinking-water treatment techniques that remove organic contaminants without affecting bromide concentrations cause a shift in the formation of DBPs towards brominated DBPs. Sketchell et al. (1995)

studied three sources containing three different DOC levels and ambient bromides, which were filtered through biologically active GAC filters. Analysis of treated waters showed no removal of bromide ion and a shift towards more brominated organo-DBPs. THM levels after treatment with GAC with no added ozone decreased from 900–1700 to 100–700 µg/litre. These water sources contained DOC levels ranging from 10 to 25 mg/litre and high concentrations of biodegradable DOC (DOC removals ranged from 60% to 80% after GAC treatment).

Table 8 summarizes the effects of ozonation and biofiltration on the formation of DBPs from various sources.

2.10 Comparative assessment of disinfectants

A comparative assessment (Table 9) of various disinfecting chemicals for pre-disinfection (or oxidation) and post-disinfection and maintaining a residual for 5 days to simulate concentrations in the distribution system showed that the use of free chlorine produces the largest concentration of halogenated DBPs (Clark et al., 1994). The concentration of DBPs may be reduced by adding ozone or chlorine dioxide as a preoxidant, although enhanced formation has been observed.

Table 10 summarizes the effects of water quality and treatment variables on the formation of DBPs.

2.11 Alternative strategies for disinfectant by-product control

The concern about chlorite, bromate, chlorate and other DBPs in drinking-water following treatment with disinfectants has stimulated research into ways to eliminate the production or enhance the removal of DBPs. Strategies for DBP control include source control, precursor removal, use of alternative disinfectants and removal of DBPs by technologies such as air stripping, activated carbon, UV light and advanced oxidation technologies. For DBPs that can arise in hypochlorite solutions (e.g., chlorate), the purity and storage conditions of the solutions are important concerns.

Table 8. Effects of ozonation and biofiltration on chlorine organic by-products

DBPs	Ozonation (% change)	Biofiltration (% change)	Ozonation + biofiltration (% change)	Reference
THMs	−20	−20	−40 (chlorine)	Speitel et al. (1993)
HAAs	−10	−13	−25 (chlorine)	Speitel et al. (1993)
Chloropicrin	+50 to +250		−50 to −100 (chlorine)	Miltner et al. (1992)
Aldehydes	+425 to +1300	−40 to −50	−92 to −98	Miltner et al. (1992)
TOX	−30		−51 (chlorine)	Miltner et al. (1992)
TOX	−10	−38	−47 (chlorine)	Shukairy & Summers (1992)
TOX	+32	−69	−60 (monochloramine)	Shukairy & Summers (1992)

Table 9. Comparative assessment of organic disinfectant by-products (µg/litre) in distribution systems[a,b]

DBPs	Sand–Cl_2	Cl_2–Sand–Cl_2	O_3–Sand–Cl_2	NH_2Cl–Sand–NH_2Cl	O_3–Sand–NH_2Cl	ClO_2–Sand–Cl_2
THMs	236.0	225.0	154.0	9.0	3.2	138.0
HAAs	60.0	146.0	82.0	14.0	9.0	44.0
HANs	3.1	2.9	2.7	<0.1	<0.1	<0.1
Haloketones	2.1	2.6	2.6	<0.1	<0.1	4.2
Chloropicrin	1.3	1.3	7.7	<0.1	<0.1	1.4
Chloral hydrate	79.0	75.0	55.0	<0.1	<0.1	45.0
TOX	557.0	540.0	339.0	59.0	27.0	379.0

[a] Clark et al. (1994).
[b] TOC = 3.0 mg/litre; pH = 7.6.

Table 10. Summary of impact of water quality and treatment variables on disinfectant by-product formation

Variable	Impact on THMs	Impact on HAAs	Impact on aldehydes	Impact on chlorate/chlorite	Impact on bromate
Contact time	Curvilinear increase with increasing contact time Rapid formation <5 h 90% formation in 24 h Levels off at 96 h	Curvilinear increase with increasing contact time Rapid formation <5 h 90% formation in 24 h Levels off at 150 h	Linear increase as long as residual chemical present Secondary reactions between disinfectants and aldehydes possible	Linear increase in bleach solutions No discernible effects in dilute solutions If oxidation of hypochlorite, contact time has a positive effect	Curvilinear increase with most bromate forming in <5 min Formation is a function of ozone residual and bromide
Disinfectant dose	Rapid and curvilinear increase after TOC demand with dose, levelling off at 2.0 mg/litre for TOC of 2.0 mg/litre	Curvilinear increase after TOC demand with increasing dose, levelling off at 2.0 mg/litre	Curvilinear with increasing ozone dose or chlorine dose No appreciable effect after ozone/DOC = 2 : 1	Concentrations related to hypochlorite doses applied Ozone oxidation of hypochlorite increases with dose	Linear increase after TOC demand and then levelling off after ozone residual disappearance
pH	Curvilinear increase with increasing pH to pH 7.0 and possible pH maximum No positive effect at pH > 9.5	Mixed, possible pH maximum for DCAA and DBAA TCAA decreases up to pH > 9 DCAA maximum at pH 7–7.5	Negative effect (forms mostly through molecular ozone) 25% decrease for pH 7–8.5	Positive effect Decomposition of hypochlorite increases with pH Oxidation of hypochlorite by ozone increases	Strong linear positive effect Hydroxyl radical generation efficiency increases

72

Table 10 (Contd).

Temperature	Linear increase with increasing temperature (10–30 °C; 15–25% increase)	Linear increase with increasing temperature (10–30 °C; 20–30% increase)	Terminal products such as carbon dioxide increase and total aldehydes slightly decrease	Positive effect Decomposition of hypochlorite increases	Curvilinear increase 20–30% increase for 15–25 °C
TOC	Increase with increasing TOC; precursor content important Humic acids more reactive than fulvic acids	Increase with increasing TOC; precursor content important Humic acids more reactive than fulvic acids	Positive effect (hydrophobic fraction mostly responsible) Doubles for every 2 mg/litre	Negative effect if ozone is used for hypochlorite oxidation Most likely no effect with hypochlorite	Decreases with increasing TOC; precursor content important Non-humic acid being less reactive with ozone
UVA$_{254}$	Increase with increasing UV absorbance; precursor content important Aromaticity of TOC being more important	Increase with increasing UV absorbance; precursor content important Aromaticity of TOC being more important	Positive effect Ozone demand increases with UV (UV absorbance is mostly due to aromaticity and hydrophobic fraction)	Negative effect if ozone is used for hypochlorite oxidation Probable negative effect with hypochlorous acid	Decreases with increasing UV absorbance; precursor content important Humic acid being more reactive with ozone
Bromide	Shift towards brominated species	Shift towards brominated species	Independent of bromide at <0.25 mg/litre At >0.25 mg/litre, aldehydes can decrease due to ozone–bromide oxidation	Shift towards more toxic bromate in hypochlorite solutions	Bromide threshold Curvilinear increase and dependent upon ozone residual
Alkalinity	No discernible effect	No discernible effect	Slight positive effect	Unknown	Positive effect

Table 10 (Contd).

Variable	Impact on THMs	Impact on HAAs	Impact on aldehydes	Impact on chlorate/chlorite	Impact on bromate
Minimization strategies	TOC removal, minimizing chlorine residual, alternative disinfectants, pH control, minimizing contact time	TOC removal, minimizing chlorine residual, alternative disinfectants, pH control, minimizing contact time	pH control, TOC removal by coagulation, GAC, optimizing doses, contact time	Avoid hypochlorite dosing solution Minimize storage Properly tune generators Use freshly made solutions	pH depression, ammonia addition, radical scavengers, minimizing and optimizing ozone residual
Removal strategies	GAC, electron beam, air stripping	GAC, electron beam	Biofiltration, advanced oxidation, GAC, nanofilters	Ferrous sulfate, GAC, electron beam, UV irradiation, nanofilters	Ferrous sulfate, UV irradiation, high-energy electron beam, GAC

74

2.11.1 Source control

Source control options involve controlling nutrient inputs to waters (e.g., algae growth control) (Hoehn et al., 1990) that are used as drinking-water sources, watershed management (e.g., constructing stormwater detention basins), saltwater intrusion control (e.g., development of structural or hydrodynamic barriers to control TOC and bromide), and using the concept known as aquifer storage and recovery (e.g., drawing water during seasons when the quality of the water is best) (Singer, 1994a).

2.11.2 Organohalogen by-products

Strategies for control of organohalogen by-products include removal of DBPs that are formed using technologies such as oxidation, aeration and carbon adsorption (Clark et al., 1994); and removal of precursors using treatment techniques such as conventional treatment, oxidation, membrane processes, carbon adsorption and biological degradation. For many organic compounds that are difficult to oxidize, such as chloroform, the kinetics of ozone oxidation are generally very slow but are faster if used in combination with UV irradiation. GAC adsorption and membrane filtration are relatively expensive processes; moreover, NOM removal by GAC cannot be accomplished to any significant degree in a filter/adsorber (i.e., GAC filter cap) mode but requires a separate post-filtration adsorber bed. The use of membranes requires pretreatment to prevent fouling, as well as processing of waste brine. The use of ozone in combination with biologically active GAC filters is a promising alternative to reduce DBP precursors.

2.11.3 Inorganic by-products

Properly designed and operated chlorine and chlorine dioxide generator systems can minimize some of the production of chlorate ion. Removal of chlorite and chlorate has been reported using reduction by Fe^{2+} or sulfite or by GAC (Voudrias et al., 1983; Lykins & Clark, 1988). GAC is seen as problematic because of chlorate production and a short bed life. A chemical process using an appropriate agent such as reduced iron (e.g., ferrous sulfate) appears to be a more promising approach (Kraft & van Eldick, 1989; Gordon et al., 1990).

If bromate is present in treated water entering the coagulation process (i.e., formed during pre-ozonation), several options exist for its removal. An aqueous-phase reducing agent (e.g., Fe^{2+}) can be added at the rapid mix step. Powdered activated carbon can likewise be added as a solid-phase reductant to remove bromate and DBP precursors. Not all utilities contemplating ozone application intend to employ pre-ozonation. Rather, they may use intermediate ozonation prior to the filtration process; in this situation, removal of bromate by activated carbon is possible. This approach has potential relevance to integration of GAC columns into a process train or, more realistically, to retro-fitting of rapid sand filters with GAC filters. For groundwaters that require no coagulation, bromate can be removed after ozonation using a GAC filter, UV irradiation or high-energy electron beam irradiation (Siddiqui et al., 1994, 1996a,b,c).

Brominated or bromochlorinated amines formed during the oxidation step of the process train using chlorine can potentially be removed using a suitable activated carbon before terminal chlorination. However, carbon that has an accumulation of surface oxides, which develop through reaction of amines, will have a diminished capacity to reduce halogenated amines to nitrogen. Organic amines can potentially be removed by activated carbon adsorption.

2.11.4 Organic by-products

There are some technologies for removing organic contaminants formed after chlorination and chloramination, a less viable option than minimizing their formation through DBP precursor removal or use of alternative disinfectants. Studies of ozone oxidation have shown that aromatic compounds, alkenes and certain pesticides (some of which have structural similarities to certain organic DBPs) are removed well by ozone treatment, but that alkanes are poorly removed. Also, removal efficiency improves for the alkenes and aromatic compounds with increasing ozone dosage and for some alkanes with increasing pH. For most compounds, the efficacy of ozone is not affected by the background water matrix if the ozone is used after coagulation. Andrews et al. (1996) showed that using hydrogen peroxide at 1.0 mg/litre in combination with UV effectively reduced or prevented the formation of aldehydes.

2.12 Models for predicting disinfectant by-product formation

The regulation of THMs and other halogenated DBPs has been complicated by findings that alternative disinfectants to free chlorine may also form by-products that are of potential health concern. Additional complicating factors impacting the regulation of DBPs have been the emergence of *Giardia* and *Cryptosporidium* as major water-borne pathogens.

In view of the finding that water chlorination produces DBPs, some of which are carcinogenic, mutagenic or possibly teratogenic, several countries have recently laid down standards for various DBP levels. This stimulated the search for mathematical models to describe or predict DBP formation in disinfected water and to evaluate the effectiveness of water treatment technologies designed to reduce DBP levels so as to comply with the standards. Most of these models are based on fitting mathematical equations to various empirical observations, rather than mechanistic and kinetic considerations. This is mainly due to the complexity of the reactions between organic precursors and disinfecting chemicals, which usually involve several parallel pathways leading to a great variety of products. The complexity of the DBP formation reactions also makes it difficult to develop universally applicable models for simulating DBP formation potential associated with disinfection of a diverse array of natural source waters. However, the analysis presented by many models suggests that many waters exhibit comparable general responses to changes in a given parameter (i.e., responses lending themselves to simulation by a particular mathematical functionality), although specific responses associated with individual waters may vary. The multiple regression models developed by many researchers represent a rational framework for modelling DBP formation in many sources. Another potential application is the modelling of DBP mixtures, e.g., predicting HAA levels from THM and water quality data.

2.12.1 Factors affecting disinfectant by-product formation and variables of interest in disinfectant by-product modelling

The information on the factors controlling DBP formation, which is available in the literature, is briefly summarized below.

The extent of formation of DBPs is dependent on several water quality parameters, such as TOC concentration, UVA_{254}, bromide concentration and temperature. It is also dependent on chlorination conditions, such as chlorine dose, pH, ammonia concentration and contact time. After the various statistically significant factors were identified, mathematical equations were developed to describe the formation of various DBPs. A least squares method was used to determine the optimum equation coefficients that best describe the experimental data. The optimum coefficients have been defined as those that produce a minimum residual error between the mathematical predictions and the experimental data.

2.12.2 *Empirical models for disinfectant by-product formation*

Numerous models for predicting THM formation through chlorination have been reported (Moore et al., 1979a; Kavanaugh et al., 1980; Engerholm & Amy, 1983; Urano et al., 1983; Amy et al., 1987, 1998; Morrow & Minear, 1987; AWWARF, 1991; Hutton & Chung, 1992). Of these, models reported by AWWARF (1991) and Amy et al. (1998) are more recent and were derived from a variety of natural source waters and more realistic treatment conditions. Not much information has been reported on the formation of other chlorination DBPs. Only Amy et al. (1998) summarized empirical models for THMs, HAAs and chloral hydrate. These chlorination by-product models can be used to assess both in-plant and distribution system formation of THMs, HAAs and chloral hydrate. Water quality conditions such as DOC, pH, temperature and bromide are needed as inputs to the models; such data then allow assessment of chlorination DBP formation as a function of reaction time:

DBP concentration (total THMs or THM species, total HAAs or HAA species, or chloral hydrate) =
f(TOC, bromide, chlorine, pH, temperature, time)

Relatively little is known about the kinetics of the formation of bromate and other DBPs during ozonation and the quantitative effects of water quality factors (temperature, pH, etc.); such an understanding is crucial for evaluating various bromate control strategies. Siddiqui & Amy (1993) and Amy et al. (1998) developed statistical relations to predict the concentrations of various ozone DBPs, including bromate, as a function of water treatment variables. Correlation matrix analysis has shown that ozone dose, dissolved ozone concentration, bromide concentration, pH and reaction time all have a positive influence on bromate formation. Von Gunten & Hoigne (1994) developed kinetic models for bromate formation.

Ozone, as a result of its strong oxidizing power, produces a variety of organic by-products, such as aldehydes and ketoacids, when used to treat natural source waters. These by-products — especially aldehydes — are highly biodegradable, and there is concern for regrowth of microorganisms following ozone treatment. They are also potentially hazardous and may produce increased amounts of chlorinated by-products upon chlorination. Siddiqui et al. (1997) developed a model to estimate the potential for total aldehyde formation in source waters upon ozonation.

2.12.3 *Models for predicting disinfectant by-product precursor removal*

It is recognized that chlorination will continue to be the most common disinfection process; hence, enhanced removal of DBP precursors present in raw sources represents a valuable option for reducing the potential for by-product formation. The removal of NOM can be achieved either by providing additional processes, such as GAC and nanofiltration, or by enhancing the existing coagulation, flocculation and sedimentation processes. Predictive models have been developed for assessing coagulation efficiency in removing NOM and reducing DBP precursor levels (AWWARF, 1991; Amy et al., 1998).

Coagulation can reduce DOC and DBP precursors but not bromide levels; hence, a greater proportion of brominated DBP species can potentially be produced in the finished water.

The effects of precursor removal by chemical coagulation can be assessed through the use of treated water models. One can either predict DBPs formed under a given degree of precursor removal or define the degree of precursor removal required to meet DBP regulations. The impact of bromide ion on meeting regulations can also be assessed. If one makes the assumption that precursor reactivity (i.e., DBP/DOC) does not change, one can also assess other precursor removal processes, such as GAC or membrane processes, through use of the raw/untreated water models. Care should be exercised when using models to approximate post-chlorination DBPs following an ozonation step.

2.13 Summary

- The primary and most important role of drinking-water treatment is to remove or inactivate harmful microorganisms. Another role is to minimize the concentrations of disinfectants and DBPs without compromising in any way the removal or inactivation of pathogens.

- Drinking-water utility managers must be more knowledgeable about options to meet regulations. It is often more practical to use treatment methods that control the concentration of several contaminants than to modify treatment practices for each new standard that is promulgated.

- A thorough understanding of DBP formation would help the successful balancing of appropriate microbial inactivation with the minimization of DBPs. Water quality variables affect DBP formation and must be considered when developing a strategy to control DBPs with various disinfectants.

- The chemistry of chlorine and its by-products has been well studied, and ozone and its by-products have recently received much attention. Studies of chlorine dioxide and chloramines and their by-products are relatively few, although more work in these areas is now being undertaken.

- One of the simplest processes to minimize halogenated DBP formation is limiting the free chlorine contact time by using monochloramine to maintain a distribution system residual following primary disinfection by chlorine or ozone. Chloramines are an effective means of controlling DBPs. However, the growth of nitrifying bacteria (and related production of nitrite) is a potential problem in chloraminated water supplies.

- Various nitrogen-containing organic compounds may be present in source waters after chlorination and chloramination. Because of analytical complexities, very few detailed studies have been undertaken to determine the individual compounds present and their concentrations.

- Many factors between the source and the tap can influence the DBPs to which consumers are exposed. Although THMs and HAAs continue to form with increasing contact time, some other halogenated DBPs, such as HANs and haloketones, form rapidly but then decay in the distribution system as a result of hydrolysis. This has major implications regarding exposure to these DBPs, depending upon their proximity to the treatment plant. For treated source waters, median levels of HAAs are often approximately one-half of the median THM levels.

- For low-bromide source waters, chloroform is normally the dominant THM species; DCA and TCA are the most prevalent HAA species; DCAN is the most prevalent HAN species; and 1,1,1-TCPN is the most prevalent of the two measured haloketones. Very low levels of chloropicrin have been observed by various researchers; this compound appears to form slowly during the incubation period, with concentrations tending to level off at 40 h. For high-bromide waters, increased levels of brominated DBPs are observed.

- Chlorine dioxide is a strong oxidant that under certain conditions surpasses chlorine in its ability to destroy pathogenic organisms. When chlorine dioxide is prepared and administered without excess free chlorine, THMs and other chlorinated by-products are not produced, but inorganic by-products are formed.

- TOC levels have been found to be correlated with halogenated DBP formation. The nature of this relationship varies with the source. TOC removal can be used as a surrogate for the reduction of DBP formation.

- Although the presence of chloral hydrate and HANs in chlorinated samples may be attributed to precursors other than amino acids, the potential for amino acids to be present in natural sources is well documented. Surface waters, but not groundwaters, tend to contain amino acids. However, the removal of these precursors during conventional water treatment is not well understood.

- The amount of chlorate that is present in delivered hypochlorite solutions depends on many factors. Freshly made hypochlorite solutions will contain less chlorate than hypochlorite that is stored without concern for temperature and pH. If a utility is using a single tank to store hypochlorite, it is likely that the level of chlorate is increasing in the tank. Thus, storage tanks should be periodically flushed and cleaned, and, if possible, the storage time should be reduced.

- Models have been developed that can be used to simulate the fate and movement of DBP precursors in distribution systems. The models can be designed as a planning tool for evaluating the impacts of source water management strategies and estimating DBP exposures. Some limitations of existing models include calibration with a limited database, application to only a specific water source or group of related sources, lack of terms to simulate important parameters, such as reaction time, and inadequate validation.

3. TOXICOLOGY OF DISINFECTANTS

In assessing the hazards associated with drinking-water disinfection, it is important not to neglect the disinfectants themselves. Adding disinfectant in excess of the demand has several practical benefits. First, it ensures that reaction of the disinfectant with DBP precursors (largely organic material and ammonia) does not shorten contact time to the point of ineffective disinfection. Second, residual disinfectant helps to prevent regrowth of organisms in the remaining portions of the treatment and distribution systems.

The result of this practice, however, is that one of the chemicals that is present in the finished water at the highest concentration is the disinfectant. In the present regulatory climate in many countries, chemicals that are introduced as direct additives to food would be subjected to a significant amount of toxicological screening before they could be used. Since the major disinfectants were introduced almost 100 years ago, they were subjected to much less thorough toxicological evaluations than would be required today. However, many of these data gaps have been addressed in the past decade.

3.1 Chlorine and hypochlorite

3.1.1 General toxicological properties and information on dose–response in animals

Chlorine gas has long been recognized as a lung irritant. This topic will not be reviewed in the present document, as it appears to be largely irrelevant to the small amounts of chlorine that are volatilized from chlorinated water in showers or other points of use in the household. In water treatment plants, however, there is a possibility of occupational exposures that could have severe sequelae. For information on these higher-level exposures, the interested reader is referred to a recent review by Das & Blanc (1993). The effects of chlorine gas that have been observed in humans will be discussed in section 3.1.3.

Sodium hypochlorite (NaOCl) or calcium hypochlorite ($Ca(OCl)_2$) solutions have also been utilized extensively in the disinfection of drinking-water. The stock solutions used for this purpose are highly caustic and are a clear concern for occupational exposures. The concentration required to produce irritation and decreased basal cell viability in the skin of guinea-pigs after an application period of 2 weeks was 0.5% sodium hypochlorite (Cotter et al., 1985). Reducing the concentration to 0.1% resulted in no effect on basal cell viability relative to control animals. Yarington (1970) demonstrated that instillation of bleach into the oesophagus of dogs produced irritation. The minimal exposure that produced oesophageal burns was 10 ml of commercial bleach with a 5-min exposure. It should be noted that the highly alkaline pH (about pH 11) of sodium hypochlorite is not likely to be encountered in drinking-water.

There have been relatively few evaluations of the effects of chlorine or hypochlorite in drinking-water. The present review will focus on studies with treatment periods longer than 4 weeks where drinking-water was the primary route of exposure. Reference to earlier studies of shorter duration and less general applicability to a safety evaluation can be found in previous reviews (Bull, 1980, 1982a,b, 1992; Bull & Kopfler, 1991).

Daniel et al. (1990a) evaluated the toxicity of solutions of chlorine prepared by bubbling chlorine gas into distilled water and adjusting the pH to 9.4. The nominal concentrations of chlorine used were 0, 25, 100, 175 or 250 mg/litre in distilled water (approximately 0, 3, 10, 16 or 21 mg/kg of body weight per day). These solutions were provided as drinking-water to both male and female Sprague-Dawley rats (10 per sex per dose) for 90 days. No deaths occurred in any treatment group. However, there were statistically significant decreases in drinking-water consumption in females treated with 100 mg/litre and higher, probably due to decreased palatability. There were no consistent effects of chlorine treatment on organ to body weight ratios or clinical chemistry parameters. A no-observed-effect level (NOEL) of 10 mg/kg of body weight per day was identified by the authors based on reduced body weight gain. However, since this was associated with reduced palatability of the drinking-water, it is not considered to be a true toxicological end-point.

The study in rats was followed up with another study in B6C3F$_1$ mice (Daniel et al., 1991a). Male and female B6C3F$_1$ mice (10 per sex per group) were administered 12.5, 25, 50, 100 or 200 mg of chlorine per litre of drinking-water for 90 days (calculated mean daily doses were 2.7, 5.1, 10.3, 19.8 or 34.4 mg/kg of body weight in males and 2.8, 5.8, 11.7, 21.2 or 39.2 mg/kg of body weight in females). Spleen and liver weights were depressed in males, but not in females, at the highest dose rates (100 and 200 mg/litre). There were no other consistent indications of target organ effects based on serum enzyme concentrations. No gross or microscopic lesions could be related to treatment with chlorine.

Several of the following studies utilized solutions of sodium hypochlorite as the treatment chemical. It is now known that such solutions can contain very high concentrations of chlorate within a short time of their preparation (Bolyard et al., 1993). The extent of this contamination has not been reported.

Hasegawa et al. (1986) examined the effects of much higher concentrations (0.025, 0.05, 0.1, 0.2 or 0.4%) of sodium hypochlorite (equivalent to 7, 14, 28, 55 and 111 mg/kg of body weight per day) administered in drinking-water to male and female F344 rats for 13 weeks. Twenty rats of each sex were assigned to each experimental group. Significant suppression of body weight (as a result of decreased consumption of water and food) occurred at 0.2% and above. The authors noted slight damage to the liver as indicated by increased levels of serum enzymes (not specified) at 0.2% and 0.4% sodium hypochlorite in both sexes. No evidence of treatment-related pathology was observed in this study or in a 2-year study in which males were subjected to 0.05% or 0.1% (13.5 or 27.7 mg/kg of body weight per day) and females to 0.1% or 0.2% (34 or 63 mg/kg of body weight per day) sodium hypochlorite. The extended exposures were conducted with 50 animals of each sex per treatment group. Analysis of dosing solutions was not reported.

In a 2-year bioassay, the National Toxicology Program (NTP) examined chlorine at 0, 70, 140 or 275 mg/litre (expressed as atomic chlorine, Cl) in drinking-water of F344 rats and B6C3F$_1$ mice (70 per sex per group) (NTP, 1992). These solutions were prepared from gaseous chlorine and neutralized to pH 9 by the addition of sodium hydroxide. Stability studies indicated that 85% of the initial target concentration remained after 3 days of preparation. Stock solutions (concentrations not specified) were prepared once weekly, and solutions for drinking were prepared 4 times weekly. Based on body weight and water consumption, doses in these studies were approximately 0,

4, 7 or 14 mg/kg of body weight per day for male rats; 0, 4, 8 or 14 mg/kg of body weight per day for female rats; 0, 7, 14 or 24 mg/kg of body weight per day for male mice; and 0, 8, 14 or 24 mg/kg of body weight per day for female mice. The only treatment-related non-tumour pathology was found to be a dilatation of renal tubules in male mice receiving 275 mg/litre for more than 66 weeks. No non-neoplastic lesions were observed in either male or female rats.

A number of immunological changes have been associated with the treatment of rodents with sodium hypochlorite in drinking-water. Water containing 25–30 mg of sodium hypochlorite per litre was found to reduce the mean number of peritoneal exudate cells recovered from female C57BL/6N mice after 2 weeks of treatment. This was, in turn, associated with a significant decrease in macrophage-mediated cyto-toxicity to melanoma and fibrosarcoma cell lines (Fidler, 1977). The treatment period was increased to 4 weeks in a subsequent study, which demonstrated that 25 mg of sodium hypochlorite per litre decreased the ability of peritoneal macrophages to phagocytose ^{51}Cr-labelled sheep red blood cells. Macrophages obtained from the mice treated with hypochlorite were found to be less effective in destroying B16-BL6 melanoma cells *in vitro*. Mice so treated were also found to have increased pulmonary metastasis of B16-BL6 cells when they were introduced by subcutaneous injection (Fidler et al., 1982).

Exon et al. (1987) examined the immunotoxicological effects of sodium hypochlorite at 5, 15 or 30 mg/litre (0.7, 2.1 or 4.2 mg/kg of body weight per day) in the drinking-water of male Sprague-Dawley rats (12 per dose) for 9 weeks. Delayed hypersensitivity reaction to bovine serum albumin was observed at the highest dose administered. Oxidative metabolism by adherent resident peritoneal cells was decreased at 15 and 30 mg/litre, and the prostaglandin E_2 levels of these cells were found to be significantly elevated. No effects on natural killer cell cytotoxicity, antibody responses, interleukin 2 production or phagocytic activity were observed. The effects on macrophage activity suggest that some impairment does occur at relatively low levels of sodium hypochlorite. As pointed out by the authors, these were relatively mild effects, the significance of which was unknown. It is not clear that these effects would be translated into a significant impairment of the immune response to a particular infectious agent. However, modification of macrophage function appears to be one of the most sensitive responses identified in studies of chlorine or hypochlorite in experimental animals. A study in which female C57BL/6 mice were administered hypochlorite in their drinking-water (7.5, 15 or 30 mg of hypochlorite per litre) for 2 weeks showed no effects on the immune system as measured by spleen and thymus weight, plaque-forming cell response, haemagglutination titre and lymphocyte proliferation (French et al., 1998).

Altered liver lipid composition has been observed as a result of acute intragastric administration of sodium hypochlorite (5 ml of a 1% solution) to rats (Chang et al., 1981). These data do not provide a clear indication of whether these effects might give rise to pathology. The concentrations of hypochlorite utilized were much greater than those that would be encountered in drinking-water.

The effects of hypochlorous acid and hypochlorite on the skin have received relatively little attention despite the current interest in bathing as a significant source of chemical exposure from drinking-water. Robinson et al. (1986) examined the effects of both hypochlorite and hypochlorous acid solutions applied to the skin of the entire body of female Sencar mice except for the head. Exposures were to 1, 100, 300 or 1000 mg/litre as hypochlorous acid at pH 6.5 for 10 min on 4 consecutive days. Hypochlorite (formed by raising the pH to 8.5) was studied only at 1000 mg/litre. Significant increases in epidermal thickness and cell counts within the epidermal layer were observed at concentrations of hypochlorous acid (pH 6.5) of 300 mg/litre and above, but the thickness of the skin was not significantly different from that in animals at 100 mg/litre. The increases in skin thickness were associated with an epidermis whose thickness was increased to 4–6 cells as compared with the normal 1–2 cells seen in mice. The effects of hypochlorite were much less marked. Following a single application, the increased thickness of the skin observed in mice exposed to hypochlorous acid (i.e., pH 6.5) did not appear until 4 days after the treatment. This differed from hypochlorite, other disinfectants and the positive control, 12-*O*-tetradecanoylphorbol-13-acetate (TPA). In the latter cases, the maximal response was observed within 24–48 h after treatment. The hyperplastic response to hypochlorous acid required 12 days to return to normal. This study suggests a considerable margin of safety between the concentrations of chlorine required to produce hyperplasia and those that are found in drinking-water.

The reactive nature of chlorine always raises questions of whether it is chlorine or a by-product that is responsible for any effect. Several studies have examined the formation of by-products in the gastro-intestinal tract following the administration of chlorine. Invariably, these studies have involved the administration of chlorine or hypo-chlorite by gavage at very high concentrations relative to the amounts that would be encountered in chlorinated drinking-water. As a consequence, the by-products formed following gavage dosing of high concentrations may not be representative of the by-products that would be seen following the consumption of modest to moderate levels of chlorine in larger volumes of water. A particular issue is that the high organic carbon concentration relative to chlorine that would be encountered in the gastrointestinal tract when water is consumed at low concentrations should dissipate disinfectant before sufficient oxidative power would be present to break down substrates to small molecules. Despite these design flaws, the data do indicate that by-products are formed. The bulk of them remain as higher molecular weight products, which may have little toxicological importance.

Vogt et al. (1979) reported that chloroform could be measured in the blood, brain, liver, kidneys and fat of rats to which sodium hypo-chlorite was administered by gavage at doses of 20, 50 or 80 mg in 5 ml of water. Thus, the by-product chloroform can be formed by the reaction of chlorine with stomach contents.

Mink and co-workers (1983) pursued this observation and found that other by-products could be detected in the stomach contents and plasma of rats that had been administered sodium hypochlorite solutions neutralized to pH 7.9. In addition to chloroform, DCAN, DCA and TCA were detected in the stomach contents analysis. DCA and TCA were also detected in blood plasma.

The third group of compounds identified as by-products of chlorination in stomach contents of the rat are the organic *N*-chloramines (Scully et al., 1990). *N*-Chloroglycine, *N*-chloroleucine or *N*-chloroisoleucine and *N*-chlorophenylalanine were confirmed prod-ucts of reactions with normal amino acids that would ordinarily be found in the gastrointestinal tract. *N*-Chlorovaline and *N*-chloroserine were also tentatively identified. Organic chloramines are reactive and could be responsible for toxic effects that may be attributed to chlorine in toxicological studies. The chlorine demand of free amino acids in stomach contents was found to be only about 4% of the total. Consequently, this process may be substrate-limited at concentrations of chlorine found as residuals in drinking-water. However, use of higher concentrations of chlorine would also lead to breakdown of proteins present in the stomach fluid. Thus, as concentrations are increased to levels that would be used in animal studies, these products would be formed at a much higher concentration, similar to the phenomena noted with THM and HAA by-products.

3.1.2 *Reproductive and developmental toxicity*

In general, animal studies have demonstrated no reproductive or teratogenic effects of chlorine. Druckrey (1968) examined the effects of water chlorinated to a level of 100 mg/litre (approximately 10 mg/kg of body weight per day) in BDII rats for seven generations. No effects were observed on fertility, growth or survival.

A number of subsequent studies have studied the effects of chlorine or hypochlorite on more specific aspects of reproduction or development. Meier et al. (1985b) reported that oral administration of sodium hypochlorite (pH 8.5) prepared from chlorine gas and administered at 4 or 8 mg/kg of body weight per day for 5 weeks increased the incidence of sperm head abnormalities in $B6C3F_1$ mice (10 animals per group). The effect was not observed when the solutions were administered at pHs at which hypochlorous acid was the predominant species (pH 6.5). However, other studies have not been able to associate adverse reproductive outcomes with the administration of chlorine or sodium hypochlorite.

Carlton et al. (1986) found no evidence of sperm head abnormalities or adverse reproductive outcomes in Long-Evans rats. Male rats were treated for 56 days prior to mating and female rats from 14 days prior to mating through gestation. Each experimental group consisted of 11–12 males and 23–24 females. Solutions of chlorine were prepared at pH 8.5, so the study evaluated hypochlorite as the dominant form in the drinking-water. Doses were as high as 5 mg/kg of body weight per day.

3.1.3   *Toxicity in humans*

There have been significant human exposures to chlorine and hypochlorite solutions. Much of that experience is with inhalation of chlorine gas, which is known to be a strong respiratory irritant. Chlorine gas is also the largest single component involved in toxic release incidents. A third major source of exposure is solutions of sodium hypochlorite, usually marketed as bleach. Bleach is frequently involved in human poisonings. These exposures are not particularly relevant to exposures to chlorine or hypochlorite in drinking-water. Therefore, only a few case reports are identified that illustrate the types of problems that have been encountered. There was no attempt to make this review comprehensive.

The irritating effects of chlorine gas have been well documented because of its use as a chemical warfare agent during World War I (Das & Blanc, 1993). In a follow-up of survivors of gassing, it was concluded that there was no evidence of permanent lung damage; however, these studies clearly indicated that survivors had breath sounds that suggested bronchitis and limited chest and diaphragmatic movement, even emphysema. Most studies suggested that there were high incidences of acute respiratory disease and a lesser prevalence of chronic sequelae. Similar sequelae have been identified following exposure of humans to accidental releases of chlorine gas. In these more modern characterizations, the acute signs and symptoms included a high incidence of pulmonary oedema and severe bronchitis. These signs and symptoms are of generally short duration and resolve themselves over the course of about 1–4 weeks. However, chronic sequelae are observed in some individuals, depending in part upon the severity of the exposure. In such cases, a decrease in the forced expiratory volume is the most consistently reported clinical sign.

Two recent reports suggest that chronic sequelae to acute exposures to chlorine gas may be more prevalent than previously appreciated. Moore & Sherman (1991) reported on an individual who was previously asymptomatic and who developed chronic, recurrent asthma after exposure to chlorine gas in an enclosed place. Schwartz et al. (1990) followed 20 individuals who had been exposed to chlorine gas in a 1975 incident. The prevalence of low residual lung volume was increased during the follow-up period. Sixty-seven per cent of those tested were found to have residual volumes below 80% of their predicted values. Five of 13 subjects tested for airway reactivity to methacholine were found to have a greater than 15% decline in forced expiratory volume.

Controlled studies have been conducted in healthy, non-smoking men exposed to chlorine gas at 1.5 and 2.9 mg/m^3 (0.5 and 1.0 ppm) for 4 or 8 h (reviewed in Das & Blanc, 1993). Four hours of exposure to 2.9 mg/m^3 (1.0 ppm) produced significant decreases in the forced expiratory volume. One individual who was found to be experiencing more difficulty than other subjects at this dose and who was later exposed to 1.5 mg/m^3 (0.5 ppm) experienced a significant decrease in forced expiratory volume. While 1.5 mg/m^3 (0.5 ppm) appears protective for most people, some more sensitive individuals may in fact have more significant responses to chlorine gas.

The effects of chronic exposure to chlorine gas have received only limited study. In one study of paper mill workers, a more rapid age-related decrease in lung volumes of workers exposed to chlorine relative to those exposed to sulfur dioxide was noted, but the trend was not statistically significant (Das & Blanc, 1993). Other studies failed to identify chronic sequelae.

There are frequent reports of human poisonings from bleach. Most often these exposures result from the mixing of bleach with acidic products or ammonia. Acidification converts hypochlorite to hypochlorous acid, which dissociates to chlorine gas, offgasses very rapidly from the solutions and presents an inhalation exposure (MMWR, 1991). Mixing bleach with ammonia results in the formation of monochloramine and dichloramine, both of which are effective respiratory irritants (MMWR, 1991).

Any potential effects of chlorine or hypochlorite in drinking-water are obscured by the fact that by-products inevitably coexist with the residual chlorine. One series of studies in which by-products formed were minimized by dissolving chlorine in distilled water attempted to identify effects of chlorine in drinking-water on humans. Chlorine in drinking-water was administered in a rising-dose tolerance study beginning with 0.1 mg/litre in two 500-ml portions and rising to a concentration of 24 mg/litre, equivalent to 0.34 mg/kg of body weight per day (Lubbers & Bianchine, 1984). No clinically important changes were observed. No findings of clinical importance were identified in a follow-up treatment with repeated dosing with 500-ml portions of a solution containing 5 mg of chlorine per litre for a 12-week period (Lubbers et al., 1984a).

Another study attempted to determine whether consumption of chlorinated drinking-water affected blood cholesterol levels (Wones et al., 1993a). The impetus for this study was a toxicological study in pigeons that suggested that chlorine raised blood cholesterol levels and modified serum thyroid levels (Revis et al., 1986a,b) and an epidemi-ological study that associated small increases in cholesterol of women with residence in communities having chlorinated water (Zeighami et al., 1990a,b; described in detail in section 5.2.2). A prior study (quoted in Wones et al., 1993a) was conducted that examined men who consumed water containing 2, 5 or 10 mg of chlorine per litre and found a small increase in serum cholesterol levels at the highest dose group. However, no control group was studied, so the changes could have been attributed to the change in diet imposed as part of the study protocol (Wones & Glueck, 1986). The longer-term study was composed of 30 men and 30 women who received a controlled diet for the duration of the study. The first 4 weeks represented an acclima-tization period during which all subjects received distilled water. Half the subjects were assigned to a group that consumed 1.5 litres of water containing 20 mg of chlorine per litre for the following 4 weeks. At the end of each 4-week period, blood was analysed for cholesterol, triglycerides, high-density lipoprotein (HDL) cholesterol, low-density lipoprotein (LDL) cholesterol or apolipoproteins A1, A2 and B. There were no significant effects. There was a slight trend towards lower thyroid hormone levels in men consuming chlorine, but this was not clinically significant (Wones et al., 1993a). These data suggest that observations obtained previously in pigeons could not be repeated under comparable conditions of chlorine consumption. It is notable that the animals utilized in the original pigeon study had consumed a modified diet (Revis et al., 1986a) that was deficient in calcium and other trace metals. A subsequent study failed to replicate the previous results in pigeons (Penn et al., 1990).

3.1.4 Carcinogenicity and mutagenicity

The International Agency for Research on Cancer (IARC) has evaluated the carcinogenicity of hypochlorite salts and concluded that there were no data available from studies in humans on their carcinogenicity and inadequate evidence for their carcinogenicity in experimental animals. Hypochlorite salts were assigned to Group 3: the compounds are not classifiable as to their carcinogenicity to humans (IARC, 1991).

Several studies have shown that sodium hypochlorite produces mutagenic responses in bacterial systems and mammalian cells *in vitro*. However, there is no evidence of activity in mammalian test systems *in vivo*. It is not clear to what extent this is influenced by the formation of mutagenic by-products as a result of reactions with components of the incubation media. Wlodkowski & Rosenkranz (1975) used short-term exposures of *Salmonella typhimurium* strain TA 1530 followed by ascorbic acid-induced decomposition to reduce the cytotoxic effects of hypochlorite. The investigators applied 0.14 µmol per tube and added ascorbic acid after intervals of 5, 10 and 15 min. At 5 min, a clear positive response was observed with minimal cytotoxicity. Significant responses were also observed in strain TA1535, but not in strain TA1538.

Rosenkranz (1973) and Rosenkranz et al. (1976) also demon-strated a positive mutagenic response in DNA polymerase A deficient *Escherichia coli* to 0.006 µmol of sodium hypochlorite. This response was unaffected by the addition of catalase, suggesting that the response was not related to the generation of hydrogen peroxide.

Matsuoka et al. (1979) reported that sodium hypochlorite at a concentration of 6.7 mmol/litre (0.5 mg/ml) produced chromosomal aberrations in Chinese hamster ovary (CHO) cells in the presence of S9 mix. This concentration was cytotoxic in the absence of S9. Some concern must be expressed about whether responses observed with such high and clearly cytotoxic concentrations in an *in vitro* system represent specific clastogenic effects. The authors report only one concentration tested with and without S9. It is probable that the positive response in the presence of S9, if it is a specific response, was a result of detoxifying hypochlorite. This protection could be non-specific as well, in that it may not have depended upon any catalytic activities present in the S9 fraction (i.e., the added protein may have acted as a reactive sink to dissipate excess hypochlorite). Conse-quently, it is difficult to use these data in interpreting the effects of chlorine or hypochlorite *in vivo*.

Ishidate (1987) studied the induction of chromosomal aberrations in cultures of Chinese hamster CHL cells at sodium hypochlorite concentrations ranging from 125 to 500 µg/ml without exogenous metabolic activation and from 31 to 125 µg/ml with and without rat liver S9 mix. A clear increase in the number of cells with structural chromosomal aberrations was observed at 500 µg/ml without S9 mix, while the results obtained in the other series, showing weakly positive responses, were considered inconclusive.

Meier et al. (1985b) evaluated the ability of hypochlorite and hypochlorous acid to induce chromosomal damage or micronuclei in the bone marrow of CD-1 mice. The samples to be tested were generated by bubbling chlorine gas into water and then adjusting the pH to 6.5 (predominantly hypochlorous acid) or 8.5 (predominantly hypochlorite). The doses administered were 1.6, 4 or 8 mg/kg of body weight for 5 consecutive days. There was no evidence of increased micronuclei or chromosomal abnormalities in bone marrow cells. Significant positive responses were observed with positive control chemicals in both assays. As reported in section 3.1.2, these authors detected a positive response in the sperm head abnormality assay in mice treated at these same doses of hypochlorite in two separate experiments. This assay is used primarily as a mutagenicity assay rather than as an assay for reproductive toxicities. Hypochlorous acid had no effect in the sperm head abnormality assay.

Tests of the ability of hypochlorite to induce cancer in rodents were conducted in F344 rats by Hasegawa et al. (1986). Sodium hypochlorite concentrations of 0, 500 or 1000 mg/litre (males) and 0, 1000 or 2000 mg/litre (females) were administered in the drinking-water for 104 weeks (equivalent to 13.5 and 27.7 mg/kg of body weight per day for males and 34.3 and 63.2 mg/kg of body weight per day for females). There were 50 male and 50 female rats assigned to each experimental group. No tumours could be attributed to sodium hypochlorite administration.

NTP (1992) conducted a 2-year bioassay of chlorine in F344 rats and B6C3F$_1$ mice. The concentrations administered in drinking-water were 0, 70, 140 or 275 mg/litre, and there were 70 animals of each sex assigned to each group (approximately 0, 4, 8 or 14 mg/kg of body weight per day for rats and 0, 7, 14 or 24 mg/kg of body weight per day for mice). There was an apparent positive trend in the induction of stromal polyps of the uterus of female mice treated with chlorine, but this was considered unlikely to be treatment-related because the incidence was below those observed in historical controls. In female rats, there was an increase in mononuclear cell leukaemia at both 140 and 275 mg/litre (8 and 14 mg/kg of body weight per day). However, the response was not considered treatment-related because it fell within the range of historical controls, there was no apparent dose–response, and there was no evidence for such an increase in male F344 rats.

A single study suggested that sodium hypochlorite could act as a promoter of skin tumours following initiation with 4-nitroquinoline-1-oxide in female ddN mice (Hayatsu et al., 1971). A solution of sodium hypochlorite that contained 10% effective concentrations of chlorine was utilized. Skin tumours were produced in 9 of 32 mice given 45 applications of sodium hypochlorite following initiation. Sodium hydroxide solutions were utilized as a control for the alkaline pH of sodium hypochlorite and produced no tumours. No tumours were observed with 60 applications of sodium hypochlorite solution in non-initiated mice. Pfeiffer (1978) conducted a much larger experiment that utilized 100 mice per group. This author found that a 1% sodium hypochlorite solution applied alternately with benzo[*a*]pyrene for 128 weeks was ineffective in producing skin tumours in female NMRI mice above those that had been initiated with benzo[*a*]pyrene alone at doses of 750 or 1500 µg. Pretreatment with the sodium hypochlorite solution before application of the benzo[*a*]pyrene actually reduced tumour yields at 128 weeks with doses of either 750 or 1500 µg of benzo[*a*]pyrene. Sodium hypochlorite used in a more traditional initiation/promotion study (i.e., sodium hypochlorite treatment following initiation with benzo[*a*]pyrene) produced a decrease in the tumour yield with the 750 µg dose of benzo[*a*]pyrene, but had no effect following 1500 µg. Thus, the ability of sodium hypochlorite to act as a tumour promoter may depend upon the initiator used, or the smaller experiment of Hayatsu et al. (1971) may simply be a false result.

As pointed out in section 3.1.1, application of solutions of hypochlorous acid to the skin of Sencar mice results in the development of hyperplasia. The concentrations required are considerably lower (300 mg/litre) (Robinson et al., 1986) than those used in the studies of either Hayatsu et al. (1971) or Pfeiffer (1978). Sodium hypochlorite was also effective at lower doses, but less so than equivalent concentrations of hypochlorous acid. These results suggest that these prior evaluations may have been conducted at too high a dose. There appear to be no reports on the effectiveness of hypochlorous acid as a tumour promoter, but the lack of activity at doses of less than 300 mg/litre would suggest that this is of no concern.

3.1.5 Comparative pharmacokinetics and metabolism

A series of pharmacokinetic studies using ^{36}Cl-labelled hypochlorous acid were conducted by Abdel-Rahman and co-workers (1983). These studies are of limited value because the form of ^{36}Cl could not be determined in various body compartments.

3.1.6 Mode of action

There are no specific toxicities of chlorine for which a mechanism needs to be proposed. It is a strong oxidizing agent, and it must be presumed that damage induced at high doses by either gaseous chlorine or solutions of hypochlorite is at least partially related to this property. In studies in which sodium hypochlorite is used without neutralization, a strong alkaline pH can also contribute to its effects. There is always the possibility that chlorine is inducing subtle effects by virtue of its reaction with organic compounds that are found in the stomach. Such reactions have been demonstrated, but there is no convincing evidence to date that any specific toxicity can be attributed to these by-products.

3.2 Chloramine

3.2.1 General toxicological properties and information on dose–response in animals

There have been relatively few evaluations of the toxic properties of chloramine in experimental animals. In large part this is because it is not marketed as a product but is created for disinfection purposes on-site and *in situ*. Chloramine is primarily used as a residual disinfectant in the distribution system. The final solution consists of mostly monochloramine, with traces of other chloramines, such as dichloramine. Chloramines, as a group, are generally recognized as potent respiratory irritants, because the formation of these compounds when household bleach and ammonia are mixed results in a number of poisoning cases each year (MMWR, 1991). In spite of this, there has been no attempt to quantify dose–response relationships in animals.

Eaton et al. (1973) investigated concerns about chloramine-induced methaemoglobin formation in kidney patients dialysed with chloramine-containing water. This was done by examining the ability of relatively large volumes of tapwater to oxidize haemoglobin in dilute suspensions of red blood cells. This circumstance is reflective of dialysis, but not of the concentrated suspension of these cells *in vivo*. Nevertheless, the authors were able to show that methaemoglobin formation occurred in a dose-related manner when 1 volume of red blood cells (human) was suspended in 100 volumes of tapwater containing 1 mg of chloramine per litre or above. This effect was not produced by comparable concentrations of sodium hypochlorite. The ability to induce methaemoglobin formation was eliminated by treating the water by reverse osmosis followed by carbon filtration. Clearly, chloramine is capable of inducing methaemoglobinaemia at low concentrations when there is a large reservoir of chloramine. This is a decidedly different exposure pattern from that of normal humans and other mammals, as they consume small volumes of water relative to the volume of red blood cells that are exposed.

Moore et al. (1980a) studied alterations of blood parameters in male A/J mice treated with 0, 2.5, 25, 50, 100 or 200 mg of mono-chloramine per litre in carbonate/bicarbonate-buffered (pH 8.9) drinking-water. Twelve animals were assigned to each group, and treatments were maintained over a 30-day period. Consistent with the inter-pretation provided above, there were no treatment-related effects on osmotic fragility, methaemoglobin levels, haemoglobin concentrations, reticulocyte counts or a number of other derived parameters. Haemato-crits of mice treated with 50, 100 or 200 mg/litre were actually higher than those observed in control mice. White blood cell counts were not altered in these animals.

Daniel et al. (1990a) conducted a more traditional 90-day study of monochloramine in Sprague-Dawley rats (10 animals per sex per dose). Treatment concentrations were 0, 25, 50, 100 or 200 mg/litre, corresponding to doses of 0, 1.8, 3.4, 5.8 or 9.0 mg/kg of body weight per day in males and 0, 2.6, 4.3, 7.7 or 12.1 mg/kg of body weight per day in females. Controls received carbonated, pH-adjusted drinking-water. A large number of haematological and clinical chemistry measures were included in the evaluation. Body weights were significantly depressed in both sexes at treatment concentrations in the 50–200 mg/litre range, but this appeared to be related to depressed water and food consumption. There were minor changes in organ to body weight ratios at the highest dose, but no evidence of treatment-related pathology was observed. Male rats were found to have decreased haematocrits at 100 mg/litre, and red blood cell counts were slightly depressed at 100 and 200 mg/litre. The authors concluded that monochloramine was more toxic than chlorine or chlorine dioxide. However, it must be noted that the changes in blood parameters were small and in themselves of no clinical significance. Other measures were not related to specific toxic reactions. Based on the decrease in organ and body weights observed in both sexes, the authors concluded that the no-observed-adverse-effect level (NOAEL) was 100 mg/litre, equivalent to 5.8 mg/kg of body weight per day.

The work in rats was followed up with a second study in B6C3F$_1$ mice (Daniel et al., 1991a). Male and female B6C3F$_1$ mice (10 per sex per group) were administered 0, 12.5, 25, 50, 100 or 200 mg of chloramine per litre of drinking-water for 90 days (calculated mean daily dose was 0, 2.5, 5.0, 8.6, 11.1 or 15.6 mg/kg of body weight for males and 0, 2.8, 5.3, 9.2, 12.9 or 15.8 mg/kg of body weight for females). Water consumption significantly decreased at 100 and 200 mg/litre in males and at 25–200 mg/litre in females. Weight gain was significantly depressed in both sexes at 100 and 200 mg/litre. Neutrophil concentrations in blood were significantly depressed in both male and female mice at the two highest doses, but other white blood cell counts were unaltered. Absolute and relative spleen and liver weights were depressed at both 100 and 200 mg/litre. No gross or microscopic evidence of target organ toxicity was observed that could be related to treatment. Based on decreased organ weights, weight gain, and food and water consumption, the authors concluded that the NOAEL was 50 mg/litre, equivalent to 8.6 mg/kg of body weight per day.

A 13-week study in which groups of 10 Sprague-Dawley rats were given drinking-water containing 200 mg of monochloramine per litre or buffered water as a control, *ad libitum* or restricted to the same consumption as the monochloramine group, was designed to resolve some of the outstanding toxicological questions. The results of this study indicated that the reduced body weight gain and the minor biochemical, haematological, immunological and histopathological changes associated with exposure to 200 mg of monochloramine per litre (equivalent to 21.6 mg/kg of body weight per day) in drinking-water were largely related to reduced water and food consumption (Poon et al., 1997).

In a 9-week study, Exon et al. (1987) examined the ability of monochloramine to modify immunological parameters in male Sprague-Dawley rats (12 per dose) exposed to concentrations of 0, 9, 19 or 38 mg of monochloramine per litre, equivalent to 0, 1.3, 2.6 or 5.3 mg/kg of body weight per day. At the middle and highest dose, chloramine treatment was observed to increase prostaglandin E_2 synthesis by adherent resident peritoneal cells (which include macrophages) in response to lipopolysaccharide stimulation. No attempt was made to relate this finding to other indices of modified macrophage function. A small depression in spleen weights was observed at the highest dose. The implications of these data for immune function are not clear. Other measures of immune function did not reveal statistically significant changes with treatment. These included a decrease in antibody formation at the lowest and middle doses in response to keyhole limpet haemocyanin injection or delayed-type hypersensitivity reactions to bovine serum albumin injected into the footpad.

The effect of monochloramine on skin irritation was tested by immersing Sencar mice into water containing chloramine at concentrations ranging from 1 to 1000 mg/litre for 10 min a day (Robinson et al., 1986). Unlike hypochlorous acid (pH 6.5) or hypochlorite (pH 8.5), chloramine did not produce hyperplasia of the skin.

3.2.2 Reproductive and developmental toxicity

Studies in laboratory animals have indicated no reproductive or developmental effects associated with chloramine. Abdel-Rahman et al. (1982a) administered monochloramine to female Sprague-Dawley rats at concentrations of 0, 1, 10 or 100 mg/litre (0, 0.15, 1.5 or 15 mg/kg of body weight per day) for 2.5 months prior to breeding and through gestation. Only six animals were assigned to each treatment group. Reproductive performance was comparable between groups, and fetal weights were not adversely affected by treatment. Between 50 and 60 fetuses were available (male and female combined) for evaluation. There was no evidence of treatment-related skeletal or soft tissue anomalies.

Carlton et al. (1986) examined the effects of monochloramine administered by gavage at doses of 0, 2.5, 5 or 10 mg/kg of body weight per day on the reproductive performance of Long-Evans rats. Males (12 per group) were treated from 56 days prior to and through mating, and females (24 per group) from 14 days prior to mating and throughout the mating period. No statistically significant effects on sperm morphology, concentration or motility were observed, nor were there any effects on fertility, viability, litter size, pup weights, day of eye opening or day of vaginal patency.

3.2.3 Toxicity in humans

The primary harmful effects of chloramine have been documented in humans poisoned by chloramine formed when household bleach was mixed with ammonia for use as a cleaning solution. Chloramine is a strong respiratory irritant. These effects were discussed in section 3.1.3.

Forty-eight men completed an 8-week protocol during which diet and other factors known to affect lipid metabolism were controlled. During the first 4 weeks of the protocol, all subjects consumed distilled water. During the second 4 weeks, one-third of the subjects were assigned randomly to drink 1.5 litres of water containing 0, 2 or 15 mg of monochloramine per litre each day. At 2 mg/litre, no significant changes were observed in total, HDL or LDL cholesterol, triglycerides or apolipoproteins A1, A2 or B. Parameters of thyroid function were unchanged. However, an increase in the level of apolipoprotein B was observed at 15 mg/litre (Wones et al., 1993b).

3.2.4 Carcinogenicity and mutagenicity

Shih & Lederberg (1976) first demonstrated that monochloramine induced mutation in a *Bacillus subtilis* reversion assay. The concentration range studied extended from 18 to 74 μmol/litre. A positive dose–response was observed through 56 μmol/litre, but 74 μmol/litre was cytotoxic. Repair-deficient mutants of *B. subtilis*, rec3, recA and polyA5, were consistently more sensitive to the cytotoxic effects of chloramine, while the uvr and recB mutants were not. The sensitivity of the polyA5 mutants parallels the observations of Rosenkranz (1973) with sodium hypochlorite and suggests that DNA polymerase A is involved in the repair of DNA lesions produced by both chemicals.

Thus, it is possible that a common intermediate or mechanism is involved in the mutagenic effects of hypochlorite and chloramine.

A broader list of chloramines was tested by Thomas et al. (1987) in *Salmonella typhimurium* tester strains TA97a, TA100 and TA102. The chloramines tested included those that could be formed at low levels from natural substrates in drinking-water or in the stomach. TA100 was found to consistently be the most sensitive strain. The most potent mutagens were the lipophilic dichloramines formed with histamine, ethanolamine and putrescine. The corresponding mono-chloramines were less potent. The more hydrophilic chloramines, such as taurine-chloramine, had little activity. Monochloramine was active in the 50 µmol/litre range, remarkably consistent with the data of Shih & Lederberg (1976). Hypochlorous acid was inactive at all concentrations that were tested, up to and including concentrations that induced cytotoxicity.

Ashby and co-workers (1987) were unable to induce clastogenic effects in the mouse bone marrow micronucleus assay when chloramine was administered orally. They suggested that the *in vitro* clastogenic effects were probably attributable to non-specific cytotoxic effects that are secondary to the release of hypochlorite to the media.

Meier et al. (1985b) found that intraperitoneal administration of monochloramine to CD-1 mice at doses of up to 8 mg/kg of body weight was without significant effect on either micronuclei or chromosomal aberrations in the bone marrow. These data would appear to be consistent with the findings of Ashby et al. (1987).

Studies on the carcinogenicity of chloramine are limited to a single set of 2-year experiments conducted by the NTP (1992). Drinking-water containing 0, 50, 100 or 200 mg of chloramine per litre was provided to F344 rats and B6C3F$_1$ mice. Seventy animals of each species and of each sex within a species were assigned to each experimental and control group. Doses in rats were 0, 2.1, 4.8 or 8.7 mg/kg of body weight per day in males and 0, 2.8, 5.3 or 9.5 mg/kg of body weight per day in females; doses in mice were 0, 5.0, 8.9 or 15.9 mg/kg of body weight per day in males and 0, 4.9, 9.0 or 17.2 mg/kg of body weight per day in females. Of some interest was the finding that two renal cell adenomas were found in male B6C3F$_1$

mice treated with the high dose of chloramine. In addition, one renal adenoma was found in one male mouse treated with 100 mg/litre and in one female mouse treated with 200 mg/litre. While this tumour site is rare in both species, there was no real dose–response trend, nor were the differences between the control and treatment groups statistically significant. A second finding of some concern was an increase in the incidence of mononuclear cell leukaemia in F344 rats. This pathology was increased in rats treated with chloramine or hypochlorite, although the effects were not clearly dose-dependent. The incidence of mono-nuclear cell leukaemia was significantly greater than in concurrent controls and was elevated above the historical incidence as well. Nevertheless, these increases were not considered to be treatment-related. In part, this conclusion arose from the lack of a clear dose–response. It was also based on the fact that there was no comparable trend in male rats.

3.2.5 Comparative pharmacokinetics and metabolism

The pharmacokinetics of ^{36}Cl derived from monochloramine have been examined in male Sprague-Dawley rats (Abdel-Rahman et al., 1983). These data are difficult to interpret because the specific form of the label is not known.

3.3 Chlorine dioxide

3.3.1 General toxicological properties and information on dose–response in animals

Despite its use as a disinfectant, there have been very few general toxicological evaluations of chlorine dioxide, because most studies have focused on its major by-product, chlorite, which is considered in section 4.6. The present review will first focus on the limited charac-terization of chlorine dioxide's general toxicology, then follow up with a discussion of its haematological and thyroid effects.

Some very cursory investigations of chlorine dioxide's effects as a respiratory irritant were published by Haller & Northgraves (1955) in an article dealing with the general chemical properties of the compound. In essence, these data suggested that exposure to chlorine dioxide in air at a concentration of more than 420 mg/m^3 (150 ppm) for longer than 15 min was fatal to guinea-pigs. The total study involved six guinea-pigs.

Rats (3–5 per group) were exposed to chlorine dioxide in various concentrations (0.28–9520 mg/m^3 [0.1–3400 ppm]) and for various periods (3 min–10 weeks). All the rats exposed daily to chlorine dioxide at 28 mg/m^3 (10 ppm) died in less than 14 days. Purulent bronchitis and disseminated bronchopneumonia were found at necroscopy. No such changes were demonstrable in rats exposed to approximately 0.28 mg/m^3 (0.1 ppm) for about 10 weeks (Dalhamn, 1957).

The LC$_{50}$ of chlorine dioxide in rats (5 per sex per group) exposed by inhalation for 4 h was 90 mg/m^3 (32 ppm) (Ineris, 1996).

Robinson et al. (1986) studied the ability of chlorine and alternative disinfectants to induce epidermal hyperplasia in the skin of Sencar mice. The thickness of the interfollicular epidermis was significantly increased by 10-min daily exposures to water containing up to 1000 mg of chlorine dioxide per litre for 4 days. The thickness of the epidermis was similar to that induced by an equivalent dose of hypochlorous acid. Unlike hypochlorous acid, however, there was no significant increase in skin thickness at concentrations of 300 mg/litre or less.

The study of Daniel et al. (1990a) was the first subchronic study that adhered to modern expectations of toxicological studies. These authors provided male and female Sprague-Dawley rats (10 per sex per treatment group) with 0, 25, 50, 100 or 200 mg of chlorine dioxide per litre of drinking-water for 90 days, equivalent to 0, 2, 4, 6 or 12 and 0, 2, 5, 8 or 15 mg/kg of body weight per day for males and females, respectively. Conventional measures of body weight, organ weights, a broad battery of clinical chemistry parameters and histopathological examinations were all included in the study design. Body and organ weights were significantly depressed at 200 mg/litre in both sexes. This appeared to be secondary to depressed water consumption, which is known to be tightly coupled to food consumption in rats. The only significant histopathological damage found was goblet cell hyperplasia and inflammation. This was observed at all doses of chlorine dioxide in both male and female rats. Presumably this inflammation occurs as a result of volatilization of chlorine dioxide from the water bottle. The amount of chlorine dioxide actually inhaled as a result of volatilization from the drinking-water containing the lowest dose of chlorine dioxide (25 mg/litre) must be extremely low. This suggests that there might be some concern for sensitive individuals showering with water containing chlorine dioxide.

The ability of chlorine dioxide to induce methaemoglobinaemia and haemolytic anaemia has received extensive study. Abdel-Rahman et al. (1980) found decreased red blood cell glutathione (GSH) concentrations and decreased osmotic fragility in Sprague-Dawley rats and white leghorn chickens given drinking-water containing chlorine dioxide concentrations of 1, 10, 100 and 1000 mg/litre for up to 4 months, but the changes were not consistently dose-related. However, the authors found that the morphology of red blood cells was modified (codocytes and echinocytes) in all dose groups, the severity increasing with increased treatment concentration. Methaemoglobin was not detected throughout these studies. However, there was no formal statistical evaluation of these results, and only four rats were assigned to each experimental group. Administration of acute doses of as little as 1 mg/kg of body weight by gavage decreased red blood cell GSH concentrations. This response was not increased as dose was increased to 4 mg/kg of body weight.

Abdel-Rahman and co-workers extended these observations to longer treatment periods in a subsequent publication (Abdel-Rahman et al., 1984a). Again, only four animals were assigned to each treatment group. At 7 and 9 months of treatment, red blood cells appeared to become resistant to osmotic shock at all treatment concentrations (1–1000 mg/litre). These data did not display a clear dose–response despite the large variation in the dose administered.

The study of Abdel-Rahman et al. (1984a) also reported changes in the incorporation of ^{3}H-thymidine into the DNA of various organs. Incorporation was significantly inhibited in testes and apparently increased in the intestinal mucosa. The effect on apparent DNA synthesis was particularly marked in the testes at 100 mg/litre, amounting to about 60% inhibition. These data are difficult to interpret for several reasons. First, rats were sacrificed 8 h after being injected with ^{3}H-thymidine. Ordinarily, sacrifices are made 30–60 min after injection because the blood is essentially depleted of ^{3}H-thymidine in an hour. Thus, it is not possible to determine if the lowered amount of label is related to decreased synthesis or to increased turnover of DNA.

Second, the result was based on total counts in DNA, which makes it impossible to determine what cell type is affected or whether the change was associated with replicative or repair synthesis. Third, only four animals were used per experimental group.

In a rising-dose protocol study, Bercz et al. (1982) evaluated the effects of chlorine dioxide on African green monkeys. These animals were provided chlorine dioxide in drinking-water at concentrations of 0, 30, 100 or 200 mg/litre, corresponding to doses of 0, 3.5, 9.5 or 11 mg/kg of body weight per day. Each dose was maintained for 30–60 days. Animals showed signs of dehydration at the highest dose (11 mg/kg of body weight per day), so exposure at that dose was discontinued. No effect was observed on any haematological parameter, including methaemoglobinaemia. However, statistically significant depressions in serum thyroxine levels were observed when animals were dosed with chlorine dioxide at a concentration of 100 mg/litre. No effect had been observed in a prior exposure of the same animals to 30 mg/litre for 30 days. The NOAEL in this study was 3.5 mg/kg of body weight per day.

The effects of chlorine dioxide on thyroid function were followed up by Harrington et al. (1986). Thyroxine levels in African green monkeys administered drinking-water containing 100 mg of chlorine dioxide per litre (4.6 mg/kg of body weight per day) were again found to be depressed at 4 weeks of treatment, but rebounded to above-normal levels after 8 weeks of treatment. These investigators also found significantly depressed thyroxine levels in rats treated with 100 or 200 mg of chlorine dioxide per litre in drinking-water (equivalent to 14 and 28 mg/kg of body weight per day) for 8 weeks. This change was dose-related. Lower doses were not examined in the rat study. The authors indicated that the results were based on 12 determinations; it was not clear if these measurements were made on individual animals.

A set of *in vivo* and *in vitro* experiments was conducted in an attempt to explain the effects of chlorine dioxide on serum thyroid hormone concentrations. The authors demonstrated that chlorine dioxide oxidizes iodide to reactive iodine species that would bind to the stomach and oesophageal epithelium. Rat chow that was treated with chlorine dioxide at approximately 80 mg/litre was found to increase the binding of iodine to chow constituents. This activation of iodine resulted in retention of labelled iodine in the ileum and colon and reduced uptake by the thyroid gland. Previous work demonstrated that chlorine dioxide was more effective than chlorine in activating iodide to a form that would covalently bind with a variety of natural foodstuffs (Bercz et al., 1986). Based on these observations, the authors concluded that the effects of chlorine dioxide were probably due to altered gastrointestinal absorption of iodide and reduced uptake into the thyroid gland.

3.3.2 *Reproductive and developmental toxicity*

A number of reproductive effects have been reported in studies with laboratory animals, but the relevance for humans of these findings remains uncertain. The reproductive effects of chlorine dioxide in Long-Evans rats were studied by Carlton et al. (1991). Chlorine dioxide was administered by gavage at doses of 2.5, 5 or 10 mg/kg of body weight per day to male rats (12 per group) for 56 days prior to and through mating and to female rats (24 per group) from 14 days prior to mating and through pregnancy. Fertility measures were not significantly different among the dose groups. There were no dose-related changes in sperm parameters (i.e., concentration, motility, progressive movement or morphology). Thyroid hormone levels were altered significantly, but not in a consistent pattern. The only significant difference was significantly depressed vaginal weights in female pups whose dams had been treated with 10 mg/kg of body weight per day.

An evaluation of the effects of chlorine dioxide on the fetal development of Sprague-Dawley rats was conducted by Suh et al. (1983). Chlorine dioxide was administered at 0, 1, 10 or 100 mg/litre (0, 0.1, 1 or 10 mg/kg of body weight per day) for 2.5 months prior to mating and throughout gestation. The total number of implants per dam was significantly reduced at the highest concentration of chlorine dioxide. The percentage of anomalous fetuses was increased in a dose-related manner, but the response was not statistically significant. These anomalies arose primarily as the percentage of abnormal or incomplete sternebrae in treated rats relative to controls. The lack of statistical significance was undoubtedly related to the relatively few female rats that were included in the study (6–8 females per treatment group). As a consequence, the results of this study must be considered inconclusive.

Orme et al. (1985) found that chlorine dioxide administered in the drinking-water of female Sprague-Dawley rats (13–16 per dose) at concentrations of 0, 2, 20 or 100 mg/litre (0, 1, 3 or 14 mg/kg of body weight per day) throughout pregnancy and through weaning decreased thyroxine levels in the serum of the pups at 100 mg/litre. This was associated with delayed development of exploratory behaviour in the pups away from their dams, and this, in turn, was probably due to an indirect effect on iodine uptake. In a second experiment, pups given 14 mg of chlorine dioxide per kg of body weight per day directly by gavage on postnatal days 5–20 showed significantly depressed activity and a decrease in serum thyroxine levels. Studies by the same group (Taylor & Pfohl, 1985) indicated that cerebellar and forebrain cell counts (based on DNA measurements) were depressed in 11-day-old pups that had been treated with chlorine dioxide at 14 mg/kg of body weight per day by gavage from 5 days of age. Cerebellar cell counts remained depressed in rats at 21 days, but forebrain counts were essentially the same as in controls. At 50–60 days of age, the locomotor activity (measured by wheel-running) of these animals was depressed relative to control animals.

The effects of chlorine dioxide on brain development were examined further by Toth et al. (1990). These authors administered chlorine dioxide by gavage at 14 mg/kg of body weight per day from postnatal day 1 to 20. Body weight was reduced, but cerebellar weight was unaltered at any age. Forebrain weight and protein content were reduced on postnatal days 21 and 35. DNA content was depressed on postnatal day 35, and the number of dendritic spines on cerebral cortical pyramidal cells was significantly reduced. No histopathological changes in the forebrain, cerebellum or brain stem were observed. There were no consistent changes in serum thyroxine or triiodo-thyronine levels in treated animals.

Collectively, these data suggest some effects of chlorine dioxide on brain development. In most studies, there are suggestions of modified thyroid function associated with these effects. It must be pointed out that the changes in thyroid hormone levels are modest, much less than are produced with classical antithyroid drugs such as propylthiouracil (Toth et al., 1990).

3.3.3   Toxicity in humans

The effects of chlorine dioxide were assessed in a two-phase study in 10 healthy male volunteers. The first study was a rising-dose tolerance study (Lubbers & Bianchine, 1984) in which doses of chlorine dioxide were increased from 0.1 to 24 mg/litre, administered in two 500-ml portions. The maximum dose for a 70-kg person was 0.34 mg/kg of body weight. The details of this study were described in section 3.1.3. Some small changes in a variety of clinical chemistry parameters were observed, but none was found to be outside the accepted range of normal. The second phase of the experiment involved the daily administration of a 500-ml portion of a solution containing 5 mg/litre to 10 healthy volunteers for a period of 12 weeks (Lubbers et al., 1984a). Again, measurement of a large battery of clinical chemistry parameters and routine physical examination failed to identify any effects of chlorine dioxide that fell outside of the normal range. Parameters yielding significant differences appeared to be primarily a result of parallel drift of values with the control group.

As with other disinfectants, it is important to recognize that chlorine dioxide is a potent respiratory irritant. No quantitative data can be used to construct a dose–response relationship for this effect.

3.3.4   Carcinogenicity and mutagenicity

The mutagenic or clastogenic effects of chlorine dioxide have received little attention. Ishidate et al. (1984) found chlorine dioxide to be positive in *Salmonella typhimurium* tester strain TA100. A linear dose–response was observed at concentrations between 2 and 20 µg per plate. Chlorine dioxide was ineffective as a clastogenic agent in a CHO system.

Meier et al. (1985b) evaluated the ability of chlorine dioxide to induce chromosomal aberrations and micronuclei in bone marrow of CD-1 mice or sperm head anomalies. Chlorine dioxide failed to produce such damage following gavage doses of up to 16 mg/kg of body weight for 5 days.

With the exception of a 1949 study by Haag (cited in TERA, 1998), which has serious limitations, no tests of the carcinogenic activity of chlorine dioxide in experimental animals were identified in the scientific literature.

3.3.5 *Comparative pharmacokinetics and metabolism*

There are significant differences in the pharmacokinetics of ^{36}Cl obtained from different disinfectants. The absorption rate for ^{36}Cl-labelled chlorine dioxide was at least 10 times that observed with chlorine, chloramine or chloride. The relative amount of ^{36}Cl that is eliminated in the urine and faeces at 24 h has a distinct pattern from that observed with other disinfectants and sodium chloride. However, the terminal half-life of the ^{36}Cl appears similar for all disinfectants. These data suggest that the form of ^{36}Cl that is being absorbed differs chemically with the different disinfectants. In the case of chlorine dioxide, this is supported by the observation that measurable amounts of chlorite (about 3% of the original dose) are eliminated in the urine during the first 24 h, and chlorite comprises about 20% of the label present in blood 72 h after administration of the test dose (Abdel-Rahman et al., 1980). However, this higher absorption rate is not explained by the absorption rates of chlorite and chlorate, which are about one-tenth as rapid (Abdel-Rahman et al., 1982b). This suggests that some of the absorption could be as chlorine dioxide itself. On the surface, this hypothesis would seem to be incompatible with the high reactivity of this disinfectant. As with other disinfectants, the terminal elimination phases observed for ^{36}Cl from chlorine dioxide seem compatible with the hypothesis that the bulk of the elimination is as chloride ion.

4. TOXICOLOGY OF DISINFECTANT BY-PRODUCTS

4.1 Trihalomethanes

As a class, the THMs are generally the most prevalent by-products of drinking-water disinfection by chlorine. A variety of non-neoplastic toxic effects have been associated with short-term and long-term exposure of experimental animals to high doses of THMs, and each of the four most common THMs — chloroform, BDCM, DBCM and bromoform — has been shown to be carcinogenic to rodents in high-dose chronic studies. Chloroform is generally the predominant THM in chlorinated water and is also the most extensively studied chemical of this class. Because the World Health Organization (WHO) recently published an Environmental Health Criteria monograph on chloroform (IPCS, 1994), this section will only update the information contained in that publication. A thorough review of findings relevant to the toxicology of the brominated THMs is included.

As with the other DBPs, the chemical and physical properties of the THMs influence their potential routes of human exposure, their pharmacokinetic behaviour, their toxicity and methods for conducting toxicological studies with these compounds. The THMs are volatile liquids at room temperature; therefore, as these chemicals vaporize during water usage (e.g., showering), inhalation becomes an important exposure route in addition to ingestion. Volatility decreases somewhat with bromine substitution, but each of the brominated THMs evaporates from drinking-water. Like that of other alkanes, the water solubility of THMs is poor, although adequate to permit dissolution of the low levels generated via water disinfection. When administered at higher levels to animals in toxicity experiments, THMs are often either emulsified in aqueous solutions or dissolved in oils. The use of oils as vehicles of administration can significantly alter the pharmacokinetics and toxicity of the THMs. Bromine substitution enhances the lipid solubility of the halomethanes (and, consequently, uptake into tissues) and generally increases their chemical reactivity and the likelihood of biotransformation to a reactive intermediate. Because toxicity is dependent upon a reactive compound actually reaching a sensitive target site, greater bromine substitution may not necessarily translate into greater *in vivo* toxicity (i.e., innocuous reactions may occur, preventing arrival at target sites). Perhaps to a greater extent than with other chemicals in this class, BDCM appears to reach a variety of target tissues where it can be readily metabolized to several intermediates, leading to adverse effects in experimental animals.

4.1.1   Chloroform

In 1994, the WHO published an Environmental Health Criteria monograph on chloroform (IPCS, 1994). The following sections will update that document with the most recent findings from health-related chloroform research. Another evaluation of chloroform was included in the 1998 Addendum to the WHO *Guidelines for drinking-water quality* (WHO, 1998).

4.1.1.1   General toxicological properties and information on dose–response in animals

1)   Acute toxicity

Keegan et al. (1998) determined the lowest-observed-adverse-effect level (LOAEL) and NOAEL for the induction of acute hepato-toxicity following oral administration of chloroform in an aqueous vehicle to male F344 rats. Based on elevations of serum clinical chemistry indicators of liver damage, a LOAEL of 0.5 mmol/kg of body weight (60 mg/kg of body weight) and a NOAEL of 0.25 mmol/kg of body weight (30 mg/kg of body weight) were established. In a corn oil gavage study of single-dose chloroform effects, an increase in renal cell proliferation was observed at doses as low as 10 mg/kg of body weight in male Osborne-Mendel rats and 90 mg/kg of body weight in male F344 rats (Templin et al., 1996a). The only increase in the hepatic labelling index was in F344 rats given 477 mg/kg of body weight. Effects in the nasal passages of both rat strains at 90 mg/kg of body weight and above included oedema and periosteal hypercellularity. Gemma et al. (1996) dosed male B6C3F$_1$ mice with chloroform (150 mg/kg of body weight) by gavage and observed increases in cell proliferation in both the liver and kidneys. The effect was more dramatic in the kidneys, where severe necrosis was also noted.

Nephrotoxicity of chloroform was evaluated in male Sprague-Dawley rats treated orally with single doses of chloroform using corn oil or an aqueous preparation (5%) of Emulphor or Tween 85 as vehicle (10 ml/kg of body weight). Comparison between gavage vehicles indicated clear trends for enhanced potency and severity of nephrotoxic effects with corn oil administration of chloroform (Raymond & Plaa, 1997).

2)   Short-term toxicity

Chloroform was administered by corn oil gavage to male $B6C3F_1$ mice at doses of 0, 34, 90, 138 or 277 mg/kg of body weight for 4 days or 3 weeks (5 days per week) (Larson et al., 1994a). Mild degenerative changes in centrilobular hepatocytes were noted in mice given 34 and 90 mg/kg of body weight per day after 4 days of treatment, but these effects were absent at 3 weeks. At 138 and 277 mg/kg of body weight per day, centrilobular necrosis was observed at 4 days and with increased severity at 3 weeks. Hepatic cell proliferation was increased in a dose-dependent manner at all chloroform doses after 4 days, but only in the 277 mg/kg of body weight dose group at 3 weeks. Renal tubular necrosis was observed in all dose groups after 4 days, while 3 weeks of exposure produced severe nephropathy at the highest dose and regenerating tubules at the lower doses. The nuclear labelling index was increased in the proximal tubules at all doses after 4 days of treatment, but was elevated only in the two highest dose groups after 3 weeks.

In a similar study (Larson et al., 1994b), female $B6C3F_1$ mice were administered chloroform dissolved in corn oil by gavage at doses of 0, 3, 10, 34, 238 or 477 mg/kg of body weight per day for 4 days or 3 weeks (5 days per week). Dose-dependent changes included centrilobular necrosis and markedly elevated labelling index in mice given 238 and 477 mg/kg of body weight per day. The NOAEL for histopathological changes was 10 mg/kg of body weight per day, and for induced cell proliferation, 34 mg/kg of body weight per day.

In an inhalation study, Templin et al. (1996b) exposed BDF_1 mice to chloroform vapour at concentrations of 0, 149 or 446 mg/m³ (0, 30 or 90 ppm) 6 h per day for 4 days or 2 weeks (5 days per week). In the kidneys of male mice exposed to 149 and 446 mg/m³ (30 and 90 ppm), degenerative lesions and 7- to 10-fold increases in cell proliferation were observed. Liver damage and an increased hepatic labelling index were noted in male mice exposed to 149 and 446 mg/m³ (30 and 90 ppm) and in female mice exposed to 446 mg/m³ (90 ppm). Both doses were lethal in groups exposed for 2 weeks (40% and 80% mortality at 149 and 446 mg/m^3 [30 and 90 ppm], respectively).

Female F344 rats were given chloroform by corn oil gavage for 4 consecutive days or 5 days per week for 3 weeks (Larson et al., 1995b). In the liver, mild degenerative centrilobular changes and dose-dependent increases in hepatocyte proliferation were noted at doses of 100, 200 and 400 mg/kg of body weight per day. At 200 and 400 mg/kg of body weight per day, degeneration and necrosis of the renal cortical proximal tubules were observed. Increased regenerative proliferation of epithelial cells lining proximal tubules was seen at doses of 100 mg/kg of body weight per day or more. Lesions of the olfactory mucosa lining the ethmoid region of the nose (new bone formation, periosteal hypercellularity and increased cell replication) were seen at all doses, including the lowest dose of 34 mg/kg of body weight per day. Larson et al. (1995a) also administered chloroform to male F344 rats by corn oil gavage (0, 10, 34, 90 or 180 mg/kg of body weight per day) or in the drinking-water (0, 60, 200, 400, 900 or 1800 mg/litre) for 4 days or 3 weeks. Gavage of 90 or 180 mg/kg of body weight per day for 4 days induced mild to moderate degeneration of renal proximal tubules and centrilobular hepatocytes — changes that were no longer present after 3 weeks. Increased cell proliferation in the kidney was noted only at the highest gavage dose after 4 days. The labelling index was elevated in the livers of the high-dose group at both time points. With drinking-water administration, rats consuming the water containing 1800 mg/litre were dosed at a rate of 106 mg/kg of body weight per day, but no increase in renal or hepatic cell prolifer-ation was observed at this or any lower dose.

In a study carried out to evaluate whether exposure to chloroform in drinking-water would interact with the activity of chloroform when administered by gavage in corn oil, female B6C3F$_1$ mice were exposed to chloroform in drinking-water for 33 days at 0, 300 or 1800 mg/litre or for 31 days at 0, 120, 240 or 480 mg/litre. Three days prior to termination, mice also received a daily dose of 263 mg of chloroform per kg of body weight per day, administered by gavage in corn oil. Exposure to chloroform in drinking-water reduced both the hepato-toxicity and the enhanced cell proliferation elicited in response to chloroform administered by gavage in corn oil (Pereira & Grothaus, 1997).

The cardiotoxicity of chloroform was examined in male Wistar rats given daily doses of 37 mg/kg of body weight (0.31 mmol/kg) by gavage in olive oil for 4 weeks (Muller et al., 1997). Chloroform caused arrhythmogenic and negative chronotropic and dromotropic effects as well as extension of the atrioventricular conduction time and depressed myocardial contractility.

A 90-day chloroform inhalation study was conducted using male and female B6C3F$_1$ mice and exposure concentrations of 0, 1.5, 10, 50, 149 and 446 mg/m^3 (0, 0.3, 2, 10, 30 and 90 ppm) for 6 h per day, 7 days per week (Larson et al., 1996). Large, sustained increases in hepatocyte proliferation were seen in the 446 mg/m^3 (90 ppm) groups at all time points (4 days and 3, 6 and 13 weeks). In the more sensitive female mice, a NOAEL of 50 mg/m^3 (10 ppm) for this effect was established. Renal histopathology and regenerative hyperplasia were noted in male mice at 50, 149 and 446 mg/m^3 (10, 30 and 90 ppm). In another 90-day inhalation study, F344 rats were exposed to chloroform at concentrations of 0, 10, 50, 149, 446 or 1490 mg/m^3 (0, 2, 10, 30, 90 or 300 ppm) for 6 h per day, 7 days per week. The 1490 mg/m^3 (300 ppm) level was extremely toxic and deemed by the authors to be inappropriate for chronic studies. Increases in renal epithelial cell proliferation in cortical proximal tubules were observed at concentrations of 149 mg/m^3 (30 ppm) and above. Hepatic lesions and increased proliferation were noted only at the highest exposure level. In the ethmoid turbinates of the nose, enhanced bone growth and hypercellularity in the lamina propria were observed at concentrations of 50 mg/m^3 (10 ppm) and above, and a generalized atrophy of the turbinates was seen at all exposure levels after 90 days (Templin et al., 1996c).

3)   Reproductive and developmental toxicity

Rat embryo culture was used to assess the developmental effects of chloroform (Brown-Woodman et al., 1998). The effect and no-effect culture medium concentrations of chloroform were 2.06 and 1.05 μmol/ml. The authors estimated that fatal or near-fatal blood levels would be required in the mother for the embryotoxic level to be reached.

4.1.1.2   Toxicity in humans

Fatal acute chloroform intoxication via inhalation was reported to cause cardiomyocyte fragmentation and waviness indicative of acute heart failure possibly caused by arrhythmias or cardiac depression (Harada et al., 1997). These observations are consistent with the results of the short-term rat study (Templin et al., 1996b) described above in section 4.1.1.1.

4.1.1.3   Carcinogenicity and mutagenicity

Jamison et al. (1996) reported that F344 rats exposed to a high concentration of chloroform vapour (1490 mg/m^3 [300 ppm]) for 90 days developed atypical glandular structures lined by intestinal-like epithelium and surrounded by dense connective tissue in their livers. These lesions appeared to arise from a population of cells remote from the bile ducts. The authors also observed a treatment-related increase in transforming growth factor-alpha (TGF-α) immunoreactivity in hepatocytes, bile duct epithelium, bile canaliculi and oval cells and an increase in transforming growth factor-beta (TGF-β) immunoreactivity in hepatocytes, bile duct epithelium and intestinal crypt-like ducts. The lesions occurred only in conjunction with significant hepatocyte necrosis, regenerative cell proliferation and increased growth factor expression or uptake.

Chloroform was tested for mutagenicity and clastogenicity by Le Curieux et al. (1995) and was negative in the SOS chromotest, the Ames fluctuation test and the newt micronucleus test. It appeared to these authors that the presence of bromine substituents was needed for genotoxic activity in the THM class. Pegram et al. (1997) examined chloroform mutagenicity in a strain of *Salmonella typhimurium* TA1535 transfected with rat glutathione-*S*-transferase (GST) T1-1. Chloroform was negative in this assay over a range of concentrations (992–23 800 mg/m^3 [200–4800 ppm]) that produced large dose-dependent increases in revertants with BDCM. A doubling of revertants was induced by chloroform in the GST-transfected strain only at the two highest concentrations tested (95 200 and 127 000 mg/m^3 [19 200 and 25 600 ppm]). Brennan & Schiestl (1998) found that chloroform induced intrachromosomal recombination in the yeast strain *Saccharomyces cerevisiae* at culture medium concentrations of 3–5.6 mg/ml.

In an *in vivo* study, Potter et al. (1996) found that chloroform did not induce DNA strand breaks in the kidneys of male F344 rats following seven daily doses of 1.5 mmol/kg of body weight. In long-term mutagenicity studies with chloroform in female *lacI* transgenic B6C3F₁ mice conducted by Butterworth et al. (1998), the mice were exposed daily by inhalation to chloroform concentrations of 0, 50, 149 or 446 mg/m³ (0, 10, 30 or 90 ppm) for 6 h per day, 7 days per week, and *lacI* mutant frequency was determined after 10, 30, 90 and 180 days of exposure. No increase in *lacI* mutant frequency was observed in the liver at any dose or time point with chloroform.

1.1.4   Comparative pharmacokinetics and metabolism

The percutaneous absorption of ¹⁴C-chloroform was examined *in vivo* using human volunteers and *in vitro* using fresh, excised human skin in a flow-through diffusion cell system (Dick et al., 1995). Aqueous and ethanol solutions of chloroform were applied to the forearm (16 and 81 g/cm) of volunteers, and absorption was determined to be 7.8% from the water vehicle and 1.6% from ethanol. More than 95% of the absorbed dose was excreted via the lungs (88% as carbon dioxide), and maximum pulmonary excretion occurred between 15 min and 2 h after dosing. *In vitro*, 5.6% of a low dose and 7.1% of a high dose were absorbed (skin plus perfusate).

The systemic uptake of chloroform during dermal exposure was also studied in hairless rats (Islam et al., 1996). Animals were immersed in water containing chloroform for 30 min, and the compound was detected in blood as early as 4 min following exposure. About 10 mg of chloroform were systemically absorbed after dermal exposure of a rat to an aqueous solution of 0.44 mg/ml.

Absorption and tissue dosimetry of chloroform were evaluated after gavage administration in various vehicles to male Fischer 344 rats and female B6C3F₁ mice (Dix et al., 1997). Animals received a single dose of chloroform (15–180 and 70–477 mg/kg of body weight for rats and mice, respectively) in corn oil, water or aqueous 2% Emulphor (dose volumes of 2 and 10 ml/kg of body weight for rats and mice, respectively). Blood, liver and kidney chloroform concentration–time courses were determined. Gavage vehicle had minimal effects on chloroform dosimetry in rats. In mice, however, tissue chloroform concentrations were consistently greater for aqueous versus corn oil vehicle. At the low vehicle volume used for rats (2 ml/kg of body weight), gavage vehicle may not play a significant role in chloroform absorption and tissue dosimetry; at the higher vehicle volume used for mice (10 ml/kg of body weight), however, vehicle may be a critical factor.

Because chloroform metabolism was reviewed in detail in the recent Environmental Health Criteria monograph (IPCS, 1994), the primary discussion of the comparative metabolism of the THMs as a class can be found in section 4.1.2.6 of the present report.

The contributions of cytochromes P450 (CYP) 2E1 and 2B1/2 to chloroform hepatotoxicity were investigated in male Wistar rats (Nakajima et al., 1995). The severity of toxicity observed in differentially induced rats suggests that CYP2E1 is a low Michaelis-Menten constant (K_m) isoform and CYP2B1/2 is a high K_m isoform for chloroform activation. A high dose of chloroform (0.5 ml/kg of body weight) induced CYP2E1 but decreased CYP2B1/2. Testai et al. (1996) generated similar results in a study examining the involvement of these isozymes in *in vitro* chloroform metabolism. At a low substrate concentration (0.1 mmol/litre), oxidative metabolism by liver microsomes was dependent primarily on CYP2E1; at 5 mmol/litre, on the other hand, CYP2B1/2 was the major participant responsible for chloroform activation, although CYP2E1 and CYP2C11 were also significantly involved. The reductive pathway was expressed only at 5 mmol/litre and was not significantly increased by any CYP inducer tested.

The reductive metabolism of chloroform by rat liver microsomes was examined by Testai et al. (1995). In hypoxic (1% oxygen partial pressure) and anoxic (0% oxygen partial pressure) incubations using microsomes from phenobarbital-induced animals, no evidence of formation of monochloromethyl carbene was found. Dichloromethane was detected as a metabolite of chloroform under variable oxygenation conditions using microsomes from phenobarbital-induced animals. With uninduced microsomes, significant levels of dichloromethane were formed only in hypoxic or anoxic incubations. In an *in vivo* study of chloroform reductive metabolism, Knecht & Mason (1991) detected no free radical adducts in the bile of rats treated with chloroform, while radicals were detected from bromoform. Lipid adducts resulting from the reductive metabolism of chloroform by hepatocytes appeared to be generated by the unspecific attack of the radical on the phospholipid fatty acyl chains (Guastadisegni et al., 1996). The primary lipid adduct has now been identified as a modified phosphatidylethanolamine, with the phosgene-derived carbonyl bound to the amine of the head group (Guastadisegni et al., 1998). Waller & McKinney (1993) found that chloroform had a lower theoretical potential to undergo reductive metabolism than the brominated THMs. Ade et al. (1994) reported that microsomes from the renal cortex of DBA/2J mice can metabolize chloroform through the reductive and oxidative pathways, as had been previously described using hepatic microsomes. However, cytolethality of chloroform to freshly isolated rodent hepatocytes was not increased under reduced oxygen tension, indicating that reductive metabolism does not contribute to chloroform-induced toxicity (Ammann et al., 1998).

The potential of chloroform to participate in the recently discovered GSH conjugation pathway for brominated THMs has been investigated (Pegram et al., 1997). The GST examined in this study has a very low affinity for chloroform compared with the brominated THMs. Chloroform conjugation with GSH occurred only at extremely high substrate concentrations.

1.1.5   Mode of action

Direct DNA reactivity and mutagenicity cannot be considered to be key factors in chloroform-induced carcinogenesis in experimental animals. A substantial body of data demonstrates a lack of direct *in vivo* or *in vitro* genotoxicity of chloroform. If THMs produce their genotoxic effects primarily via the GSH conjugation mechanism, the results of Pegram et al. (1997) indicate that chloroform would be mutagenic in mammals only at lethal doses.

There is, however, compelling evidence to support a mode of action for tumour induction based on metabolism of chloroform by the target cell population, followed by cytotoxicity of oxidative metabo-lites and regenerative cell proliferation. The evidence for the link with cytotoxicity is strongest for hepatic and renal tumours in the mouse and more limited for renal tumours in the rat (ILSI, 1997). A number of recent studies support the hypothesis that chloroform acts to produce cancer in rodents through a non-genotoxic/cytotoxic mode of action, with carcinogenesis resulting from events secondary to chloroform-induced cytolethality and regenerative cell proliferation (Larson et al., 1994a,b, 1996; Pereira, 1994; Templin et al., 1996a,b,c, 1998). These studies have shown that organ toxicity and regenerative hyperplasia are associated with the tumorigenicity of chloroform and are apparently the key steps in its carcinogenic mode of action. Thus, sustained toxicity would result in tumour development. Chloroform induces liver and kidney tumours in long-term rodent cancer bioassays only at doses that induce frank cytotoxicity in these target organs. Furthermore, there are no instances of chloroform-induced tumours that are not preceded by this pattern of dose-dependent toxic responses (Golden et al., 1997).

The organ toxicity and carcinogenicity of chloroform are dependent on oxidative metabolism and levels of CYP2E1. Numerous studies have also shown that oxidative metabolism by CYP2E1 generates highly reactive metabolites (phosgene and hydrogen chloride), which would lead to cytotoxicity and regenerative hyperplasia.

4.1.2 Bromodichloromethane

4.1.2.1 General toxicological properties and information on dose–response in animals

1) Acute toxicity

The acute oral lethality of the brominated THMs has been determined in ICR Swiss mice (Bowman et al., 1978) and Sprague-Dawley rats (Chu et al., 1980). The resulting LD_{50}s for BDCM were 450 and 900 mg/kg of body weight for male and female mice, respectively, and 916 and 969 mg/kg of body weight for male and female rats, respectively. Clinical observations of animals dosed with high levels of BDCM in these studies and others (NTP, 1987) included ataxia, sedation, laboured breathing and anaesthesia (500 mg/kg of body weight), as well as gross evidence of liver and kidney damage. Hewitt et al. (1983) gave single doses of BDCM to male Sprague-Dawley rats by corn oil gavage and found doses of 1980 mg/kg of body weight and above to be lethal. Little clinical evidence of hepatic or renal toxicity was observed at doses below 1980 mg/kg of body weight.

Acute hepatotoxic and nephrotoxic responses to orally dosed BDCM and various factors affecting these toxicities (e.g., gavage vehicle and glutathione status) have been studied in male F344 rats.

Lilly et al. (1994, 1997a) examined the time course of toxicity and dose–response relationships following oral administration of aqueous solutions of BDCM. BDCM-induced liver toxicity was maximal at 24 h after dosing with 1–3 mmol/kg of body weight (164–492 mg/kg of body weight), as indicated by elevations in serum levels of aspartate aminotransferase (ASAT), alanine aminotransferase (ALAT), sorbitol dehydrogenase (SDH) and lactate dehydrogenase (LDH) and histopathological observations of centrilobular vacuolar degeneration and hepatocellular necrosis. Significant abatement of hepatic toxicity was noted by 48 h post-dosing. The acute oral NOAEL and LOAEL for liver toxicity following aqueous delivery of BDCM, based on elevations in serum enzymes, were determined to be 0.25 and 0.5 mmol of BDCM per kg of body weight (41 and 82 mg/kg of body weight), respectively (Keegan et al., 1998). BDCM and chloroform appear to be equipotent hepatotoxicants in rats at 24 h after exposure, but BDCM causes more persistent damage to the liver, based on observations at 48 h post-dosing (Lilly et al., 1997a; Keegan et al., 1998).

Kidney toxicity after corn oil or aqueous dosing of BDCM (1.5–3 mol/kg of body weight) peaked between 24 and 48 h, as indicated by elevations in kidney weight, urinary N-acetyl-β-glucosaminidase, ASAT, ALAT, LDH and protein, serum urea and creatinine, and histopathological findings of renal tubule degeneration and necrosis (Lilly et al., 1994, 1997a). The actual time of peak renal effects was dose-dependent; in contrast to findings in the liver, toxicity was increasingly prolonged in the kidney with increasing dose. Nephrotoxicity has been noted in rats given single BDCM doses as low as 200 mg or 1.2 mmol/kg of body weight (Lilly et al., 1994, 1997a), and BDCM is a slightly more potent acute oral renal toxicant than chloroform (based on the magnitude of the responses), especially at lower doses (Lilly et al., 1997a). Kroll et al. (1994a,b) found that among the THMs that occur in drinking-water, BDCM was the most potent inducer of renal dysfunction in rats following intraperitoneal injection of single 3 mmol/kg of body weight doses. Glomerular filtration, renal concentrating ability, and proximal tubular secretion and reabsorption were all more severely affected by BDCM than by chloroform.

Several factors have been found to influence dose–response relationships for BDCM toxicity. Acute hepatotoxicity and nephrotoxicity were more severe after administration of 400 mg of BDCM per kg of body weight in corn oil than when the same dose was given in an aqueous vehicle (Lilly et al., 1994). However, vehicle differences at a lower dose (200 mg/kg of body weight), although less pronounced, were reversed: greater renal toxicity at this dose was associated with the aqueous vehicle. The adverse renal and hepatic effects of BDCM were also exacerbated in GSH-depleted rats (Gao et al., 1996) and in rats that were dosed during the active period of their diurnal cycle (Pegram et al., 1993). Induction of the cytochrome P-450 isozymes CYP2E1 and CYP2B1/2 also potentiated acute liver toxicity, but not renal toxicity, following dosing with BDCM (Thornton-Mannning et al., 1994).

2)   Short-term toxicity

Studies employing repeated daily BDCM dosing regimens have also yielded results demonstrating liver and kidney toxicity. Thornton-Manning et al. (1994) administered five consecutive daily BDCM doses to female F344 rats and female C57BL/6J mice by aqueous gavage and found that BDCM is both hepatotoxic and nephrotoxic to female rats (150–300 mg/kg of body weight per day), but only hepatotoxic to female mice (75–150 mg/kg of body weight per day). Hepatic cytochrome P450 activities were decreased in rats, but not in mice, in this study. Munson et al. (1982) administered BDCM (50, 125 or 250 mg/kg of body weight per day) to male and female CD-1 mice by aqueous gavage for 14 days and reported evidence for hepatic and renal toxicity as well as effects on the humoral immune system. Nephrotoxicity, as reflected by significant elevations of blood urea nitrogen (BUN), occurred only at the highest dose in both males and females. Male mice appeared more sensitive than females to BDCM-induced hepatotoxicity; 2- to 3-fold elevations in ASAT and ALAT (although not significant, according to the authors' statistical analysis) occurred at the lowest dose only in males. Based on the degree of these elevations, BDCM was the most potent hepatotoxicant compared with chloroform, DBCM and bromoform, which were also tested in this study. Immunotoxic effects described in the study included decreases in both antibody-forming cells and haemagglutination titres at the 125 and 250 mg/kg of body weight per day doses, although a recent investigation found no effects of BDCM on immune function (French et al., 1999). Condie et al. (1983) conducted a similar 14-day comparative dosing study with THMs and male CD-1 mice, but used corn oil as the vehicle of administration for doses of BDCM of 37, 74 and

147 mg/kg of body weight per day. Evidence of renal damage was observed at the mid and high doses, whereas liver toxicity occurred only at the high dose. A 14-day corn oil gavage study by NTP (1987) demonstrated the greater sensitivity of the B6C3F$_1$ mouse to BDCM: all male mice that received 150 or 300 mg/kg of body weight per day died before the end of the study. Aida et al. (1992a) incorporated microencapsulated BDCM into the diet of Wistar rats for 1 month, and a LOAEL of 66 mg/kg of body weight per day and a NOAEL of 21 mg/kg of body weight per day were determined based on histopathological findings of hepatocellular vacuolization.

In a 13-week corn oil gavage study, NTP (1987) administered BDCM doses of 0, 19, 38, 75, 150 or 300 mg/kg of body weight per day, 5 days per week, to F344/N rats (10 per sex per dose). The highest dose was lethal to 50% of males and 20% of females, and body weight depression was observed at the two highest doses. BDCM-induced lesions were found only at 300 mg/kg of body weight per day; these included hepatic centrilobular degeneration in both sexes and renal tubular degeneration and necrosis in males. Additional findings included mild bile duct hyperplasia and atrophy of the thymus, spleen and lymph nodes in both sexes. B6C3F$_1$ mice were also dosed with BDCM in this study, and doses of 50 mg/kg of body weight per day and below produced no compound-related effects. Degeneration and necrosis of the kidney were observed in male mice at 100 mg/kg of body weight per day, whereas centrilobular degeneration of the liver was noted in females at 200 and 400 mg/kg of body weight per day.

3) Chronic toxicity

Moore et al. (1994) administered BDCM in drinking-water (containing 0.25% Emulphor) to male F344 rats and B6C3F$_1$ mice for 1 year and evaluated clinical indicators of kidney toxicity. Water containing BDCM concentrations of 0.08, 0.4 and 0.8 g/litre for rats and 0.06, 0.3 and 0.6 g/litre for mice resulted in average daily doses of 4.4, 21 and 39 mg/kg of body weight for rats and 5.6, 24 and 49 mg/kg of body weight for mice. A urinary marker for renal proximal tubule damage, N-acetyl-β-glucosaminidase, was elevated above controls in each dose group in rats and at the highest treatment level in mice. Significant increases in urinary protein, indicative of glomerular damage, were also noted in low- and mid-dose rats as well as high-dose mice.

In an NTP (1987) study, BDCM was administered by corn oil gavage for 102 weeks, 5 days per week, to F344/N rats (50 per sex per dose) at doses of 0, 50 or 100 mg/kg of body weight per day and to B6C3F$_1$ mice at doses of 0, 25 or 50 mg/kg of body weight per day (50 males per group) and 0, 75 or 150 mg/kg of body weight per day (50 females per group). In male rats, compound-related non-neoplastic lesions included renal cytomegaly and tubular cell hyperplasia and hepatic necrosis and fatty metamorphosis. Kidney tubule cell hyperplasia was also observed in female rats, as well as eosinophilic cytoplasmic change, clear cell change, focal cellular change and fatty metamorphosis of the liver. Histopathological changes were noted at both doses in rats. BDCM-induced non-neoplastic lesions in male mice included hepatic fatty metamorphosis, renal cytomegaly and follicular cell hyperplasia of the thyroid gland, all observed in both dose groups. In female mice, hyperplasia of the thyroid gland was observed at both doses.

Microencapsulated BDCM was fed in the diet to Wistar rats for 24 months, resulting in average daily doses of 6, 26 or 138 mg/kg of body weight for males and 8, 32 or 168 mg/kg of body weight for females (Aida et al., 1992b). Relative liver weight was increased in both sexes of all dose groups, as was relative kidney weight in the high-dose group. BDCM induced hepatic fatty degeneration and granuloma in all dose groups and cholangiofibrosis in the high-dose groups. Therefore, this study identified a LOAEL for chronic liver toxicity of 6 mg/kg of body weight per day.

4.1.2.2 Reproductive and developmental toxicity

Klinefelter et al. (1995) studied the potential of BDCM to alter male reproductive function in F344 rats. BDCM was consumed in the drinking-water for 52 weeks, resulting in average dose rates of 22 and 39 mg/kg of body weight per day. No gross lesions in the reproductive organs were revealed by histological examination, but exposure to the high BDCM dose significantly decreased the mean straight-line, average path and curvilinear velocities of sperm recovered from the cauda epididymis. These effects of BDCM on sperm motility occurred at a lower exposure level than was observed for other DBPs that compromised sperm motility.

A teratological assessment of BDCM was conducted in Sprague-Dawley rats by administering the compound by gavage from day 6 to day 15 of gestation (Ruddick et al., 1983). Doses of 50, 100 and 200 mg of BDCM per kg of body weight per day did not produce any teratogenic effects or dose-related histopathological changes in either the dams or fetuses, but sternebra aberrations were observed with a dose-dependent incidence in all dose groups. The increased incidence of these variations appeared to be significant, but no statistical analysis of the data was performed. Maternal weight gain was depressed in the high-dose group, and maternal liver and kidney weights were increased. Narotsky et al. (1997) employed a similar experimental model to test BDCM in F344 rats using doses of 0, 25, 50 or 75 mg/kg of body weight per day in aqueous or oil gavage vehicles. BDCM induced full-litter resorptions in the 50 and 75 mg/kg of body weight per day dose groups with either vehicle of administration. For dams receiving corn oil, full-litter resorptions were noted in 8% and 83% of the litters at 50 and 75 mg/kg of body weight per day, respectively. With the aqueous vehicle, 17% and 21% of the litters were fully resorbed at 50 and 75 mg/kg of body weight per day, respectively. All vehicle control litters and litters from the group given 25 mg/kg of body weight per day survived the experimental period. BDCM had been shown to cause maternal toxicity at these doses in a previous study (Narotsky et al., 1992).

1.2.3 Neurotoxicity

Neurotoxicological findings for the brominated THMs are limited to various observations of anaesthesia associated with acute high-dose exposures and results from a behavioural study conducted by Balster & Borzelleca (1982). Adult male ICR mice were dosed by aqueous gavage for up to 90 days. Treatments of 1.2 or 11.6 mg/kg of body weight per day were without effect in various behavioural tests, and dosing for 30 days with 100 mg/kg of body weight per day did not affect passive avoidance learning. Animals dosed with either 100 or 400 mg/kg of body weight per day for 60 days exhibited decreased response rates in an operant behaviour test; these effects were greatest early in the regimen, with no evidence of progressive deterioration.

4.1.2.4   Toxicity in humans

Clinical case findings resulting from human exposure to BDCM have not been reported.

4.1.2.5   Carcinogenicity and mutagenicity

IARC has evaluated the carcinogenicity of BDCM and concluded that there is sufficient evidence for its carcinogenicity in experimental animals and inadequate evidence for its carcinogenicity in humans. On this basis, BDCM was assigned to Group 2B: the agent is possibly carcinogenic to humans (IARC, 1991, 1999).

Among the four THMs commonly found in drinking-water, BDCM appears to be the most potent rodent carcinogen. BDCM caused cancer at lower doses and at more target sites than for any of the other THMs. In the NTP (1987) 2-year bioassay, a corn oil gavage study (50 animals per sex per group, dosed 5 days per week), compound-related tumours were found in the liver, kidneys and large intestine. Daily doses were 0, 50 or 100 mg/kg of body weight (male and female rats), 0, 25 or 50 mg/kg of body weight (male mice) and 0, 75 or 150 mg/kg of body weight (female mice). NTP (1987) concluded that there was clear evidence of carcinogenic activity for both sexes of F344 rats and B6C3F$_1$ mice, as shown by increased incidences of tubular cell adenomas and adenocarcinomas in the kidney and adeno-carcinomas and adenomatous polyps in the large intestine of male and female rats, increased incidences of tubular cell adenomas and adeno-carcinomas in the kidney of male mice, and increased incidences of hepatocellular adenomas and carcinomas in female mice (Table 11).

Aida et al. (1992b) maintained Slc:Wistar rats on diets containing microencapsulated BDCM for 24 months and examined the animals for neoplastic lesions. The only significant finding was a slight increase in the incidence of liver tumours in females receiving the high dose (168 mg/kg of body weight per day). These included cholangio-carcinomas and hepatocellular adenomas.

To date, effects following chronic BDCM administration via drinking-water have not been described in the literature. However, two separate drinking-water studies are currently being conducted by the US Environmental Protection Agency (EPA) and the NTP.

Table 11. Tumour frequencies in rats and mice exposed to
bromodichloromethane in corn oil for 2 years[a]

Animal/tissue/tumour	Tumour frequency at control, low and high doses (mg/kg of body weight per day)		
Male rat	0	50	100
Large intestine[b]			
Adenomatous polyp	0/50	3/49	33/50
Adenocarcinoma	0/50	11/49	38/50
Combined	0/50	13/49	45/50
Kidney[b]			
Tubular cell adenoma	0/50	1/49	3/50
Tubular cell adenocarcinoma	0/50	0/49	10/50
Combined	0/50	1/49	13/50
Large intestine and/or kidney combined[b]	0/50	13/49	46/50
Female rat	0	50	100
Large intestine[c]			
Adenomatous polyp	0/46	0/50	7/47
Adenocarcinoma	0/46	0/50	6/47
Combined	0/46	0/50	12/47
Kidney			
Tubular cell adenoma	0/50	1/50	6/50
Tubular cell adenocarcinoma	0/50	0/50	9/50
Combined	0/50	1/50	15/50
Large intestine and/or kidney combined[d]	0/46	1/50	24/48
Male mouse	0	25	100
Kidney[e]			
Tubular cell adenoma	1/46	2/49	6/50
Tubular cell adenocarcinoma	0/46	0/49	4/50
Combined	1/46	2/49	9/50
Female mouse	0	75	150
Liver			
Hepatocellular adenoma	1/50	13/48	23/50
Hepatocellular carcinoma	2/50	5/48	10/50
Combined	3/50	18/48	29/50

[a] Adapted from NTP (1987).
[b] One rat died at week 33 in the low-dose group and was eliminated from the cancer risk calculation.
[c] Intestine not examined in four rats from the control group and three rats from the high-dose group.
[d] One rat in the high-dose group was not examined for intestinal tumours and kidney tumours.
[e] In the control group, two mice died during the first week, one mouse died during week 9 and one escaped in week 79. One mouse in the low-dose group died in the first week. All of these mice were eliminated from the cancer risk calculations.

Although BDCM has given mixed results in bacterial assays for genotoxicity, the results have tended to be positive in tests employing closed systems to overcome the problem of the compound's volatility (IARC, 1991, 1999; Pegram et al., 1997). Pegram et al. (1997) tested the THMs using a TA1535 strain transfected with rat GST T1-1 and found that the mutagenicity of the brominated THMs, but not chloroform, was greatly enhanced by the expression of the transferase. BDCM was mutagenic in this assay at medium concentrations below 0.1 mmol/litre. Mutation spectra of the brominated THMs at the *hisG46* allele were characterized by DeMarini et al. (1997) using revertants induced in the GST-transfected strain. The overwhelming majority (96–100%) of the mutations induced by the brominated THMs were GC to AT transitions, and 87–100% of these were at the second position of the CCC/GGG target. BDCM produced primary DNA damage in the SOS chromotest (*Escherichia coli* PQ37), but was negative in the Ames fluctuation test with *Salmonella typhimurium* TA100 (Le Curieux et al., 1995). A mixture of BDCM and benzo[*a*]pyrene was tested in an Ames mutagenicity test with *S. typhimurium* strains TA98 and TA100 plus S9 (Kevekordes et al., 1998). BDCM in combination with benzo[*a*]pyrene caused a 25% increase in revertants in both strains compared with benzo[*a*]pyrene alone.

BDCM was also positive in the majority of *in vitro* genotoxicity tests employing eukaryotic systems, but the responses with and without an exogenous metabolizing system are less consistent. This may be due to the fact that the reactive intermediates suspected to be involved in THM mutagenicity must be generated within the target cells (Thier et al., 1993; Pegram et al., 1997). Moreover, extensive metabolism of the THMs by the supplemental S9 outside of the cells would greatly diminish the intracellular dose. Many of the positive studies are for the induction of sister chromatid exchange (SCE) (IARC, 1991, 1999). Morimoto & Koizumi (1983) found that BDCM induced SCEs in human lymphocytes *in vitro* in the absence of S9 activation at concentrations greater than or equal to 0.4 mmol/litre, and Fujie et al. (1993) reported increased SCEs in rat erythroblastic leukaemia cells under similar conditions. Metabolically activated BDCM also increased SCEs *in vitro* in human lymphocytes (at 1 mmol/litre) and in rat hepatocytes (at 100 mmol/litre) (Sobti, 1984).

In vivo, doses of 50 mg of BDCM per kg of body weight and above produced SCEs in male CR/SJ mice (Morimoto & Koizumi,

1983). BDCM was negative in *in vivo* clastogenicity tests (micro-nucleus formation) in mice and rats (Ishidate et al., 1982; Hayashi et al., 1988). Fujie et al. (1990) reported that BDCM induced bone marrow chromosomal aberrations (primarily chromatid and chromosome breaks) in Long-Evans rats following oral or intraperitoneal dosing at doses as low as 16.4 mg/kg of body weight. Potter et al. (1996) found that BDCM did not induce DNA strand breaks in the kidney of male F344 rats following seven daily doses of 1.5 mmol/kg of body weight (246 mg/kg of body weight). Stocker et al. (1997) studied the effect of gastric intubation of aqueous solutions of BDCM on unscheduled DNA synthesis (UDS) in the liver of male rats. BDCM did not cause UDS in hepatocytes isolated after administration of single doses of 135 or 450 mg/kg of body weight. The *in vivo* mutagenicity studies of BDCM and the other brominated THMs are summarized in Table 12.

In comparison with other chemicals known to produce mutations via direct DNA reactivity such as aflatoxin B1 and ethylene dibromide, BDCM is a relatively weak mutagen.

1.2.6 Comparative pharmacokinetics and metabolism

Bromine substitution would be expected to confer greater lipophilicity on the brominated THMs compared with chloroform, which would affect tissue solubility and other factors that can influence pharmacokinetics. Because metabolism of each THM is qualitatively similar (with one known exception), this section addresses key features of the metabolism of all four THMs.

The absorption, distribution and elimination of BDCM have been studied in rats and mice, and more recent work has led to the development of a physiologically based pharmacokinetic (PBPK) model for BDCM in rats. Mink et al. (1986) compared the pharmacokinetics of orally administered ^{14}C-BDCM in male B6C3F$_1$ mice and Sprague-Dawley rats. The animals received single doses of 100 mg/kg of body weight (rats) or 150 mg/kg of body weight (mice) in corn oil by gavage, and tissue levels of radioactivity were determined after 8 h. Absorption of BDCM appeared to be rapid and fairly complete, as would be expected for small halocarbons. This was especially true in the mouse, where 93% of the dose was recovered within 8 h as carbon dioxide (81%), as expired volatile organics assumed to be unmetabolized parent compound (7.2%), in urine (2.2%) or in organs (3.2%).

Table 12. Dose information for selected *in vivo* mutagenicity studies of brominated trihalomethanes

End-point	Assay system	Dose[a]	Result	Reference
Sister chromatid exchange	Male CR/SJ mice, gavage, 4 days	50 mg BDCM/kg bw per day	positive	Morimoto & Koizumi (1983)
Sister chromatid exchange	Male CR/SJ mice, gavage, 4 days	25 mg DBCM/kg bw per day	positive	Morimoto & Koizumi (1983)
Sister chromatid exchange	Male CR/SJ mice, gavage, 4 days	25 mg bromoform/kg bw per day	positive	Morimoto & Koizumi (1983)
Sister chromatid exchange	B6C3F$_1$ mice, i.p.[b]	200 mg bromoform/kg bw	positive	NTP (1989a)
Micronucleus formation	ddY mice, MS mice, Wistar rats, i.p. in olive oil	500 mg BDCM/kg bw per day	negative	Ishidate et al. (1982)
Micronucleus formation	ddY mice, MS mice, Wistar rats, i.p. in olive oil	500 mg DBCM/kg bw per day	negative	Ishidate et al. (1982)
Micronucleus formation	ddY mice, MS mice, Wistar rats, i.p. in olive oil	500 mg bromoform/kg bw per day	negative	Ishidate et al. (1982)
Micronucleus formation	ddY mice, i.p., single dose in corn oil	500 mg BDCM/kg bw	negative	Hayashi et al. (1988)
Micronucleus formation	ddY mice, i.p., single dose in corn oil	1000 mg DBCM/kg bw	negative	Hayashi et al. (1988)
Micronucleus formation	ddY mice, i.p., single dose in corn oil	1400 mg bromoform/kg bw	negative	Hayashi et al. (1988)
Chromosomal aberrations	Long-Evans rats, bone marrow, i.p., single dose	16.4 mg BDCM/kg bw	positive	Fujie et al. (1990)
Chromosomal aberrations	Long-Evans rats, bone marrow, i.p., single dose	20.8 mg DBCM/kg bw	positive	Fujie et al. (1990)
Chromosomal aberrations	Long-Evans rats, bone marrow, i.p., single dose	25.3 mg bromoform/kg bw	positive	Fujie et al. (1990)

Table 12 (Contd.)

End-point	Assay system	Dose[a]	Result	Reference
Chromosomal aberrations	Long-Evans rats, bone marrow	253 mg bromoform/kg bw per day	positive	Fujie et al. (1990)
Unscheduled DNA synthesis	Rat liver, gavage	450 mg BDCM/kg bw per day	negative	Stocker et al. (1997)
Unscheduled DNA synthesis	Rat liver, gavage	2000 mg DBCM/kg bw per day	negative	Stocker et al. (1997)
Unscheduled DNA synthesis	Rat liver, gavage	1080 mg bromoform/kg bw per day	negative	Stocker et al. (1997)
Micronucleus formation	Mouse, bone marrow, gavage, single dose	1000 mg bromoform/kg bw	negative	Stocker et al. (1997)
DNA strand break	Male F344 rats, kidney, gavage, 7 days	1.5 mmol BDCM/kg bw per day	negative	Potter et al. (1996)
DNA strand break	Male F344 rats, kidney, gavage, 7 days	1.5 mmol DBCM/kg bw per day	negative	Potter et al. (1996)
DNA strand break	Male F344 rats, kidney, gavage, 7 days	1.5 mmol bromoform/kg bw per day	negative	Potter et al. (1996)
Sex-linked recessive mutation	Drosophila	1000 ppm solution	positive	NTP (1989a)

[a] Doses listed are the lowest at which an effect was observed or, in the case of negative results, the highest dose tested. bw = body weight.
[b] Intraperitoneal.

Much more of the ^{14}C dose was expired as the assumed parent compound by the rat (42%) than by the mouse, but total recovery after 8 h was less (63%) because of lower conversion to carbon dioxide (14%). The liver, stomach and kidneys were the organs with the highest residual radioactivity levels. The authors estimated BDCM half-lives of 1.5 and 2.5 h in the rat and mouse, respectively.

Mathews et al. (1990) studied the disposition of ^{14}C-BDCM in male F344 rats after single oral (corn oil gavage) doses of 1, 10, 32 or 100 mg/kg of body weight and 10-day repeat oral dosing of 10 or 100 mg/kg of body weight per day. The doses of BDCM were well absorbed from the gastrointestinal tract, as demonstrated by 24-h recoveries exceeding 90% in non-faecal excreta samples and tissues. Persistence of radiolabelled residues in tissues after 24 h was low (3–4% of dose), with the most marked accumulation in the liver (1–3% of dose). The kidneys, particularly cortical regions, also contained significant concentrations of radiolabelled residues. Approximately 3–6% of the dose was eliminated as volatile organics in the breath (primarily the parent compound, presumably), much less than in Sprague-Dawley rats (Mink et al., 1986). Urinary and faecal elimination were low at all dose levels, accounting for 4% and 1–3% of the administered doses, respectively. Repeated doses had no effect on the tissue distribution of BDCM, and significant bioaccumulation was not observed (0.9–1.1% total retention of the label).

Lilly et al. (1998) examined absorption and tissue dosimetry of BDCM in male F344 rats after doses of 50 or 100 mg/kg of body weight were given orally using either an aqueous emulsion or corn oil as the vehicle of administration. After delivery in the aqueous vehicle, concentrations of BDCM in venous blood peaked at about 6 min, with maximum concentration (C_{max}) values of 16 and 26 mg/litre for the low and high doses. With corn oil dosing, C_{max} occurred at 15–30 min, with lower peak blood levels attained (5 and 9 mg/litre). The time required for blood concentrations to decline to half-C_{max} was about 1 h with the 50 mg/kg of body weight dose and 1.5 h with the 100 mg/kg of body weight dose. Tissue partition coefficient determinations confirmed the anticipated effect of bromine substitution on THM tissue solubility. BDCM partition coefficients for fat and liver were 526 and 30.6 (Lilly et al., 1997b), compared with 203 and 21.1 for chloroform (Corley et al., 1990). Lilly et al. (1998) found slightly higher maximum concentrations of BDCM in the liver and kidneys after aqueous administration compared with corn oil delivery. With the 100 mg/kg of body weight aqueous dose, hepatic and renal levels peaked at about 15 mg/litre at 5 min after dosing in the liver and at 5–30 min in the kidneys. At 6 h after dosing, concentrations of BDCM in the liver and kidneys were less than 1 mg/litre. More of the parent compound was eliminated unmetabolized via exhaled breath after aqueous dosing (8.9%, low dose; 13.2%, high dose) than after corn oil gavage (5.3%, low dose; 5.8%, high dose).

The elimination kinetics of BDCM have been studied in humans who had swum in chlorinated pools (Lindstrom et al., 1997; Pleil & Lindstrom, 1997). BDCM half-lives of 0.45–0.63 min for blood were estimated using breath elimination data.

The deleterious effects of the THMs result from reactive metabolites generated by biotransformation. Two isoenzyme groups of cytochrome P450, CYP2E1 and CYP2B1/2, as well as a θ-class GST, have been implicated in the metabolism of BDCM to toxic species in rats (Thornton-Manning et al., 1993; Pegram et al., 1997). No specific information is available regarding human metabolism of brominated THMs. In rats, P450-mediated metabolism of BDCM (Figure 1) is believed to proceed by the same two pathways established for chloroform: oxidation with phosgene the proposed active metabolite, and reduction with the dichloromethyl free radical proposed as the reactive product (Tomasi et al., 1985; IPCS, 1994; Gao et al., 1996). Most investigations of THM metabolism and reaction mechanisms have focused on chloroform, and a detailed review of chloroform biotransformation has been published recently (IPCS, 1994). Although the qualitative aspects of the cytochrome P450-mediated metabolism of brominated THMs are similar to those for chloroform, numerous studies have demonstrated that brominated THMs are metabolized to a greater extent and at faster rates than chloroform. There is evidence to suggest that both CYP2E1 and CYP2B1/2 can catalyse the oxidative pathway and that CYP2B1/2 catalyses the reductive metabolism of haloforms, but it has also been postulated that either isoform can catalyse both routes (Tomasi et al., 1985; Testai et al., 1996). CYP2E1 is clearly involved in the hepatotoxicity induced by BDCM in rats, but its role in the nephrotoxic response is less certain (Thornton-Manning et al., 1993). Because CYP2E1 is highly conserved across mammalian species, it seems likely that this isoform metabolizes BDCM in

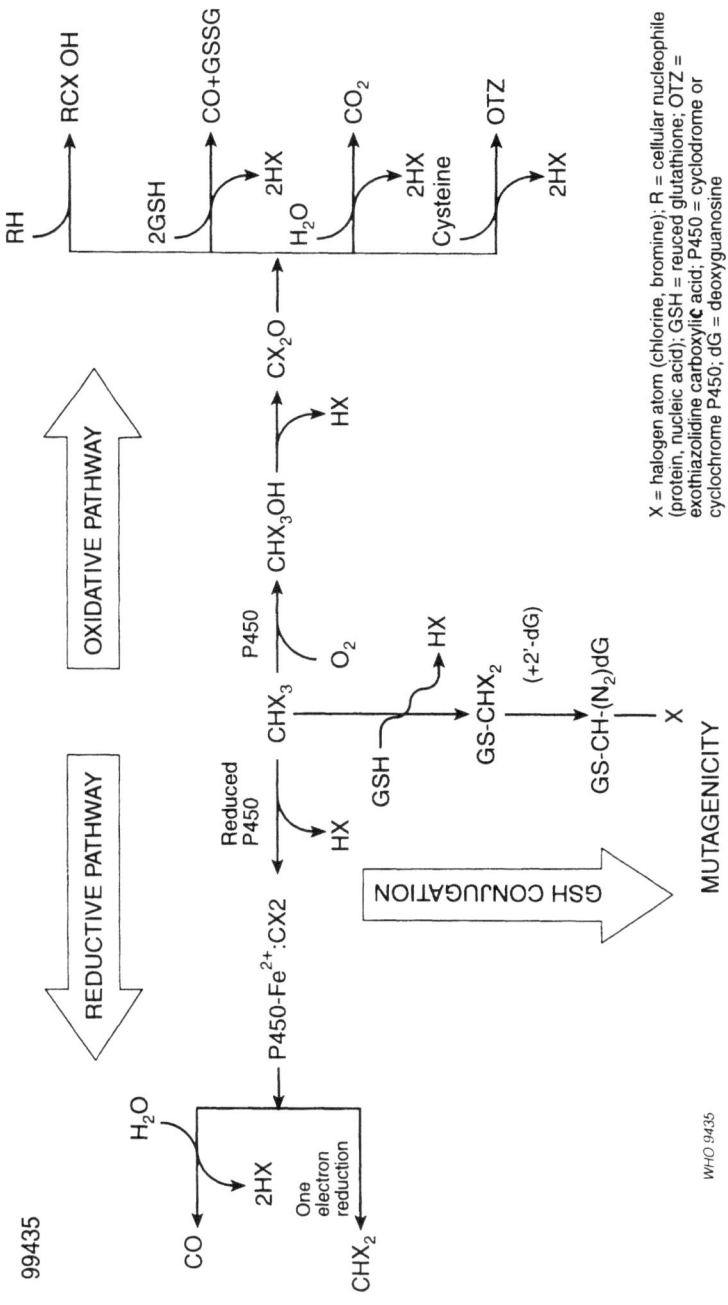

Fig. 1. Metabolic pathways of trihalomethane biotransformation
(adapted from Wolf et al., 1977; Stevens & Anders, 1981; Tomasi et al., 1985; Pegram et al., 1997).

X = halogen atom (chlorine, bromine); R = cellular nucleophile (protein, nucleic acid); GSH = reuced glutathione; OTZ = exothiazolidine carboxyliC acid; P450 = cyclodrome or cyclochrome P450; dG = deoxyguanosine.

WHO 9435

133

humans, although this has not yet been demonstrated. CYP2B1/2 are not expressed in humans, and there is no direct analogue for their catalytic activity; however, based on substrate similarities with CYP2B1/2, human forms CYP2A6, CYP2D6 and CYP3A4 appear to be possibilities.

Gao et al. (1996) demonstrated that GSH affords protection against the toxicity and macromolecular binding of BDCM, indicating that oxidative metabolism of BDCM, like that of chloroform, generates phosgene, which can then react with GSH (Stevens & Anders, 1981). *In vitro* binding of a BDCM-derived intermediate to microsomal protein under aerobic conditions and the prevention of this binding by GSH supplementation provide further evidence for the production of phosgene from BDCM (Gao et al., 1996). The reaction of GSH with phosgene forms *S*-(chlorocarbonyl)-GSH, which may react with a second GSH molecule to produce diglutathionyl dithiocarbonate (Pohl et al., 1981) or to give glutathione disulfide and carbon monoxide as minor products (Stevens & Anders, 1981). Anders et al. (1978) and Mathews et al. (1990) reported that carbon monoxide is a product of BDCM metabolism. The most likely outcome for phosgene is hydrolysis to carbon dioxide and hydrogen chloride (Brown et al., 1974), and, in fact, 70–80% of ^{14}C-BDCM doses administered to F344 rats or B6C3F$_1$ mice appeared as expired ^{14}C-labelled carbon dioxide (Mink et al., 1986; Mathews et al., 1990), which also shows the predominance of oxidative biotransformation as a metabolic route in these animals. Sprague-Dawley rats were much less efficient metabolizers of THMs, disposing of only 14% of a BDCM dose as carbon dioxide. In both rats and mice, BDCM was more extensively metabolized to carbon dioxide than was chloroform or bromoform (Mink et al., 1986). *In vitro* binding assays with rat hepatic microsomes have also shown that BDCM has a greater capacity than chloroform to be metabolized to intermediates (presumably phosgene) that bind protein under aerobic conditions (Gao & Pegram, 1992; Bull et al., 1995). Similar tests with kidney microsomes have shown that GSH is much less effective in preventing renal protein binding than in preventing liver protein binding, suggesting that a significant portion of this binding in the kidney may have resulted from generation of a reactive intermediate via a different pathway (Gao et al., 1996).

Cytochrome P450-mediated reductive dehalogenation of BDCM to form a dichloromethyl radical has been demonstrated *in vivo* in phenobarbital-treated rats using an electron spin resonance (ESR) spin-trapping technique (Tomasi et al., 1985). These authors reported that more free radical was derived from BDCM than from chloroform and that more radical was trapped from bromoform than from BDCM. Waller & McKinney (1993) conducted a theoretical investigation into the potential of halogenated methanes to undergo reductive metabolism using density-functional theory-based computational chemistry. The estimated reductive potentials for the THMs were in agreement with the reaction order described in the ESR study. The dichloromethyl radical reacts preferentially with the fatty acid skeleton of phospholipids to give covalently bound adducts (De Biasi et al., 1992). *In vitro* binding of metabolically activated THMs to hepatic microsomal lipids, presumably by the radical, has also been investigated, and lipid binding by BDCM was found to exceed that of chloroform by more than 300% (Gao & Pegram, 1992; Gao et al., 1996). Free radical generation by this pathway may explain the loss of CYP2B1/2 in rats treated with BDCM (Thornton-Manning et al., 1994). Finally, carbon monoxide has also been postulated to be a product of the reductive pathway (Wolf et al., 1977).

Although the reactions of GSH with phosgene are protective against THM-induced hepatic and renal toxicity, direct conjugation of the brominated THMs to GSH may lead to genotoxicity. A GST-mediated mutagenic pathway of brominated THM metabolism has recently been identified using a *Salmonella* strain transfected with rat GST T1-1 (Pegram et al., 1997). Base substitution revertants were produced in this strain by BDCM (at medium concentrations of less than 0.1 mmol/litre) and the other brominated THMs, but not by chloroform (De Marini et al., 1997; Pegram et al., 1997). The propensity for GSH conjugation may therefore explain the different results noted in mutagenicity tests with chloroform and the brominated THMs. Currently, it is not known if GSH conjugation leading to genotoxicity occurs in mammalian cells. However, it is likely that the analogous human GST T1-1 will also activate the brominated THMs, because similar substrate specificities have been demonstrated for the rat and human GST isoforms (Thier et al., 1993, 1996). Human GST T1-1 is expressed polymorphically and could therefore be a critical determinant of susceptibility to the genotoxicity of the brominated THMs.

A PBPK model has recently been developed to describe the absorption, distribution, tissue uptake and dosimetry, metabolism and elimination of BDCM in rats (Lilly et al., 1997b, 1998). Metabolism was characterized directly by measuring production of bromide ion, which is liberated by all known biotransformation reactions of BDCM, and indirectly by gas uptake techniques. Determinations of plasma bromide concentrations after constant-concentration inhalation exposures of rats to BDCM provided evidence for metabolic saturation at concentrations of 1340 mg/m³ (200 ppm) and greater. Total *in vivo* metabolism of BDCM was accurately described by the model as a saturable process using metabolic rate constant values of 12.8 mg/h for maximum rate of metabolism (V_{max}) and 0.5 mg/litre for K_m. This compares with a V_{max} value for chloroform of 6.8 mg/h (Corley et al., 1990), providing additional evidence for more rapid metabolism and greater generation of reactive intermediates from BDCM than from chloroform. Production of bromide from BDCM following treatment with an inhibitor of CYP2E1, *trans*-dichloroethylene, increased the apparent K_m from 0.5 to 225 mg/litre, further demonstrating that CYP2E1 is a major isoform involved in BDCM metabolism. The metabolism model, derived from inhalation exposure data, was subsequently linked to a multicompartment gastrointestinal tract submodel using estimates of oral absorption rate constants determined by fitting blood and exhaled breath chamber concentration–time curves obtained after gavage of rats with BDCM. This model accurately predicted tissue dosimetry and plasma bromide ion concentrations following oral exposure to BDCM and can be utilized in estimating rates of formation of reactive intermediates in target tissues.

1.2.7 Mode of action

As stated above, the metabolism of the THMs is believed to be a prerequisite for the toxicity and carcinogenicity associated with exposure to these DBPs. The primary target tissues for the THMs are active sites of their metabolism, and treatments that increase or decrease biotransformation also tend to cause parallel increases or decreases in the toxicity induced by the THMs (Thornton-Manning et al., 1993; US EPA, 1994b). The reactive intermediates generated from the three brominated THM metabolic pathways react with macromolecules to elicit both cytotoxic and genotoxic responses.

The cytotoxicity of the brominated THMs observed in the liver and kidneys of exposed animals has been proposed to result from covalent adducts formed between cellular proteins and lipids and dihalocarbonyls or dihalomethyl free radicals. The adducts presumably impair the function of these molecules and cause cell injury. BDCM produced these adducts in *in vitro* incubations with hepatic and renal microsomes to a significantly greater extent than did chloroform (Gao & Pegram, 1992; Gao et al., 1996). Induction of lipid peroxidation by free radical metabolites of reductive metabolism has been proposed as another mechanism underlying THM cytotoxicity. Each of the brominated THMs induced lipid peroxidation in rat liver microsomes *in vitro*, which was maximal at low oxygen tensions (de Groot & Noll, 1989).

As described above (section 4.1.2.6), it appears that direct conjugation of BDCM and the other brominated THMs with GSH generates mutagenic intermediates (Pegram et al., 1997), but this process has not yet been demonstrated in mammals. However, the reaction was dependent on a transfected rat enzyme (GST T1-1), and the human GST T1-1 has been shown to catalyse GSH conjugation with the dihalomethanes (Thier et al., 1996). The GC to AT transitions observed in the *Salmonella* strain expressing GST T1-1 indicate that DNA lesions on either guanine or cytosine occurred after exposure to brominated THMs (De Marini et al., 1997). Based on similar reactions by dihalomethanes, it can be proposed that S-(1,1-dihalomethyl)-GSH is the product of GSH conjugation of brominated THMs, which then reacts directly with guanine. Dechert & Dekant (1996) found that S-(1-chloromethyl)-GSH reacts with deoxyguanosine to produce S-[1-(N^2-deoxyguanosinyl)-methyl]-GSH, and a methylguanosine adduct was also formed from reactions of S-(1-acetoxymethyl)-GSH with model nucleosides (Thier et al., 1993). *In vivo* covalent DNA binding by ^{14}C-BDCM has been observed in each of the cancer target tissues for BDCM in the rat, but the nucleoside adducts have not yet been identified (Bull et al., 1995).

An interplay of direct mutagenicity with cytotoxic responses leading to regenerative hyperplasia may explain some, but not all, of the carcinogenic effects of the brominated THMs. For example, renal tubular cell hyperplasia coincident with tubular cell cancers was observed in rats gavaged with BDCM for 2 years (NTP, 1987), but necrosis and hyperplasia were not associated with the liver neoplasms induced by BDCM in mice (NTP, 1987). Melnick et al. (1998) recently revisited this issue and noted that high incidences of liver tumours were observed with BDCM and DBCM at doses that had little or no effect on hepatic regenerative hyperplasia. No evidence for cytotoxic responses in the intestine was noted in the NTP study with BDCM, but high incidences of intestinal carcinomas were reported (NTP, 1987). Therefore, while cytotoxic effects of BDCM may potentiate tumorigenicity in certain rodent tissues at high dose levels, direct induction of mutations by BDCM metabolites may also play a carcinogenic role. The extent to which each of these processes contributed to the induction of tumours observed in chronic animal studies is at present unclear. Additional *in vivo* studies are required to confirm the mechanism or mechanisms underlying brominated THM-induced carcinogenesis.

4.1.3 Dibromochloromethane

1.3.1 General toxicological properties and information on dose–response in animals

1) Acute toxicity

Acute oral LD_{50}s of 800 and 1200 mg of DBCM per kg of body weight were reported by Bowman et al. (1978) for male and female ICR Swiss mice, respectively, whereas Chu et al. (1980) found LD_{50}s of 1186 and 848 mg/kg of body weight for male and female Sprague-Dawley rats, respectively. A DBCM dose of 500 mg/kg of body weight produced ataxia, sedation and anaesthesia in mice (Bowman et al., 1978). Hewitt et al. (1983) dosed male Sprague-Dawley rats with DBCM by corn oil gavage and found doses of 2450 mg/kg of body weight and above to be lethal. No clinical evidence for significant liver or kidney toxicity was found at sublethal doses.

Induction of acute renal toxicity by DBCM was studied by Kroll et al. (1994a,b); a single intraperitoneal dose of 3 mmol/kg of body weight resulted in elevated BUN, reductions in glomerular filtration rate and renal concentrating ability, and interference with proximal tubular secretion and reabsorption.

2) Short-term toxicity

Daily gavage of male and female CD-1 mice with DBCM in an aqueous vehicle for 14 days produced hepatotoxicity in both sexes at the highest dose of 250 mg/kg of body weight per day (Munson et al.,

1982). Depressed immune function was also observed in both sexes at doses of 125 and 250 mg/kg of body weight per day, whereas the 50 mg/kg of body weight per day dose was without effect. Corn oil gavage of DBCM to male CD-1 mice for 14 days (Condie et al., 1983) led to observations of kidney and liver toxicity at a lower dose (147 mg/kg of body weight per day) than had been observed with aqueous delivery (Munson et al., 1982). In another 14-day corn oil gavage study, NTP (1985) found that a dose of 500 mg/kg of body weight per day was lethal to B6C3F$_1$ mice, and doses of 500 and 1000 mg/kg of body weight per day were lethal to F344/N rats. Dietary administration of microencapsulated DBCM to Wistar rats for 1 month caused liver cell vacuolization, with a LOAEL of 56 mg/kg of body weight per day and a NOAEL of 18 mg/kg of body weight per day (Aida et al., 1992a).

DBCM-induced cardiotoxicity was reported in male Wistar rats after short-term exposure (4 weeks of daily dosing with 0.4 mmol/kg of body weight). Arrhythmogenic and negative chronotropic and dromotropic effects were observed, as well as extension of atrio-ventricular conduction times. Inhibitory actions of DBCM on calcium ion dynamics in isolated cardiac myocytes were also noted.

In the NTP (1985) study, DBCM was administered by corn oil gavage to F344/N rats and B6C3F$_1$ mice (10 per sex per dose) for 13 weeks (5 days per week) at doses of 0, 15, 30, 60, 125 or 250 mg/kg of body weight per day. The highest dose was lethal to 90% of the rats, producing severe lesions and necrosis in kidney, liver and salivary glands. Hepatocellular vacuolization indicative of fatty changes was observed in male rats at doses of 60 mg/kg of body weight per day and higher. In the mice, no DBCM-related effects were reported at doses of 125 mg/kg of body weight per day or lower. At the highest dose, fatty liver and toxic nephropathy were noted in males, but not in females. A NOAEL of 30 mg/kg of body weight per day can be derived from this study.

A 90-day corn oil gavage study was conducted using Sprague-Dawley rats and doses of 0, 50, 100 or 200 mg/kg of body weight per day (Daniel et al., 1990b). Body weight gain was significantly depressed in the high-dose groups to less than 50% and 70% of the controls in males and females, respectively. Observations of liver damage included elevated ALAT in mid- and high-dose males, centrilobular lipidosis (vacuolization) in males at all doses and high-dose females, and centrilobular necrosis in high-dose males and females. Kidney proximal tubule cell degeneration was induced by DBCM in all high-dose rats and to a lesser extent at 100 mg/kg of body weight per day in males and at both 50 and 100 mg/kg of body weight per day in females.

3) Chronic toxicity

The chronic oral toxicity of DBCM was studied by NTP (1985) in F344/N rats and B6C3F₁ mice using corn oil gavage (5 days per week for 104 weeks) and doses of 0, 40 or 80 mg/kg of body weight per day for rats and 0, 50 or 100 mg/kg of body weight per day for mice. Liver lesions, including fat accumulation, cytoplasmic changes and altered basophilic staining, were observed in male and female rats at both dose levels. The low-dose male mice in this study were lost as a result of an overdosing accident. Compound-related hepatocyto-megaly and hepatic focal necrosis were observed in high-dose male mice, and liver calcification (high dose) and fatty changes (both low and high doses) were noted in female mice. Renal toxicity (nephrosis) was also observed in male mice and female rats.

1.3.2   Reproductive and developmental toxicity

Borzelleca & Carchman (1982) conducted a two-generation reproductive study of DBCM in ICR Swiss mice. Male and female mice at 9 weeks of age were maintained on drinking-water containing 0, 0.1, 1.0 or 4.0 mg of DBCM per ml, leading to average doses of 0, 17, 171 or 685 mg/kg of body weight per day. Fertility and gestational index were reduced in the high-dose group for the F_1 generations. Only fertility was decreased (high-dose) in the F_2 generation. At the mid and high doses in both generations, litter size and the viability index were decreased. Other effects included decreased lactation index and reduced postnatal body weight. No dominant lethal or teratogenic effects were observed in the F_1 or F_2 generations.

In a developmental study in rats conducted by Ruddick et al. (1983), gavage of DBCM (0, 50, 100, or 200 mg/kg of body weight per day) on gestational days 6–15 caused a depression of maternal weight gain, but no fetal malformations.

4.1.3.3   Neurotoxicity

DBCM was tested for behavioural effects in male ICR mice by Balster & Borzelleca (1982), who found no effect of treatments up to 100 mg/kg of body weight per day for 60 days. Dosing for 60 days with 400 mg/kg of body weight per day produced decreased response rates in an operant behaviour test. Korz & Gattermann (1997) observed DBCM-induced behavioural alterations in male golden hamsters exposed either for 14 days to a dose of 5 mg/kg of body weight per day or acutely to a single dose of 50 mg/kg of body weight. At the low dose, subchronic treatment caused reduced aggressive behaviour during social confrontation on day 14 as compared with vehicle-dosed controls. Following the acute dose, increased locomotor activity on days 3–6 and decreased wheel running on days 6–9 were observed, but no effects were noted after day 9.

4.1.3.4   Toxicity in humans

Clinical case findings resulting from human exposure to DBCM have not been reported.

4.1.3.5   Carcinogenicity and mutagenicity

IARC has evaluated the carcinogenicity of DBCM and concluded that there is inadequate evidence for its carcinogenicity in humans and limited evidence for its carcinogenicity in experimental animals. The compound was assigned to Group 3: DBCM is not classifiable as to its carcinogenicity to humans (IARC 1991, 1999).

In a 104-week corn oil gavage study, DBCM was not carcinogenic in F344 rats (50 per sex per dose) at doses of 0, 40 or 80 mg/kg of body weight given 5 days per week (NTP, 1985). In female B6C3F$_1$ mice, however, DBCM significantly increased the incidence of hepato-cellular adenomas and the combined incidences of hepatocellular adenomas and carcinomas at the high dose (100 mg/kg of body weight per day) (Table 13). The incidence of hepatocellular carcinomas was significantly increased in male mice at the same dose. The low-dose (50 mg/kg of body weight per day) male mice were lost midway through the study as a result of an inadvertent overdose. NTP judged that these results provided equivocal evidence of DBCM

Table 13. Frequencies of liver tumours in mice administered
dibromochloromethane in corn oil for 104 weeks[a]

Treatment (mg/kg of body weight per day)	Sex	Adenoma	Carcinoma	Adenoma or carcinoma (combined)
Vehicle control	M	14/50	10/50	23/50
	F	2/50	4/50	6/50
50	M	—[b]	—	—
	F	4/49	6/49	10/49
100	M	10/50	19/50[c]	27/50[d]
	F	11/50[c]	8/50	19/50[e]

[a] Adapted from NTP (1985).
[b] Male low-dose group was inadequate for statistical analysis.
[c] P < 0.05 relative to controls.
[d] P < 0.01 (life table analysis); P = 0.065 (incidental tumour tests) relative to controls.
[e] P < 0.01 relative to controls.

carcinogenicity in male mice and some evidence of carcinogenicity in female mice.

Based on *in vitro* studies, mutagenic potency appears to increase with the degree of bromine substitution in the THMs. DBCM is mostly positive in tests employing closed systems to overcome the problem of volatility (IARC, 1991, 1999; Pegram et al., 1997). In the GST-transfected TA1535 strain (see section 4.1.1.3), DBCM is the most potent THM, inducing greater than 10-fold more revertants per plate than BDCM after exposure to THM vapour (3400 mg/m^3 for DBCM; 2680 mg/m^3 for BDCM [400 ppm]) (Pegram et al., 1996; DeMarini et al., 1997). DBCM has given mostly positive results in eukaryotic test systems (Loveday et al., 1990; IARC, 1991, 1999; McGregor et al., 1991; Fujie et al., 1993), although there is less consistency in results between the different assays when considered with or without an exogenous metabolic system.

Data from *in vivo* studies are more equivocal. DBCM was positive for SCE and chromosomal aberrations in mouse bone marrow (Morimoto & Koizumi, 1983; Fujie et al., 1990) and in a newt micro-nucleus assay (Le Curieux et al., 1995), but was negative for micro-nuclei and UDS in the liver of rats (Ishidate et al., 1982; Hayashi et al., 1988; Stocker et al., 1997). Potter et al. (1996) found that DBCM did not induce DNA strand breaks in the kidneys of male F344 rats following seven daily doses of 1.5 mmol/kg of body weight.

These studies are summarized in Table 12.

4.1.3.6 *Comparative pharmacokinetics and metabolism*

The pharmacokinetics of DBCM have been studied the least among the THMs. Mink et al. (1986) compared the absorption, distribution and excretion of DBCM with those of the other THMs. A dose of 100 mg/kg of body weight was administered orally in corn oil to male Sprague-Dawley rats by gavage, and 150 mg/kg of body weight was administered similarly to male $B6C3F_1$ mice. The pattern of distribution and elimination of DBCM was very similar to that observed with BDCM: rats expired more of the dose than mice as a trapped organic component presumed to be the parent compound (48% vs. 12%) and expired less as carbon dioxide (18% vs. 72%) after 8 h. Total recovery from excised organs was 1.4% in rats and 5.0% in mice, whereas less than 2% of the dose was excreted in the urine in both species. Half-lives of DBCM in rats and mice were estimated to be 1.2 h and 2.5 h, respectively.

The cytochrome P450-mediated metabolism of DBCM has not been directly investigated. Presumably, metabolism proceeds via the same routes of biotransformation as described for BDCM (section 4.1.2.6) and chloroform (IPCS, 1994). Oxidative metabolism of DBCM would be expected to yield a bromochlorocarbonyl rather than phosgene, and reductive dehalogenation would produce a bromochloromethyl radical. Anders et al. (1978) demonstrated *in vivo* carbon monoxide production from DBCM in male Sprague-Dawley rats at a rate intermediate to those of BDCM and bromoform. DBCM was very reactive in the *Salmonella*-GST mutagenicity assay, indicating that it has greater potential for GSH conjugation than BDCM (De Marini et al., 1997).

Pankow et al. (1997) reported the metabolism of DBCM to bromide and carbon monoxide in rats after gavage of olive oil solutions (0.4–3.1 mmol/kg of body weight). The DBCM concentrations in blood and fat 6 h after the last of seven consecutive daily doses (0.8 mmol/kg of body weight) were lower than at 6 h after a single gavage of this dose, suggesting that more of the chemical was metabolized after the seventh dose than after the single dose. The seven-dose regimen also caused a 2-fold induction of a CYP2E1-specific activity. The involvement of CYP2E1, CYP2B1/2 and GSH in DBCM metabolism was also demonstrated.

1.3.7 Mode of action

Mechanistic issues for DBCM are similar to those addressed for BDCM (sections 4.1.2.6 and 4.1.2.7). The greater propensity for the metabolism of this compound and bromoform as compared with BDCM is difficult to reconcile with its lower carcinogenicity in the NTP (1985) bioassay. A possible explanation is less bioavailability resulting from the greater lipophilicity of this compound and the use of corn oil as the vehicle of administration. Greater lipophilicity and reactivity of this compound or its metabolites (i.e., the bromochloro-carbonyl metabolite) may also prevent it from reaching critical target sites. It is also of note that DBCM did not induce carcinomas of the large intestine in rats in the NTP studies using corn oil vehicle, whereas both BDCM and bromoform did induce these tumours.

4.1.4 Bromoform

1.4.1 General toxicological properties and information on dose–response in animals

1) Acute toxicity

Among the brominated THMs, bromoform is the least potent as a lethal acute oral toxicant. The acute oral LD_{50}s for bromoform were 1400 and 1550 mg/kg of body weight in male and female mice, respectively (Bowman et al., 1978), and 1388 and 1147 mg/kg of body weight in male and female rats, respectively (Chu et al., 1980). Bromoform was also a less potent anaesthetic than BDCM and DBCM: a 1000 mg/kg of body weight dose was required to produce this effect in mice. Intraperitoneal administration of bromoform in a corn oil vehicle at doses of 25–300 µl/kg of body weight produced no signifi-cant elevations of serum enzymes indicative of liver damage (Agarwal & Mehendele, 1983).

Bromoform was included in the acute renal toxicity studies of Kroll et al. (1994a,b) but was ranked as the least potent among the

THMs in general disruption of renal function. A single intraperitoneal dose (3 mmol/kg of body weight) did, however, induce significant decreases in glomerular filtration rate, renal concentrating ability, and tubular secretion and reabsorption. Tubule function was affected as early as 8 h after dosing, whereas the other effects were observed at 24–48 h.

2)   Short-term toxicity

Male and female CD-1 mice were gavaged daily with bromoform (50, 125 or 250 mg/kg of body weight) in an aqueous vehicle for 14 days, leading to liver toxicity and a decrease in antibody-forming cells only at the highest dose (Munson et al., 1982). The magnitude of the liver effects was less than that observed with the other THMs, and BUN was not elevated by bromoform. Condie et al. (1983) noted both liver and kidney toxicity in CD-1 mice after dosing with 289 mg of bromoform per kg of body weight per day in corn oil for 14 days, whereas no significant effects were found at 72 and 145 mg/kg of body weight per day. NTP (1989a) also conducted a 14-day corn oil gavage study with bromoform and found that doses of 600 and 800 mg/kg of body weight per day were lethal to both sexes of F344/N rats. Mice given doses of 400 mg/kg of body weight and higher had raised stomach nodules. Microencapsulated bromoform was added to the diet of Wistar rats for 1 month, producing liver damage (Aida et al., 1992a).

Bromoform was given to F344/N rats (10 per sex per dose) and B6C3F$_1$ mice (10 per sex per dose) by corn oil gavage for 13 weeks (5 days per week) at doses of 0, 25, 50, 100 or 200 mg/kg of body weight per day, with an added dose of 400 mg/kg of body weight per day for mice only (NTP, 1989a). The only significant finding, hepatic vacuolation, was observed in male rats, but not in female rats, at doses of 50 mg/kg of body weight per day and higher, and in male mice, but not in female mice, at doses of 200 and 400 mg/kg of body weight per day. The NOAEL in the rat study was 25 mg/kg of body weight per day, whereas that in the study in mice was 100 mg/kg of body weight per day.

3) Chronic toxicity

Bromoform was administered in drinking-water (containing 0.25% Emulphor) to male F344 rats and B6C3F$_1$ mice for 1 year, and clinical indicators of kidney toxicity were examined (Moore et al., 1994). Water containing bromoform concentrations of 0.12, 0.6 and 1.2 g/litre for rats and 0.08, 0.4, and 0.8 g/litre for mice resulted in average daily doses of 6.2, 29 or 57 mg/kg of body weight for rats and 8.3, 39 or 73 mg/kg of body weight for mice. Several indicators of tubular and glomerular damage were elevated at each treatment level in mice, and mice appeared more susceptible to the nephrotoxic effects of bromoform than to those of BDCM (see section 4.1.2.1). As in mice, urinary protein was increased in all rat dose groups, but little evidence of loss of tubule function was observed in rats.

Two-year investigations of bromoform toxicity were conducted by administering doses of 0, 100 or 200 mg/kg of body weight by corn oil gavage, 5 days per week for 103 weeks, to F344/N rats (50 per sex per dose) and female B6C3F$_1$ mice (50 per dose) (NTP, 1989a). Male mice (50 per dose) received doses of 0, 50 or 100 mg/kg of body weight per day. Survival of high-dose male rats and both dose groups of female mice was significantly lower than that of the vehicle controls. Focal or diffuse fatty change of the liver was observed in a dose-dependent fashion in both sexes of rats, and active chronic hepatic inflammation was found in male and high-dose female rats. Minimal necrosis of the liver was noted in high-dose male rats. In mice, the incidence of fatty changes of the liver was increased in females, but not in males, at both dose levels. Follicular cell hyperplasia of the thyroid gland was observed in high-dose female mice. The different target organ (liver) in this study as compared with the drinking-water study of Moore et al. (1994), in which renal effects predominated, suggests that the vehicle and mode of administration can affect which tissues are affected by bromoform.

1.4.2 *Reproductive and developmental toxicity*

Ruddick et al. (1983) conducted a teratological investigation of bromoform in Sprague-Dawley rats (15 per group). Bromoform was administered by gavage at doses of 50, 100 or 200 mg/kg of body weight per day on gestation days 6–15. Evidence of a fetotoxic response was observed, but there were no fetal malformations.

Interparietal deviations were, however, noted in the mid- and high-dose groups. NTP (1989b) utilized the same bromoform doses given by gavage for 105 days to 20 male–female pairs of Swiss CD-1 mice to examine effects on fertility and reproduction. There was no detectable effect of bromoform on fertility, litters per pair, live pups per litter, proportion of pups born alive, sex of live pups or pup body weights. Bromoform was also found to induce full-litter resorptions in pregnant F344 rats when administered orally on gestation days 6–15, but at higher doses (150 and 200 mg/kg of body weight per day) than those required to produce the same effect for BDCM (Narotsky et al., 1993).

4.1.4.3 Neurotoxicity

Bromoform was included in the mouse behavioural study of Balster & Borzelleca (1982). Doses of 9.2 mg/kg of body weight per day for up to 90 days had no effect on the outcome of several behavioural tests, and 100 mg/kg of body weight per day for 30 days did not deter passive avoidance learning. However, mice receiving either 100 or 400 mg/kg of body weight per day for 60 days exhibited decreased response rates in an operant behaviour test.

4.1.4.4 Toxicity in humans

Bromoform was used in the late 19th and early 20th centuries as a sedative for children with whooping cough. Patients were typically given doses of one drop (approximately 180 mg) 3–6 times per day (Burton-Fanning, 1901), which usually resulted in mild sedation in the children. A few rare instances of death or near-death were reported but were believed to be due to accidental overdoses (Dwelle, 1903). These clinical observations have been used to estimate a lethal dose for a 10- to 20-kg child to be about 300 mg/kg of body weight and an approximate minimal dose for sedation to be 50 mg/kg of body weight per day (US EPA, 1994b).

4.1.4.5 Carcinogenicity and mutagenicity

IARC has evaluated the carcinogenicity of bromoform and concluded that there is inadequate evidence for its carcinogenicity in humans and limited evidence for its carcinogenicity in experimental animals. The compound was assigned to Group 3: bromoform is not classifiable as to its carcinogenicity to humans (IARC, 1991, 1999).

Two-year studies of bromoform carcinogenicity were conducted by administering doses of 0, 100 or 200 mg/kg of body weight in corn oil by gavage, 5 days per week, to groups of F344/N rats (50 per sex per group) and female B6C3F₁ mice (50 per group) and doses of 0, 50 or 100 mg/kg of body weight to male mice (NTP, 1989a). No neoplastic effects were associated with the exposure of mice to bromoform. In rats, however, intestinal carcinomas were induced by bromoform, as had also been observed with BDCM. The uncommon adenomatous polyps or adenocarcinomas (combined) of the large intestine (colon or rectum) were observed in 3 out of 50 high-dose male rats and in 8 out of 50 high-dose female rats as compared with 0 out of 50 rats in the male controls and 0 out of 48 rats in the female controls (Table 14). Because these tumours are very rare in the rat, these findings were considered significant, and the NTP therefore concluded that there was clear evidence for carcinogenic activity in female rats and some evidence in male rats.

Table 14. Tumour frequencies in rats exposed to bromoform in corn oil for 2 years[a]

Animal/tissue/tumour	Tumour frequency		
	Control	100 mg/kg of body weight per day	200 mg/kg of body weight per day
Male rat			
Large intestine			
Adenocarcinoma	0/50	0/50	1/50
Polyp (adenomatous)	0/50	0/50	2/50
Female rat			
Large intestine			
Adenocarcinoma	0/48	0/50	2/50
Polyp (adenomatous)	0/48	1/50	6/50

[a] Adapted from NTP (1989a).

Bromoform, in common with the other brominated THMs, is largely positive in bacterial assays of mutagenicity conducted in closed systems (Zeiger, 1990; IARC, 1991, 1999). In the GST-transfected *Salmonella typhimurium* TA1535 strain (see section 4.1.2.5), bromoform produced about 5 times more revertants than BDCM at comparable exposure levels (Pegram et al., 1997). As with BDCM, the mutations were almost exclusively GC to AT transitions (DeMarini et al., 1997). In prokaryotic tester strains, bromoform induced mutations without metabolic activation in *S. typhimurium* strain TA100 (Simmon & Tardiff, 1978; Ishidate et al., 1982; NTP, 1989a; Le Curieux et al., 1995), with and without activation in TA98 (NTP, 1989a; Zeiger, 1990) and with microsomal activation in TA97 (NTP, 1989a). In eukaryotic test systems, bromoform is largely positive (IARC, 1991; Fujie et al., 1993). As with bacterial assays, bromoform appeared more potent than the other brominated THMs (Morimoto & Koizumi, 1983; Banerji & Fernandes, 1996).

In vivo studies (summarized in Table 12) have given contradictory results. Bromoform was positive and negative in *Drosophila* (Woodruff et al., 1985). It was positive in the newt micronucleus test (Le Curieux et al., 1995) and gave increased SCE and chromosomal aberrations in mouse and rat bone marrow cells (Morimoto & Koizumi, 1983; Fujie et al., 1990). It gave negative results in mouse bone marrow (Hayashi et al., 1988; Stocker et al., 1997), in the rat liver UDS assay (Pereira et al., 1982; Stocker et al., 1997) and in the dominant lethal assay (Ishidate et al., 1982). In the studies carried out by the NTP (1989a), it was positive for micronuclei and SCE, but negative for chromosomal aberrations in mouse bone marrow. Potter et al. (1996) found that bromoform did not induce DNA strand breaks in the kidneys of male F344 rats following seven daily doses of 1.5 mmol/kg of body weight.

4.1.4.6   Comparative pharmacokinetics and metabolism

^{14}C-Bromoform pharmacokinetics were examined in Sprague-Dawley rats and B6C3F$_1$ mice in a study that included all four of the common THMs that occur as DBPs (Mink et al., 1986). Recoveries of ^{14}C-label 8 h after gavage dosing were 79% in rats and 62% in mice. The distribution and elimination of bromoform resembled those of chloroform rather than those of the other brominated THMs. The percentage of ^{14}C-label recovered from excised organs and tissues was 2.1% in rats and 12.2% in mice. Tissue levels of ^{14}C in mice were substantially greater than those observed for the other brominated THMs. Urinary excretion of label after 8 h (2.2–4.6%) was also greater for bromoform than for BDCM and DBCM. Bromoform (and organic metabolite) elimination via exhaled breath was greater than that for all other THMs in the rat (67%), but less than that for all other THMs in the mouse (6%). The estimated half-life of bromoform was 0.8 h in rats and 8 h in mice.

The cytochrome P450-dependent metabolism of bromoform was studied by Anders et al. (1978), who found that bromoform was converted to carbon monoxide *in vivo* in male Sprague-Dawley rats at a rate significantly greater than were the other three THMs. Evidence was presented suggesting that some of the carbon monoxide arose from the oxidative metabolism of bromoform to a dibromocarbonyl and subsequent reactions with GSH. It is possible that some of the carbon monoxide was also generated from reductive metabolism of bromo-form, as indicated by *in vitro* results of Wolf et al. (1977) from anaerobic incubations using hepatic preparations derived from pheno-barbital-treated rats. Carbon monoxide was produced from anaerobic bromoform metabolism in this study at much greater levels than from chloroform metabolism. Among the four THMs tested by Mink et al. (1986), bromoform exhibited the least metabolism to carbon dioxide (4% in rats and 40% in mice in 8 h). Free radicals from the *in vivo* reductive metabolism of bromoform were detected by ESR spin-trapping after dosing phenobarbital-treated rats (Tomasi et al., 1985). More radicals were generated from bromoform *in vivo* than from any other bromochlorinated THM, which is consistent with computational chemistry predictions that bromoform would have the greatest reduc-tive potential of the THMs (Waller & McKinney, 1993). Knecht & Mason (1991) also detected the *in vivo* production of radicals from bromoform in the bile of rats, but only after the induction of hypoxia.

Bromoform, like DBCM, has a much greater potential than BDCM to be conjugated by GSH to form a mutagenic intermediate. Base pair revertants were produced in a dose-dependent fashion in GST-transfected *Salmonella typhimurium* strain TA1535 by bromo-form and BDCM, but not by chloroform (Pegram et al., 1996, 1997; De Marini et al., 1997). At an exposure concentration of 33 100 mg/m^3 for bromoform and 22 800 mg/m^3 for BDCM (3200 ppm), GST-dependent revertants per plate induced by bromoform and BDCM averaged 373 and 1935, respectively, compared with a control rate of 23 per plate (Pegram et al., 1996).

The basic mechanisms of action for bromoform are similar to those described for BDCM (section 4.1.2.7). Although bromoform seems to have a greater propensity for metabolism and is a more potent mutagen than BDCM, it appears to be a less potent toxicant and carcinogen based on the results of the NTP (1985, 1987) bioassays and numerous other *in vivo* studies of toxicity. As with DBCM, a possible explanation is less bioavailability resulting from the greater lipophilicity of this compound and the use of corn oil as the vehicle of administration. This concept may be supported by the occurrence of bromoform-induced tumours in the intestinal tract, but not in the liver or kidneys. Greater lipophilicity and reactivity of bromoform metabolites may also prevent it from reaching critical target sites. Moreover, when bromoform was injected intraperitoneally, its metabolism was greater than that of the other THMs (Anders et al., 1978; Tomasi et al., 1985); when administered by corn oil gavage, however, bromoform was the least metabolized THM (Mink et al., 1986). Data from studies of oral exposure to bromoform in aqueous solutions are therefore required.

4.2   Haloacids

Like the THMs, the haloacids produced in the chlorination of drinking-water consist of a series of chlorinated and brominated forms. To date, the chlorinated acetic acids have been more thoroughly characterized toxicologically than their brominated analogues. As discussed in earlier chapters, the dihaloacetates and trihaloacetates occur in significantly higher concentrations than the monohaloacetates. The present review will emphasize the di- and trihaloacetates as the dominant forms of the haloacids found in drinking-water and the ones for which extensive toxicological data have been developed. The probable existence of many longer-chain halogenated acids in chlorinated drinking-water may be surmised from studies of chlorinated humic acids (reviewed by Bull & Kopfler, 1991). Few of these compounds have been extensively studied toxicologically. However, brief reference will be made to those compounds that are known to share some of the effects of the HAAs on intermediary metabolism.

4.2.1 Dichloroacetic acid (dichloroacetate)

Before beginning discussions of available toxicological evaluations of DCA, it is important to point out that this compound exists in drinking-water as the salt, despite the fact that it is widely referred to as dichloroacetic acid. DCA has a pK_a of 1.48 at 25 °C (IARC, 1995). As a consequence, it occurs almost exclusively in the ionized form at the pHs found in drinking-water (broadly speaking, a pH range of 5–10). Failure to recognize this has resulted in a number of studies that have employed the free acid in test systems. At low doses, the buffering capacity of the physiological system can neutralize acid, and the measured activity may in fact be representative. However, most of the experimentation has been conducted using doses ranging from 50 to 1000 mg/kg of body weight *in vivo* or in the mmol/litre range *in vitro*. Therefore, the applicability of the results of such studies to estimating human risks will be uncertain because of the large pH artefacts that can be expected when administering these quantities of a strong acid.

DCA has been shown to produce developmental, reproductive, neural and hepatic effects in experimental animals. In general, these effects occur when the compound has been administered at high dose rates, at which there is evidence to indicate that the metabolic clearance of DCA is substantially inhibited. This has important implications in attempting to associate these toxicities with the low doses that are obtained in drinking-water.

Because it was being developed as a potential therapeutic agent, there is a toxicological literature that precedes DCA's discovery as a by-product of chlorination. The present review discusses these early, more general explorations of DCA's effects on intermediary metabolism before proceeding to descriptions of studies designed to more specifically study its toxicology.

2.1.1 General toxicological properties and information on dose–response in animals

1) Acute toxicity

DCA is not very toxic when administered acutely to rodents. Woodard et al. (1941) reported LD_{50}s of 4.5 and 5.5 g/kg of body weight in rats and mice, respectively, for DCA administered as the sodium salt. This is roughly in the same range as the LD_{50}s for acetic acid. There is reason to believe that other species, most specifically the dog, may be more sensitive because of some repeated-dose experiments discussed below; however, no specific data seem to have been reported in the literature.

2) Short-term toxicity

Katz et al. (1981) published the first substantive evaluation of DCA's subchronic toxicity in rats and dogs. DCA was administered by gavage at 0, 125, 500 or 2000 mg/kg of body weight per day to rats (10–15 per sex per group) and at 0, 50, 75 or 100 mg/kg of body weight per day to dogs (3–4 per sex per group) for 3 months. One of three female dogs died at 75 mg/kg of body weight per day, and one of four male dogs died at 100 mg/kg of body weight per day. The most overt toxicity in rats was hindlimb paralysis at the highest dose. Clinical chemistry indicated significant increases in total and direct bilirubin at 500 and 2000 mg/kg of body weight per day in rats, and relative liver weights were significantly increased at all doses. In dogs, an increase in the incidence of haemosiderin-laden Kupffer cells was noted at all dose rates. Histopathological changes were observed in the brain and testes of both species. In rats, oedematous brain lesions were seen at 60% incidence (primarily in the cerebrum, but also in the cerebellum) at the lowest dose and at 100% in the two higher doses in both sexes. Slight to moderate vacuolation of myelinated tracts was observed at all doses in both rats and dogs. Testicular germinal epithelial degeneration was observed in rats at doses of 500 mg/kg of body weight per day and above and at all doses in dogs, with severity increasing with dose. In dogs, a high incidence of ocular anomalies was observed, and lenticular opacities were found to be irreversible upon suspension of treatment with DCA. In both rats and dogs, glucose and lactate levels were suppressed in a dose-related manner.

Bull et al. (1990) examined the effects of DCA on the liver of B6C3F$_1$ mice administered 1 or 2 g of DCA per litre (approximately 170 and 300 mg/kg of body weight per day) in their drinking-water, with exposure lasting up to 1 year. As had been at least alluded to in earlier studies, DCA was found to produce a severe hepatomegaly in mice at concentrations in drinking-water of 1 g/litre and above. The hepatomegaly could be largely accounted for by large increases in cell size (cytomegaly). In shorter-term experiments, it was determined that treatment with DCA produced only minor changes in the labelling index of hepatocytes using a pulse dose of tritiated thymidine (Sanchez & Bull, 1990). In general, increases in labelling indices were seen in areas of acinar necrosis in the liver. Hepatocytes from these mice stained very heavily for glycogen using periodic acid/Schiff's reagent (PAS). The accumulation of glycogen began to occur with as little as 1–2 weeks of treatment (Sanchez & Bull, 1990), but became progressively more severe with time (Bull et al., 1990). Sanchez & Bull (1990) noted that these effects could not be replicated by exposing mice to the metabolites of DCA — glycolate, glyoxylate or oxalate — in the drinking-water.

Davis (1990) investigated the effects of DCA and TCA treatments on male and female Sprague-Dawley rats for up to 14 days. The authors reported decreased plasma glucose and lactic acid concentrations in both plasma and liver. There were some inconsistencies in the reporting of the doses in this study. However, the author has provided the correct doses, which were 120 and 316 mg/kg of body weight per day (M.E. Davis, personal communication, 1996). This places the results in a context that is more consistent with those of other studies (e.g., Katz et al., 1981).

Mather et al. (1990) found increases in liver weight in rats treated with DCA at 5 g/litre (350 mg/kg of body weight per day) in their drinking-water for 90 days. Relative liver and kidney weights were increased at concentrations of 0.5 g/litre (35 mg/kg of body weight per day) and above. PAS staining of liver sections revealed accumulation of glycogen in severely swollen hepatocytes, which was quite marked with 5 g DCA/litre. The treatment caused small, statistically significant increases in alkaline phosphatase (AP) and ALAT in serum. However, these changes were too small to be of clinical importance. DCA was found to approximately double the activity of cyanide-insensitive acyl coenzyme A (CoA) activity in the liver at 5 g/litre, indicating some induction of peroxisome synthesis.

Cicmanec et al. (1991) examined the subchronic effects of DCA in dogs. DCA was administered at doses of 0, 12.5, 39.5 or 72 mg/kg of body weight per day for 90 days to groups of five males and five females. Liver weights were significantly increased in a dose-related manner, beginning with the lowest dose, and kidney weight was increased at the highest dose. This was accompanied by histopathological observation of vacuolar changes in the liver and haemosiderosis. The pancreas displayed evidence of chronic inflammation and acinar degeneration at the two highest doses. Testicular degeneration was observed in virtually all the male dogs administered DCA. This pathology was not observed in the control animals. Vacuolization of white myelinated tracts in the cerebrum or cerebellum was observed at all doses, and vacuolar changes were observed in the medulla and spinal cord of male dogs. Although the vacuolization was present in all dose groups, the authors described it as being mild. These authors failed to find evidence of the lenticular opacities that had been previously reported by Katz et al. (1981) under very similar treatment conditions. They also found fairly consistent decreases in erythrocyte counts and haemoglobin concentrations at 72 mg/kg of body weight per day in both male and female dogs. As found by others in rat studies, evidence of hindlimb paralysis was reported, but the effect was expressed only sporadically in dogs.

A number of other studies are consistent with the pattern of toxicological effects produced by DCA described above. Included in this group are the study of Bhat et al. (1991), which adds observations of enlarged portal veins, deposition of collagen in the area of the portal triads and some similar lesions in the vasculature of the lung in rats. This study also noted atrophic testes and focal vacuolation and gliosis in the brain. Only a single dose level of 10.5 g/litre of drinking-water (approximately 1100 mg/kg of body weight per day) was utilized in this 90-day study, a level that substantially exceeds concentrations reported to reduce water and food consumption in other studies (Bull et al., 1990).

More recent studies have more closely examined the dose–response relationships involved in the accumulation of glycogen in the liver of male B6C3F$_1$ mice treated with DCA in drinking-water at levels ranging from 0.1 to 3 g/litre (approximately 20–600 mg/kg of body weight per day) for up to 8 weeks (Kato-Weinstein et al., 1998). Significant increases in the glycogen content of the liver of mice were seen with concentrations as low as 0.5 g/litre (100 mg/kg of body weight per day) in their drinking-water, with a small, but insignificant, increase being observed at 0.2 g/litre (40 mg/kg of body weight per day). Glycogen concentrations in the liver reached maximum levels within 1 week of treatment with concentrations in drinking-water of 1 g/litre and above. At this early stage, the glycogen that accumulates is subject to mobilization by fasting. With continued treatment, the glycogen that is deposited becomes increasingly resistant to mobilization until approximately 8 weeks of treatment, when the glycogen contents of the livers of DCA-treated mice are not different in fasted and non-fasted states.

The enzymatic basis of hepatic glycogen accumulation remains unclear. DCA treatment has no effect on the total amount of either form of glycogen synthase in the liver (e.g., glucose-6-phosphate-dependent vs. glucose-6-phosphate-independent activity). The proportion of glycogen synthase in the active form was significantly decreased in mice treated with DCA for as little as 1 week. The amount of phosphorylase in the active form appeared unaltered by treatment. Such changes could indicate that a feedback inhibition may have developed on the synthesis of glycogen as a result of its accumulation in hepatocytes.

Carter et al. (1995) examined the time course of DCA's effects in the liver of B6C3F$_1$ mice at concentrations of 0, 0.5 or 5 g/litre in drinking-water for up to 30 days. As reported in prior studies, the high-dose group displayed severe liver hypertrophy. However, a smaller, but consistent, increase in liver weight became evident with as little as 10 days of treatment at 0.5 g/litre. Even at this relatively low dose, some hepatocytes appeared to have lost nuclei or possessed nuclei that had undergone some degree of karyolysis. These experiments also appeared to rule out cytotoxicity and reparative hyperplasia as consistent features of DCA's effects. The authors suggested that this was in apparent contrast to the earlier observations of Sanchez & Bull (1990). However, Sanchez & Bull (1990), in a 14-day study in mice, noted that these effects were closely associated with what appeared to be infarcted areas in the liver of mice treated with high doses of DCA rather than cytotoxicity. These infarcts are thought to be secondary to the severe swelling of hepatocytes that results from DCA treatment. This interpretation is supported by the apparent lack of cytotoxic effects of DCA in isolated hepatocytes of both mice and rats at concentrations in the mmol/litre range (Bruschi & Bull, 1993). Subsequently, these infarcted areas have been identified as acinar necrosis (ILSI, 1997), which occurs in a somewhat random fashion when high concentrations of DCA (≥ 2 g/litre) are administered for prolonged periods of time (Stauber & Bull, 1997).

It is important to note that the dog appears to be very sensitive to the effects of DCA on the liver; substantial increases in liver weights are observed at daily doses as low as 12.5 mg/kg of body weight per day for a 90-day period (Cicmanec et al., 1991). By comparison, the lowest effect level noted in mice is 0.5 g/litre of drinking-water, which approximates 70–100 mg/kg of body weight per day (Carter et al. 1995), and the lowest effect level noted in rats is 125 mg/kg of body weight per day (Katz et al., 1981).

4.2.1.2   *Reproductive effects*

DCA produces testicular toxicity when administered at high doses in drinking-water. These effects were first noted in studies of the general toxicity of DCA (Katz et al., 1981) and were discussed above (section 4.2.1.1). Cicmanec et al. (1991) followed up on these original observations in dogs and detected degeneration of the testicular epithelium and syncytial giant cell formation at doses as low as 12.5 mg/kg of body weight.

Toth et al. (1992) examined DCA's ability to modify male reproductive function in Long-Evans rats given 0, 31, 62 or 125 mg/kg of body weight per day by gavage for 10 weeks. Reduced weights of accessory organs (epididymis, cauda epididymis and preputial gland) were observed at doses as low as 31 mg/kg of body weight per day. Epididymal sperm counts were found to be depressed and sperm morphology was increasingly abnormal at doses of 62 mg/kg of body weight per day and above. These latter effects were accompanied by changes in sperm motion. Fertility was tested in overnight matings and was found to be depressed only at the highest dose evaluated, 125 mg/kg of body weight per day.

The testicular toxicity of DCA was evaluated in adult male rats given both single and multiple (up to 14 days) oral doses. Delayed spermiation and altered resorption of residual bodies were observed in rats given single doses of 1500 or 3000 mg/kg of body weight; these effects persisted to varying degrees on post-treatment days 2, 14 and 28. Delayed spermiation and formation of atypical residual bodies were also observed on days 2, 5, 9 and 14 in rats dosed daily with 54, 160, 480 or 1440 mg/kg of body weight per day. Distorted sperm heads and acrosomes were observed in step 15 spermatids after administration of doses of 480 and 1440 mg/kg of body weight per day for 14 days.

Decreases in the percentage of motile sperm occurred after 9 days at doses of 480 and 1440 mg/kg of body weight per day and after 14 days at 160 mg/kg of body weight per day. Increased numbers of fused epididymal sperm were observed on days 14, 9 and 5 in rats dosed with 160, 480 or 1440 mg/kg of body weight per day, respectively; other morphological abnormalities occurred at 160 mg/kg of body weight per day and higher. On day 14, a significant decrease in epididymis weight was observed at 480 and 1440 mg/kg of body weight per day, and epididymal sperm count was decreased at 160 mg/kg of body weight per day and higher. These studies demonstrate that the testicular toxicity induced by DCA is similar to that produced by the analogue DBA (see section 4.2.3.2). However, the testicular toxicity of DCA is less severe at equal mol/litre concentrations. Moreover, the DCA-induced testicular lesions occur at lower doses as the duration of dosing increases, indicating the importance of using low-dose subchronic exposures to assess the health risk of prevalent DBPs (Linder et al., 1997a).

DCA was found to be more potent than TCA in inhibiting *in vitro* fertilization of B5D2F$_1$ mouse gametes (Cosby & Dukelow, 1992). For DCA, the percentage of gametes fertilized dropped from 87.0% to 67.3% at the lowest concentration tested, 100 mg/litre. No effects were noted for TCA at 100 mg/litre; at 1000 mg/litre, however, 71.8% of the gametes were fertilized. Both responses were statistically different from those of their concurrent control groups.

4.2.1.3   Developmental effects

DCA has been shown to induce soft tissue abnormalities in fetal rats when administered by gavage in a water vehicle to their dams during gestation days 6–15 (Smith et al., 1992). These effects were observed at doses of 140 mg/kg of body weight per day and above and were not observed at 14 mg/kg of body weight per day. The heart was the most common target organ. An interventricular septal defect between the ascending aorta and the right ventricle was most commonly observed. Urogenital defects (bilateral hydronephrosis and renal papilla) and defects of the orbit were also observed. In a subsequent publication, these authors identified the most sensitive period to be days 12–15 of gestation (Epstein et al., 1992).

Some limited experimentation has been conducted to evaluate the developmental effects of DCA in rat whole embryo culture (Saillenfait et al., 1995). The applicability of these data to the *in vivo* situation is difficult to evaluate based on the very high concentrations that were utilized in these studies. At a concentration of 1 mmol/litre, DCA retarded growth of the embryos by a variety of measures. It required 2.5 mmol/litre to induce brain and eye defects and 3.5 mmol/litre to produce abnormalities in other organ systems.

4.2.1.4   Neurotoxicity

Yount et al. (1982) demonstrated that DCA administered to rats in their feed at doses of 2.5–4 mmol/kg of body weight per day (322–716 mg/kg of body weight per day) produced hindlimb weakness and abnormal gait within 2–4 weeks of treatment. These effects were associated with significant reductions in nerve conduction velocity and a decrease in the cross-sectional area of the tibial nerve.

4.2.1.5   Toxicity in humans

DCA was first investigated as a potential orally effective hypo-glycaemic agent. Stacpoole et al. (1978) found that DCA, administered in doses of 3–4 g of dichloroacetate as the sodium salt per day for 6–7 days (43–57 mg/kg of body weight per day for a 70-kg person), significantly reduced fasting hyperglycaemia in patients with diabetes mellitus alone or in combination with hyperlipoproteinaemia by 24%. In addition, plasma lactic acid concentrations dropped by 73% and plasma alanine concentrations by 82%. Only mild sedation was noticed by some of the patients, and there was no evidence of altered blood counts or prothrombin time. There was a slower, but significant, decline in plasma triglyceride levels and less consistent effects on plasma cholesterol. β-Hydroxybutyrate concentrations in plasma increased significantly and continuously over the 6 days of adminis-tration. Uric acid concentrations in serum increased and those in urine decreased, reflecting a 50% decrease in urinary clearance.

Further details on the early investigations of DCA as an oral antidiabetic agent have been reviewed extensively (Crabb et al., 1981; Stacpoole, 1989; Stacpoole & Greene, 1992) and will not be dwelt on extensively in the present review. The main reason that DCA was not fully developed for this application was that longer-term administration to patients induced a reversible polyneuropathy (Moore et al., 1979b; Stacpoole, 1989). As discussed above, similar pathology was reported in experimental animals by several authors, which added significant weight to this observation. Subsequent work in rats suggested that thiamine deficiency contributed to the development of peripheral neuropathy (Stacpoole et al., 1990). However, a recent report (Kurlemann et al., 1995) indicated that supplementing the diet with 100 mg of thiamine daily did little to ameliorate the development of polyneuropathy of a patient treated with DCA at a dose of 100 mg/kg of body weight for 20 weeks.

Subsequently, DCA has been investigated extensively in the treatment of congenital lactic acidosis (Coude et al., 1978; Stacpoole & Greene, 1992; Toth et al., 1993), a disease that is frequently fatal. More recently, DCA has been evaluated with success in the treatment of lactic acidosis associated with severe malaria in children (Krishna et al., 1995). It is also apparently effective in treatment of lactic acidosis associated with liver transplantation (Shangraw et al., 1994). DCA has been reported to improve psychiatric symptoms, as well as to markedly decrease elevated lactic acid levels in an individual with mitochondrial myopathy (Saijo et al., 1991). Doses of up to 100 mg/kg of body weight per day were administered. In a second study, DCA was shown to reverse lesions to the basal ganglia in a patient with complex I deficiency as measured by computerized tomography (CT) scan and magnetic resonance imaging (MRI) (Kimura et al., 1995). However, a second patient with pyruvate dehydrogenase complex deficiency displayed only transient improvement.

Based on work done in animals, several studies have examined the effects of DCA on cardiovascular function under a variety of disease conditions and altered physiological states. DCA was found to stimulate myocardial lactate consumption and improve left ventricular efficiency in 10 patients with congestive heart failure (Bersin et al., 1994). On the other hand, although DCA decreased blood lactate levels in patients with congestive heart failure, it had no effect on exercise time, peak exercise oxygen consumption or flow to the exercising leg (Wilson et al., 1988). In normal individuals, DCA decreased blood lactate levels when exercising at less than 80% of average maximal oxygen consumption, but it did not affect blood lactate concentrations at exhaustion (Carraro et al., 1989).

These studies show that DCA has some beneficial effects in a variety of metabolic diseases. Acutely, DCA produces little in the way of risk, because short exposures are without apparent adverse effect. However, despite the limited number of subjects that have been studied, the results, when coupled with the results of animal experiments, indicate relatively strongly that DCA is neurotoxic in humans. The delayed induction of these toxicities may be attributable in part to the fact that systemic concentrations of DCA can be expected to sharply increase with prolonged treatment, at least at the high doses used therapeutically, typically in the range 25–100 mg/kg of body weight. There is no human evidence of adverse effects at lower exposures to DCA (e.g., those that would be derived from drinking chlorinated water).

4.2.1.6 Carcinogenicity and mutagenicity

IARC has evaluated the carcinogenicity of DCA and, based on the data available at the time, concluded that there is inadequate evidence for its carcinogenicity in humans and limited evidence for its carcinogenicity in experimental animals. The compound was assigned to Group 3: not classifiable as to its carcinogenicity to humans (IARC, 1995).

DCA is a very effective inducer of hepatic tumours in both mice and rats at high doses. Several studies in male and female B6C3F$_1$ mice found multiple tumours per animal with treatment concentrations of 2 g/litre and above with as little as 1 year of treatment (Herren-Freund et al., 1987; Bull et al., 1990; DeAngelo et al., 1991; Daniel et al., 1992a; Pereira, 1996). These studies are summarized in Table 15. Early in treatment (i.e., 52 weeks), the dose–response curve is very steep, with essentially no response observed at concentrations of 1 g/litre, but as many as four tumours per liver in mice treated with 2 g/litre (Bull et al., 1990). However, concentrations as low as 0.5 g/litre will result in a hepatic tumour incidence of approximately 80% in a full 2-year study (Daniel et al., 1992a).

Hepatic tumours are also induced by DCA in male F344 rats (Richmond et al., 1995). High doses of DCA given to rats also produce overt signs of peripheral neuropathy. Nevertheless, increased incidences of hyperplastic nodules, hepatocellular adenoma and hepatocellular carcinoma were observed at 60 weeks of treatment at 2.4 g/litre

Table 15. Carcinogenic effects of dichloroacetate in rodents

Species (sex)	Dose (g/litre)	Duration (weeks)	Tumour site	HN & HA[a]		HC[b]		Reference
				Incidence	Tumour/n (multiplicity)	Incidence	Tumour/n (multiplicity)	
Mice								
B6C3F$_1$ (M)	0	61						Herren-Freund et al. (1987)
	5	61	Liver	25/26	(4.6)	21/26	(1.7)	
B6C3F$_1$ (M)	1	52	Liver	2/11	0.3	–	–	Bull et al. (1990)
	2	52	Liver	23/24	3.6	5/24	0.25	
	2	37	Liver	7/11	2.2	0/11	0	
B6C3F$_1$ (M)	0	60	Liver	0/10	0	0/10	0	DeAngelo et al. (1991)
	0.5	60	Liver					
	3.5	60	Liver	12/12	2.3	8/12	1.7	
	5	60	Liver	27/30	2.3	25/30	2.2	
	0	75	Liver	2/28	0.07			
	0.05	75	Liver	4/29	0.31			
	0.5	75	Liver	3/27	0.11			

Table 15 (Contd).

B6C3F$_1$ (F)							Daniel et al. (1992a)
0	104	Liver	1/20	0.05	2/20	0.1	
0.5	104	Liver	12/24	0.5	15/24	0.63	
							Pereira (1996)
0	52	Liver	1/40	0.03	0/40	0	
0.28	52	Liver	0/40	0	0/40	0	
0.93	52	Liver	3/20	0.20	0/20	0	
2.8	52	Liver	7/20	0.45	1/20	0.1	
0	81	Liver	2/90	0.02	2/90	0.02	
0.28	81	Liver	3/50	0.06	0/50	0	
0.93	81	Liver	7/28	0.32	1/28	0.04	
2.8	81	Liver	16/19	5.6	5/19	0.37	
Rats							
F344 (M)							Richmond et al. (1995)
0	60	Liver	0/7	0	0/7	0	
0.05	60	Liver	0/7	0	0/7	0	
0.5	60	Liver	0/7	0	0/7	0	
2.4	60	Liver	(26/27)	0.96	1/27	0.04	

292

Table 15 (Contd).

Species (sex)	Dose (g/litre)	Duration (weeks)	Tumour site	HN & HA[a]		HC[b]		Reference
				Incidence	Tumour/n (multiplicity)	Incidence	Tumour/n (multiplicity)	
	0	104	Liver	1/23	0.04	0/23	0	
	0.05	104	Liver	0/26	0	0/26	0	
	0.5	104	Liver	(9/29)	0.31	3/29	0.1	
	2.4	104	Liver	NR[c]	NR	NR	NR	
F344 (M)	0	104	Liver	1/33	0.03	1/33	0.03	DeAngelo et al. (1996)
	0.05	104	Liver	0/26	0	0/26	0	
	0.5	104	Liver	5/29	0.17	3/29	0.10	
	1.6[d]	104	Liver	4/28	0.14	6/28	0.24	

[a] Combined hepatocellular nodules and hepatocellular adenomas.
[b] Hepatocellular carcinoma.
[c] NR = not reported.
[d] Concentration was 2.6 g/litre of drinking-water for 18 weeks and then lowered to 1 g/litre to give a mean daily concentration of 1.6 g/litre.

(Table 15). As in mice, if DCA treatment was extended to 104 weeks, the incidence of these lesions was 41% in a group of 29 rats at a treatment concentration of 0.5 g/litre. No tumours were observed at 0.05 g/litre, and only one hepatic tumour was observed in 23 control rats.

Estimated doses of DCA in mg/kg of body weight per day for the studies in Table 15 were as follows (ILSI, 1997; US EPA, 1998a):

Herren-Freund et al. (1997): 5 g/litre = 1000 mg/kg of body weight per day

Bull et al. (1990): 1 or 2 g/litre = 140 or 300 mg/kg of body weight per day

DeAngelo et al. (1991): 0.05, 0.5, 3.5 or 5 g/litre = 7.6, 77, 410 or 486 mg/kg of body weight per day

Daniel et al. (1992a): 0.5 g/litre = 95 mg/kg of body weight per day

Pereira (1996): 0.26, 0.86 or 2.6 g/litre = 40, 120 or 330 mg/kg of body weight per day

Richmond et al. (1995): 0.05, 0.5 or 2.4 g/litre = 4, 40 or 300 mg/kg of body weight per day

DeAngelo et al. (1996): 0.05, 0.5 or 1.6 g/litre = 4, 40 or 140 mg/kg of body weight per day.

Male F344 rats were exposed for 2 years to DCA in their drinking-water at concentrations of 0.05, 0.5 or 1.6 g/litre. Based upon the pathological examination, DCA induced observable signs of toxicity in the nervous system, liver and myocardium. However, treatment-related neoplastic lesions were observed only in the liver. A statistically significant increase in carcinogenicity (hepatocellular carcinoma) was noted at 1.6 g/litre. Exposure to 0.5 g/litre increased hepatocellular neoplasia (carcinoma and adenoma) at 100 weeks. Calculation of the time-weighted mean daily dose at which 50% of the animals exhibited liver neoplasia indicated that the F344 male rat (approximately 10 mg/kg of body weight per day) is 10 times more sensitive than the $B6C3F_1$ male mouse (approximately 100 mg/kg of body weight per day) (DeAngelo et al., 1996).

The ability of DCA to induce damage to DNA that could give rise to mutations or chromosomal damage has been studied both *in vivo* and *in vitro*. Classical evaluations of DCA in *Salmonella typhimurium* tester strains, both with and without metabolic activation, have been largely negative if held to the standard of at least a 2-fold increase in apparent mutation frequency (Waskell, 1978; Herbert et al., 1980). However, a number of more recent studies have suggested some potential for DCA-induced modifications in DNA. DeMarini et al. (1994) reported that DCA induced prophage in *Escherichia coli* at a concentration of 0.26 mmol/litre and produced 2.7 and 4.2 revertants per ppm in *S. typhimurium* strain TA100 with and without S9 addition, respectively. There are some difficulties in interpreting this report, as the authors introduced DCA as a vapour, and it is not clear whether the concentrations reported (i.e., ppm) refer to air or medium concentrations. Second, at least in the case of the *Salmonella* assay, the DCA was introduced as the free acid and allowed to vaporize and partition into the incubation medium. Because DCA is a strong acid, and if sufficient time is allowed, such conditions could result in near-quantitative transfer of DCA to the medium. The amount volatilized in this case was approximately 60–600 mmol. Therefore, it is likely that the pH of this small amount of medium (2.5 ml) was substantially modified, even if only a fraction of this relatively large amount of strong acid was indeed transferred to the medium. The amount of DCA introduced into the prophage assay was unclear because the method of addition was not described, although the introduction to the journal article implied that it was again being tested as a volatile.

Fox et al. (1996) recently published an evaluation of the muta-genic effects of sodium dichloroacetate. These investigations found no evidence of increased mutation rates in *Salmonella typhimurium* tester strains TA98, TA100, TA1535 or TA1537; *Escherichia coli* strain WP2urvA; or the mouse lymphoma forward mutation assay, whether incubated in the presence or absence of rat liver S9 fraction for metabolic activation. These authors found no evidence that DCA was capable of inducing chromosomal aberrations in CHO cells *in vitro* at doses of up to 1100 mg/kg of body weight for 3 days. These studies utilized neutralized DCA, supporting the contention that positive results in prior studies may have been due to artefactual results obtained by testing of the free acid or because various sources of DCA have greater amounts of impurities.

Giller et al. (1997) examined the mutagenicity of DCA in the SOS chromotest, the Ames fluctuation assay and the newt micronucleus assay. DCA induced a positive response at 500 μg/ml (approximately 3.5 mmol/litre) in the SOS chromotest and at concentrations ranging from 100 to 1500 μg/ml (approximately 1–10 mmol/litre) in the Ames fluctuation assay. The effects were observed at a lower concentration in the absence of S9. The concentrations used in these studies exceed the peak systemic concentrations of DCA that produce a high incidence of liver tumours in mice by approximately 3 orders of magnitude (Kato-Weinstein et al., 1998). Moreover, it appears that the authors utilized the free acid in these experiments, raising the possibility of a pH artefact. The newt micronucleus assay was found to be negative.

DCA has been shown to produce a mutagenic and clastogenic response in the *in vitro* mouse lymphoma assay, but only at doses at or above 1 mmol/litre (Harrington-Brock et al., 1998).

Analogous difficulties have been encountered when attempting to document the mutagenic effects of DCA *in vivo*. Nelson & Bull (1988) and Nelson et al. (1989) reported that DCA induced single strand breaks (SSB) in hepatic DNA when administered by gavage to both mice and rats. Subsequent investigators were unable to replicate these results in detail (Chang et al., 1992; Daniel et al., 1993a). However, a small transitory increase in SSB was observed with doses of 5 and 10 mmol/kg of body weight in male B6C3F$_1$ mice (Chang et al., 1992). The bases of the discrepancies in these results are not clear, but could, in part, be attributed to slightly different methods. As noted in the subsequent section on TCA (section 4.2.2), the Nelson & Bull (1988) results were not replicated by Styles et al. (1991), although there was greater similarity in the methods used. More recently, Austin et al. (1996) showed that acute doses of DCA oxidatively damage nuclear DNA, measured as increases in the 8-hydroxy-2-deoxyguanosine (8-OH-dG) relative to 2-deoxyguanosine content of the isolated DNA. The time course of this damage is more consistent with the development of SSB breaks reported by Chang et al. (1992) and could represent the repair process that involves strand scission. There are two important points that must be made: (i) the induction of SSB by Chang et al. (1992) was very small relative to that seen with the positive controls, diethylnitrosamine and methylmethane sulfonate; and (ii) although increased 8-OH-dG was observed with acute treatments with DCA, there was not a sustained elevation of this adduct in nuclear

DNA of mice when treatments were extended to 3 or 10 weeks in drinking-water (Parrish et al., 1996).

Fuscoe et al. (1996) reported results obtained with the mouse peripheral blood micronucleus assay. They found a small, but statistically significant, increase in polychromatic erythrocytes containing micronuclei in male B6C3F$_1$ mice treated for 9 days with 3.5 g of DCA per litre of drinking-water. However, this response was not maintained through 28 days of exposure. These investigators also examined DNA migration in the single-cell gel assay. In this case, DCA appeared to retard migration of DNA, suggesting the possibility of DNA cross-linking after 28 days of treatment at 3.5 g/litre. Neither assay revealed significant effects of DCA at concentrations of 2 g/litre or below. DCA induces 3–4 tumours per animal within 1 year at 2 g/litre in drinking-water (Bull et al., 1990). The higher dose adds little to the tumorigenic response. More information with regard to the possibility that DCA can cause mutations in liver cells is found in a recent study using the *lacI* locus in the Big Blue® transgenic mouse mutagenesis assay (Leavitt et al., 1997). These investigators used a drinking-water route and the same doses of DCA as were used in the rodent bioassay. After 10 and 60 weeks of DCA administration, an increased frequency of mutants was observed at the high dose (3.5 g/litre). Mutational spectral analysis of these mutations revealed a different spectrum in the mutants from DCA-treated animals than was seen in the untreated animals. At this high dose of DCA, a large portion of the liver can actually be tumour tissue. Because tumours result from clonal expansion, the presence of tumour tissue in the evaluated sample would give a falsely high mutation frequency if a *lacI* mutation occurred in the rapidly expanding tumour clone. Thus, these indications of genotoxic activity may have little to do with the induction of hepatic cancer by DCA.

DCA appears to specifically stimulate outgrowth of hepatocellular adenomas, rather than hepatocellular carcinomas. Pereira & Phelps (1996) examined the role of DCA as a promoter of methylnitrosourea (MNU)-initiated hepatic tumours in female B6C3F$_1$ mice. These data are provided in graphic form in Figure 2. At a concentration of 2.6 g/litre of drinking-water, DCA induced a very large increase in the number of hepatocellular adenomas, but had no significant effect on the induction of hepatocellular carcinomas. These data would appear to be consistent with the stop experiments of Bull et al. (1990), who found that suspension of treatment with DCA appeared to arrest progression

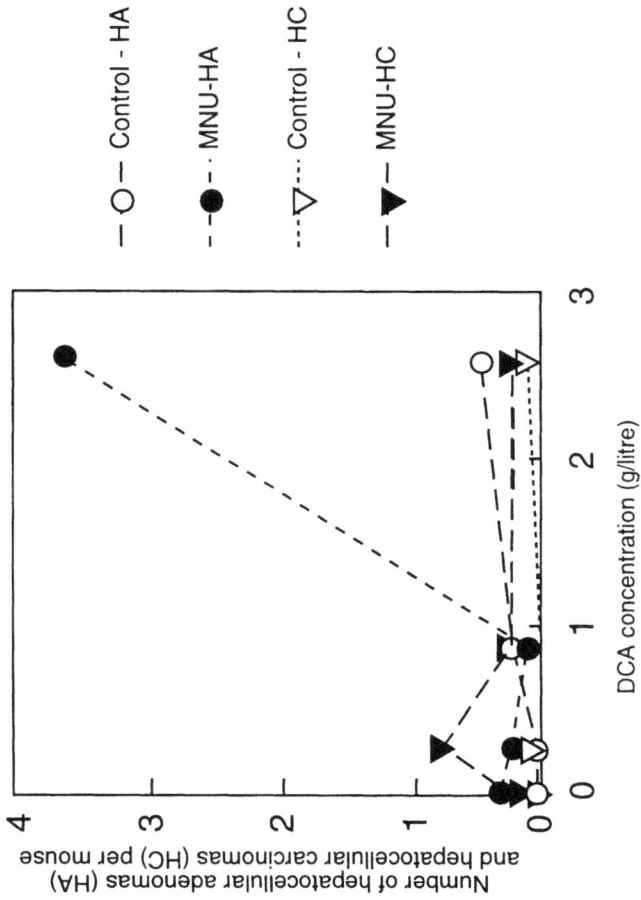

Fig. 2. The ability of DCA to promote the formation of liver tumours in B6C3F₁ mice that have been previously exposed to methylnitrosourea as an initiator (adapted from the results of Pereira & Phelps, 1996).

WHO 99406

of liver tumours, but resulted in a yield of hepatocellular adenomas and nodules that was proportional to the total dose of DCA administered. In contrast, most of the tumours that remained after the suspension of TCA treatment for 3 months were hepatocellular carcinomas.

More recent studies on the effects of DCA on cell replication within normal hepatocytes and hyperplastic nodules and tumours (predominantly adenomas) indicate that DCA has selective effects. Stauber & Bull (1997) found that DCA had a small, stimulatory effect on the replication rate of normal hepatocytes over the first 14 days of treatment. As treatment was extended to 28 days and beyond, these effects became inhibitory at concentrations in drinking-water of 0.5 g/litre and above. In contrast, hepatocytes within nodules and tumours appeared to be resistant to the inhibitory effects of DCA. At a concentration of 2 g/litre, DCA doubled the rate at which c-Jun immunoreactive hepatocytes replicated within hyperplastic nodules and adenomas. This strong stimulation of tumour cell replication would appear to be responsible for the very rapid induction of tumours in mice treated with DCA in drinking-water at concentrations of 2 g/litre and above. It would appear that the slower induction of liver tumours at lower doses of DCA depends primarily on the selective suppression of the replication of normal hepatocytes relative to that of initiated cells.

The inhibitory effect of DCA on replication of normal hepatocytes has been observed by a number of investigators (Carter et al., 1995). The rate of replication is sharply inhibited within 5 days at concentrations of DCA of 5 g/litre. At 0.5 g/litre, the replication rate becomes inhibited to the same extent as observed with 5 g/litre after 20 days of treatment. These decreases in replication were accompanied by an increase in the percentage of the cells that were mononucleated, which is probably associated with an increase in tetraploid cells.

The suppression of cell replication by DCA in normal hepatocytes of treated mice is accompanied by decreases in apoptosis (Snyder et al., 1995). At concentrations of 5 g/litre, the frequency at which apoptotic cells are observed drops by 60–75% with as few as 5 days of treatment. At 0.5 g/litre, there is a downward trend that is observed over the period from 5 to 30 days such that the frequency of apoptotic bodies at this low dose approaches that observed at the highest dose at 30 days. This result essentially parallels that described above for suppression of the rates of cell replication. This raises a dilemma as to whether the driver of the response is suppressed replication or suppressed apoptosis. Whichever is the case, this has to translate into suppressed turnover of normal hepatocytes. The question is whether this suppressive effect on cell turnover increases the probability of transformation of hepatocytes.

Small, but statistically significant, increases in the rate of DNA synthesis in primary cultures of rat hepatocytes have been reported at a concentration of 1 mmol of DCA per litre (Reddy et al., 1992). This is indirect evidence of an effect on the rate of cell division, because replication rates were not actually measured in this study. Nevertheless, it seems probable that DCA does act as a weak mitogen. Adaptation or down-regulation of this response has been consistently observed *in vivo* as described above. The key observation appears to be that the mitogenic response is not down-regulated in hyperplastic nodules or tumours (Stauber & Bull, 1997).

Hyperplastic nodules and tumours induced by DCA have some common characteristics that distinguish them from nodules and tumours that are induced by TCA. In female mice, Pereira (1996) indicated that liver tumours induced by DCA tended to be eosinophilic, whereas those induced by TCA were basophilic. In male B6C3F$_1$ mice treated with 2 g of DCA per litre, a substantial fraction (66%) of the altered hepatic foci found and nodules were reported to be eosinophilic. However, the larger lesions tend to be basophilic (Stauber & Bull, 1997). These larger lesions included hyperplastic nodules, adenomas and carcinomas. These data suggest that there are some differences in tumour induction by DCA based on sex. However, this difference appears to be important primarily at high doses (≥ 2 g/litre), where the rate of cell replication is enhanced in a set of basophilic lesions. The development of these lesions may account for the much shorter latencies observed in male mice as compared with female mice at high doses.

As pointed out by previous investigators examining responses in male mice (Bull et al., 1990; DeAngelo et al., 1991), Pereira (1996) found the dose–response curves describing the induction of total lesions by DCA to be non-linear in female mice. Conversely, the effects of TCA are essentially linear with dose.

Stauber & Bull (1997) found that DCA-induced liver tumours in male mice were immunoreactive to c-Jun and c-Fos antibodies, whereas TCA-induced liver tumours were not. This difference would appear consistent with the observation that DCA-induced tumours in female mice expressed the GST-π at high levels, whereas TCA-induced tumours were largely GST-π negative. The expression of GST-π is dependent on AP-1 transcription factor binding sites in the promoter region of the gene. Thus, elevations of c-Jun and c-Fos would be expected to increase GST-π expression (Angel & Karin, 1991). Conversely, peroxisome proliferator activated receptor (PPAR)-α is known to interfere with the c-Jun activity (Sakai et al., 1995). As a consequence, GST-π is generally not observed in tumours induced by peroxisome proliferators.

Tao et al. (1996) reported a further differentiation of DCA- and TCA-induced tumours. Non-neoplastic hepatocytes observed in mice treated with DCA were found to have high levels of TGF-α, whereas cells within the tumour expressed much lower levels. The opposite was observed with TGF-β expression, which was high in tumours and low in normal tissues. This differential distribution of expression was not observed in non-involved tissue and tumours from TCA-treated mice. The precise involvement of these growth factors in the growth and development of tumours cannot be stated. However, both TGF-α and TGF-β are known to be intimately involved with cell birth and cell death processes. In liver tissue, TGF-β expression is associated with apoptosis (programmed cell death) and TGF-α expression is associated with proliferative states. It should be noted that it is not known whether these differences reflect characteristics of the neoplastic cells or are actually responses induced by DCA.

Anna et al. (1994) and Ferreira-Gonzalez et al. (1995) independently assessed the frequency and spectra of H-*ras* mutations in DCA-induced tumours. These data and those of historical controls for male B6C3F$_1$ mice (Maronpot et al., 1995) specifically at codon-61 of H-*ras* are displayed in Table 16. The mutation frequency in DCA-induced tumours does not differ significantly from that observed in spontaneous tumours. However, there is an obvious change in the mutation spectra in codon 61, involving a significant increase in the H-*ras*-61(CTA) mutation largely at the expense of the H-*ras*-61(AAA) lesion. A traditional interpretation of changes in mutation spectra would be that

Table 16. Mutation frequency and spectra with codon 61 of H-ras of B6C3F$_1$ mice treated with dichloroacetate and trichloroacetate[a]

Chemical	No. of H-ras 61/ no. of tumours	Fraction	CAA	AAA	CGA	CTA
Spontaneous hepatocellular carcinomas[b]	183/333	0.56	150 (0.45)	106 (0.32)	50 (0.15)	21 (0.06)
Dichloroacetate[b,c,d]	61/110	0.55	48 (0.44)	15 (0.14)	25 (0.22)	22 (0.20)
Trichloroacetate[c]	5/11	0.45	6 (0.55)	4 (0.36)	1 (0.09)	0 (0)

[a] Mutations at other codons are not included, although these tumours are kept as part of the denominator. Therefore, all mutants and wild-type at codon 61 do not add up to the total number of tumours.

[b] Anna et al. (1994).

[c] Ferreira-Gonzalez et al. (1995).

[d] Maronpot et al. (1995).

this is evidence of mutation (Reynolds et al., 1987). As pointed out by Anna et al. (1994), however, such an effect could be accounted for if cells expressing a particular mutation were selected for by treatment. Since the H-*ras*-61(CTA) mutation codes for leucine, a neutral amino acid, whereas the H-*ras*-61(AAA) mutation codes for lysine, a charged amino acid in this position, the structures of these two mutant proteins are potentially quite different in the Switch 2 region of the *ras* protein. Alterations in structure within this region could significantly affect the affinity of H-*ras* binding to *raf*-1 and other proteins involved in signal transduction (Drugan et al., 1996).

4.2.1.7   Comparative pharmacokinetics and metabolism

The mammalian metabolism of DCA has received relatively little study. However, there is sufficient information to show that its metabolism is very dose-dependent and is dramatically affected by prior exposure. While some significant differences in the details of metabolism appear between species, these general statements hold for both rodents and humans.

A proposed metabolic scheme for DCA, adapted from Larson & Bull (1992), is provided in Figure 3. Oxalate, glyoxylate, MCA and carbon dioxide have all been established as metabolites of DCA (Stacpoole, 1989; Larson & Bull, 1992; Lin et al., 1993; Gonzalez-Leon et al., 1997). In addition to the metabolites depicted, thiodiacetate has been observed in small amounts in the urine of mice and rats (Larson & Bull, 1992). This may arise from the reaction of MCA with GSH (Yllner, 1971), but other mechanisms are also possible. The intermediates indicated are hypothetical but reasonable in terms of the end-products observed. The extent to which reductive dehalogenation and peroxy radical formation play a role in the metabolism of DCA is unclear. As discussed later, such reactions clearly play a role in the metabolism of trihaloacetates, and they are included here for completeness. An additional pathway to glycolate could also be rationalized by the oxidative metabolism of MCA.

The human metabolism of DCA first came under study because of its proposed use as an oral hypoglycaemic agent. Lukas et al. (1980) studied intravenously infused (over a 20-min interval) doses of 10 and 20 mg/kg of body weight in two human volunteers at each dose. The low and high doses led to mean half-lives of 0.34 and 0.51 h,

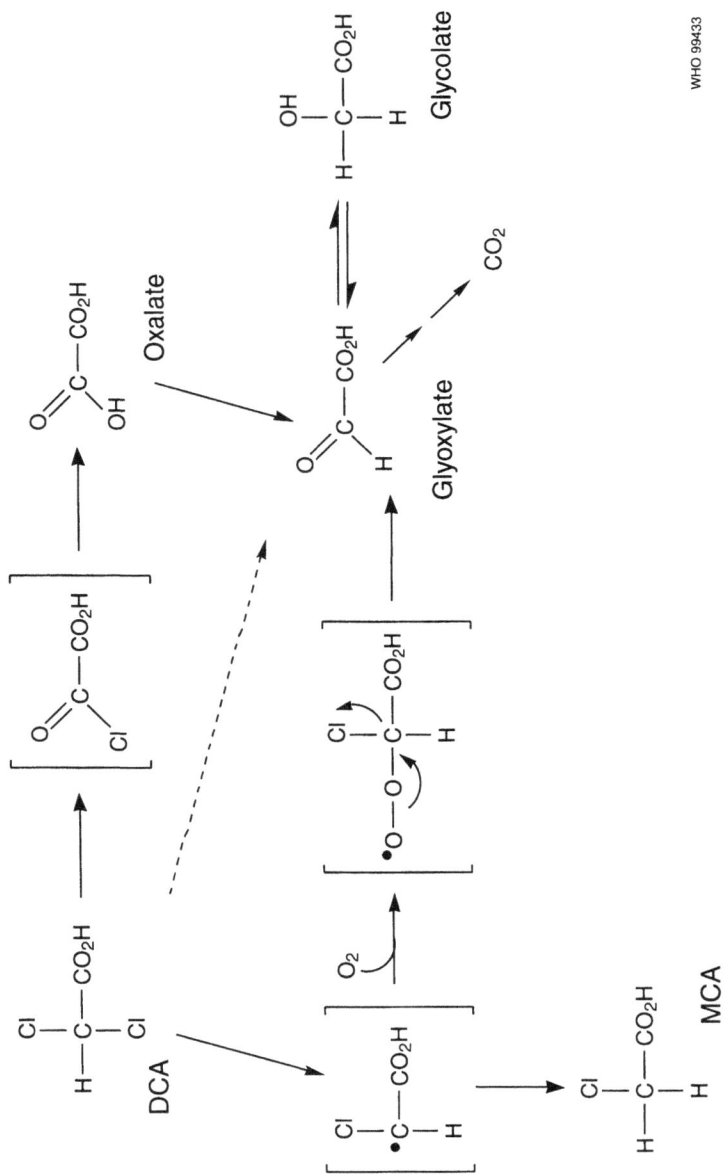

Fig. 3. Metabolic scheme for the metabolism of DCA (adapted from Larson & Bull, 1992).

WHO 99433

175

respectively. Wells et al. (1980) noted that the peak concentration increased disproportionately when intravenous doses (30-min infusion) of DCA increased from 1 to 50 mg/kg of body weight and departed from linearity as doses approached 30 mg/kg of body weight. Whereas the half-life of DCA in this study was seen to be approximately 20 min at doses below 25 mg/kg of body weight, the half-life at higher doses was closer to 40 min, and the mean half-life was 31.8 ± 10.9 (standard deviation [SD]) for all 11 subjects. The authors also noted that the effects of DCA on plasma lactate and alanine persisted several days after cessation of repeated oral treatment with DCA, but ended within 12 h after administering a single intravenous dose. Curry et al. (1985) found that the mean half-life of DCA increased from 63.3 min to an average of 374 min following the fifth of a series of 50 mg/kg of body weight doses of DCA administered intravenously at 2-h intervals. These data suggest that high repeated doses of DCA appear to hinder the metabolic clearance of DCA.

There are substantial species differences in the metabolism of DCA. Dogs, in particular, clear DCA from blood at a very low rate. Lukas et al. (1980) found that the half-life of DCA administered as a single 100 mg/kg of body weight dose was between 17.1 and 24.6 h. In contrast, the clearance of the same dose in rats occurred with a half-life of 2.1–4.4 h. The very much lower metabolic clearance of DCA in the dog is probably responsible for its much greater acute toxicity in this species (Katz et al., 1981). However, the half-life of DCA in humans is much closer to that in rats than to that in dogs (Curry et al., 1991).

Larson & Bull (1992) studied the metabolism of DCA in mice and rats. These authors estimated a half-life of 1.5 h in mice and 0.9 h in rats following oral doses. The estimates of half-life in mice in this study were problematic, because it was clear that there is a tremendous first-pass effect on DCA's absorption from the gastrointestinal tract, which was particularly marked in mice. These authors also estimated a maximum concentration of DCA from oral doses of 20 and 100 mg/kg of body weight. In mice, the C_{max} was found to be 4 and 20 nmol/ml, respectively. In rats, the C_{max} was found to be 15 and 380 at the same doses. These authors also found that significant amounts of DCA were metabolized to carbon dioxide and the non-halogenated acids — glycolate, glyoxylate and oxalate. The fraction of DCA that was metabolized to carbon dioxide was substantially underestimated in these studies, as was shown in the more recent study of Xu et al.

(1995), in which approximately 45% of an oral dose of DCA was metabolized to carbon dioxide in mice within 24 h. Lin et al. (1993) also provided more definitive analyses of the production of glycolate, glyoxylate and oxalate as major urinary metabolites of DCA in the F344 rat. It is notable for later discussions that these authors found a smaller percentage of the dose of $1\text{-}^{14}\text{C}$-DCA ending up in glycolate than was observed with $2\text{-}^{14}\text{C}$-DCA. This was offset by a somewhat greater yield (not statistically significant) of carbon dioxide from $1\text{-}^{14}\text{C}$-DCA than from $2\text{-}^{14}\text{C}$-DCA. These data would suggest that there are alternative pathways from DCA to carbon dioxide in the rat besides the conversion to glyoxylate.

The decreases in DCA clearance with repeated doses appear to be largely due to the inactivation of one enzyme involved in its metabolism. There appear to be subtle differences in the metabolism of mice and rats that lead to different manifestations of this inhibition. In experiments that involved pretreatment of F344 rats at a level of 0.2 or 2 g/litre in their drinking-water for a 14-day period, it was found that the conversion of an oral dose of DCA to carbon dioxide was substantially inhibited. Similar pretreatment of male B6C3F$_1$ mice did not affect carbon dioxide production from DCA. However, in both cases, it is apparent that the metabolic clearance of DCA from blood was affected by the DCA pretreatment. In rats, the kinetics of DCA disappearance were studied with intravenous dosing, which allows more precise definition of the kinetics. This pretreatment led to an increase in the half-life of DCA in the blood of rats from 2.4 ± 0.8 h to 10.8 ± 2.0 h when animals were administered a dose of 100 mg/kg of body weight intravenously. Oral dosing was used in mice, and the major impact of pretreatment was to increase the C_{max} from 2.6 ± 2.6 µg/ml in naive mice to 129.9 µg/ml in mice that had DCA in their drinking-water at 2 g/litre until the prior day (16 h before administration of the test dose). Therefore, the phenomenon that DCA treatment inhibited its own metabolism, which was originally observed in humans, could be replicated in both mice and rats.

The mechanism by which this tremendous change in metabolism occurs has not been established. It has been shown by Lipscomb et al. (1995) that the bulk of the metabolism of DCA occurs in cytosolic fractions. Very little DCA is metabolized in microsomes. It is apparent that the metabolism of DCA in cytosolic preparations from rodent liver is dependent upon nicotinamide cofactor and GSH. However, the metabolism is not mediated by enzymes that can be recovered on a GSH-sepharose column. Glutathione transferase activities towards chlorodinitrobenzene were observed in the column. Subsequent work has shown that it is the activity in the cytosol, however, that is eliminated by DCA treatment (Gonzalez-Leon et al., 1997). Tong et al. (1998) showed that a substantial fraction of DCA's metabolism is mediated by a novel GST, GST-ζ. This enzyme appears to be subject to autoinhibition by DCA.

4.2.1.8   Mode of action

Some indication of mechanisms by which DCA produces its effects can be gleaned from studies cited in previous sections of this document. While DCA produces many different types of toxicological effects (i.e., neurotoxicity, reproductive and developmental toxicities and carcinogenicity), there may be some features that are common to the mechanisms that produce all these effects. The particulars of those mechanisms remain to be established. What follows is a brief outline of what is known and some speculation on how new research may be applied to developing this information to better assess the risks associated with the production of DCA as a by-product of the chlorination of drinking-water.

Given the lack of evidence that induction of DNA damage by DCA is involved in liver cancer induction, are there plausible alternative mechanisms that may be invoked? The most common alternative mode of action would be evidence that carcinogenic doses of DCA induce cytotoxic damage in the target organ, which leads to reparative hyperplasia. Although there is some evidence of single-cell necrosis with chronic exposure (Stauber & Bull, 1997) and infarcts are occasionally observed (Sanchez & Bull, 1990) in the livers of B6C3F$_1$ mice, this mode of action plays a negligible role at the lowest doses that induce liver cancer. Small and variable initial increases in replication rates of hepatocytes in treated mice are reversed with continued treatment, with the dominant effect becoming inhibition of replication within a 4- to 8-week period (Carter et al., 1995; Stauber & Bull, 1997). These observations indicate that necrosis followed by reparative hyperplasia do not explain the rapid carcinogenic responses to DCA.

Additional data add support to the hypothesis that DCA does in fact act largely by a "non-genotoxic" mode of action. Early data indicated that DCA was capable of inducing peroxisome proliferation (Nelson & Bull, 1988; DeAngelo et al., 1989). While these effects have been observed by others, they are clearly of short duration, disappearing within a few months (DeAngelo et al., 1989). Moreover, it has become apparent that DCA induces hepatic tumours at dose rates that are significantly below those required to induce peroxisome proliferation (cf. DeAngelo et al., 1989 and Daniel et al., 1992a).

New research has shown that DCA acts primarily to increase the growth rate of pre-initiated cells in the liver. Stauber et al. (1998) found that DCA induces growth of colonies on soft agar when cell suspensions were obtained from the liver of neonatal mice. The most impressive aspect of these studies was that the colonies expressed the same phenotype (c-Jun+) as was found in DCA-induced tumours *in vivo*. Similar experiments produced a c-Jun− phenotype when TCA was incorporated into the soft agar. A concentration of 0.5 mmol of DCA per litre was required in the medium to produce a significant increase in the number of colonies formed in a 10-day interval when the cells were derived from naive mice. However, if mice were pretreated with 0.5 g of DCA per litre in their drinking-water prior to the isolation of the cells, 0.02 mmol of DCA per litre was as effective as 0.5 mmol/litre. Moreover, the yield of colonies was increased by this pretreatment. The increased sensitivity to DCA appears closely related to the finding that pretreating animals with low levels of DCA (<0.2 g/litre of drinking-water) reduces its metabolism by more than 90% (Gonzalez-Leon et al., 1997). The increased number of colonies produced by pretreatment appears to be due to clonal expansion of these cells. It appears that this activity accounts for the tumours induced by DCA at higher doses (≥2 g/litre) where blood concentrations are found to be in the 100–500 μmol/litre range. However, blood concentrations ranging from 1 to 7 μmol/litre produced in mice treated with 0.5 g/litre (Kato-Weinstein et al., 1998) result in an 80% incidence of liver tumours (Daniel et al., 1992a), suggesting that a second mechanism may be involved at lower doses.

At all carcinogenic doses studied, DCA increases the deposition of glycogen in the liver (Kato-Weinstein et al., 1998). This suggests that DCA is modifying cell signalling pathways. Low intraperitoneal doses of DCA produce increases in serum insulin concentrations in response to glucose challenge (Kato-Weinstein et al., 1998). In contrast, decreases in serum insulin concentrations have been observed in mice chronically administered DCA at either 0.5 or 2 g/litre (Smith et al., 1997). However, these measurements were made during the daylight hours when both serum glucose and blood DCA concentrations are low. Clearly, the involvement of insulin in DCA-induced liver tumorigenesis needs to be studied further.

Recent studies have provided more substantive evidence that DCA at very high levels possesses some ability to induce genotoxic effects. Of particular note are the studies of Harrington-Brock et al. (1998), who found significant increases in mutant frequencies in mouse lymphoma cells *in vitro* at concentrations in excess of 1 mmol/litre. Similar potency of DCA has been observed in the Ames fluctuation assay by Giller et al. (1997). Previous studies were largely negative or made use of the free acid form of DCA. Brusick (1986) had previously documented that low pH produces increased evidence of genotoxic damage in cultured mammalian cells.

Leavitt et al. (1997) reported increased recovery of mutant cells from the *lacI* transgenic mouse with varying periods of treatment with DCA in drinking-water. Significant increases were observed only when mice had been treated with 3.5 g/litre for 60 weeks, but not for shorter time intervals. No significant increases were noted at 1 g/litre. Although the authors took care to ensure that nodules and tumours were excluded from the sampling, Stauber & Bull (1997) demonstrated that there are numerous lesions that are smaller than nodules in B6C3F$_1$ mice maintained on 2 g of DCA per litre for only 40 weeks. It was inevitable that some of these microscopic lesions were included within the tissue samples described. Given the marked stimulation of cell replication that occurs within lesions in mice, it is not possible to determine if the effect reported by Leavitt et al. (1997) is due to mutagenic effects of DCA or its demonstrated ability to selectively stimulate the growth of tumour phenotype.

Based on the available evidence, it is probable that genotoxic effects of DCA play little, if any, role in the induction of liver cancer in rodents at low doses. This conclusion is based on clear evidence that DCA is capable of acting as a tumour promoter and produces effects on cell replication or apoptosis at all carcinogenic doses (Snyder et al.,

1995; Pereira & Phelps, 1996; Stauber & Bull, 1997). The concentrations of DCA required to produce genotoxic effects *in vitro* and the blood levels necessary to detect minimal genotoxic effects *in vivo* are 3 orders of magnitude higher than those necessary for induction of an 80% tumour incidence. The recent evaluation by ILSI (1997) also concluded that the mechanism by which DCA increased liver tumours was non-genotoxic. However, new data indicate that the actual mechanism is by tumour promotion rather than by cytotoxicity and reparative hyperplasia.

The metabolism of DCA is very dose-dependent, with metabolism and clearance of the chemical being inhibited sharply with high dose rates. Most data now suggest that it is the parent compound that is responsible for the effects related to carcinogenicity. Thus, simply on the basis of considerations of target organ dosimetry, the effects of DCA would be predicted to increase sharply at chronic dosing levels that approach or exceed 30 mg/kg of body weight per day rather than being simple linear functions of dose. Unfortunately, the available data do not allow the systemic dose versus external dose relationships to be determined with any precision on the basis of current information. In rats, the full inhibition was observed at concentrations of DCA in drinking-water as low as 0.2 g/litre (Gonzalez-Leon et al., 1997). The minimum treatment level for DCA's inhibition of its own metabolism in mice has not been established. However, blood concentrations of DCA increase from 2–4 μmol/litre when the mice are treated with 0.5 g/litre in drinking-water to approximately 300 μmol/litre when the treatment concentration is 2 g/litre (Kato-Weinstein et al., 1998). These are peak concentrations measured during the night when mice are consuming the DCA-containing water. This 100-fold increase in blood concentrations with a mere 4-fold increase in dose undoubtedly contributes to the highly non-linear tumorigenic response for DCA reported previously (Bull et al., 1990). The effect in humans has been documented to occur with doses in a similar range, 30 mg/kg of body weight (Wells et al., 1980). The animal data need to be extended to lower dosing rates or the human treatments need to be extended in time to more precisely define the level of chronic exposure that is required to produce this phenomenon. Alternatively, a better understanding of the mechanism of this inhibition should allow the critical question of whether the inhibition is a function of cumulative dose or daily dose to be answered.

The available data indicate that DCA differentially affects the replication rates of normal hepatocytes and hepatocytes that have been initiated. The dose–response relationships are complex, with DCA initially stimulating division of normal hepatocytes. However, at the lower chronic doses used in animal studies (but still very high relative to those that would be derived from drinking-water), the replication rate of normal hepatocytes is eventually sharply inhibited. This indicates that normal hepatocytes eventually down-regulate those pathways that are sensitive to stimulation by DCA. However, altered cells, particularly those that express high amounts of a protein that is immunoreactive to a c-Jun antibody, do not seem to be able to down-regulate this response. Thus, the rates of replication in the preneoplastic lesions with this phenotype are very high at the doses that cause DCA tumours to develop with a very low latency. Preliminary data suggest that this continued alteration in cell birth and death rates is also necessary for the tumours to progress to malignancy (Bull et al., 1990). This interpretation is supported by studies that employ initiation/promotion designs as well (Pereira, 1996).

On the basis of the above considerations, it is suggested that the currently available cancer risk estimates for DCA should be modified by incorporating newly developing information on its comparative metabolism and modes of action to formulate a biologically based dose–response model. These data are not available at the time of this writing, but should become available within the next 2–3 years.

The dose–response data for effects other than cancer vary significantly, with dogs being extraordinarily sensitive (Katz et al., 1981). However, inhibition of the metabolism of DCA in chronically treated rodents (Gonzalez-Leon et al., 1997) and humans (Wells et al., 1980; Curry et al., 1985) may cause differences in sensitivities between species to converge somewhat with repeated treatment or exposure. However, a significant difference in species sensitivity remains. Cicmanec et al. (1991) identified a LOAEL of 12.5 mg/kg of body weight per day in dogs treated for 90 days. NOAELs for hepatomegaly in mice appear to be in the neighbourhood of 0.2 g/litre, which is approximately 40 mg/kg of body weight per day. On the basis of the rates of metabolic clearance and the assumption that the intrinsic sensitivities of different species are similar, the average human would seem to more closely approximate rats than dogs. To obtain more accurate pictures of human sensitivity at low doses, however, it is clear that future work must focus more specifically on toxicodynamic variables.

4.2.2 Trichloroacetic acid (trichloroacetate)

Like DCA, TCA exists almost exclusively in the salt form at pHs found in drinking-water because of its very low pK_a of 0.70 (IARC, 1995).

4.2.2.1 General toxicological properties and information on dose–response in animals

1) Acute toxicity

Very little information exists on the mammalian toxicology of TCA before it was discovered as a by-product of drinking-water chlorination. Woodard et al. (1941) determined the oral LD_{50} of tri-chloroacetate (i.e., neutralized to pH 6–7) to be 3.32 g/kg of body weight in rats and 4.97 g/kg of body weight in albino mice when the compound was administered in aqueous solution. These values were in the same general range as those for neutralized acetic acid.

Davis (1990) examined the effects of TCA on blood glucose and lactate levels following a dosing regimen of total doses of 0.92 or 2.45 mmol/kg of body weight administered 3 times in 1 day to Sprague-Dawley rats by gavage. A typographical error in dosage was suspected and confirmed with the author (M.E. Davis, personal communication, 1996). Reductions in plasma glucose concentrations were observed in females at the high dose, and lactic acid levels were decreased at 0.92 and 2.45 mmol/kg of body weight doses in females, but only at the high dose in males. The authors noted that these high concentrations were neutralized with sodium hydroxide. However, these are very low doses of TCA relative to those found to produce similar effects in other studies. These initial experiments were followed by a study of the effects of TCA administered in drinking-water for 14 days at 0.04, 0.16, 0.63 or 2.38 g/litre. Effects on urine volume and osmolality were reported to occur at the highest dose, but not at 0.63 g/litre. Effects on glucose and lactate were not reported.

2)   Short-term toxicity

Mather et al. (1990) administered TCA to male Sprague-Dawley rats in drinking-water at concentrations of 0, 50, 500 or 5000 mg/litre (0, 4.1, 36.5 or 355 mg/kg of body weight per day) for 90 days. Small, but statistically insignificant, decreases in body weight were observed at the highest dose. TCA produced a significant increase in the liver to body weight ratio at this dose, but not at 500 mg/litre. This effect was associated with a small, but statistically significant, increase in cyanide-insensitive acyl CoA oxidase activity in the liver, an indicator of peroxisome proliferation.

Unlike DCA and MCA, TCA does not appear to be a substrate for the mitochondrial pyruvate carrier (Halestrap, 1975). TCA does appear to inhibit the pig heart pyruvate dehydrogenase kinase at approximately the same concentrations as for DCA (Whitehouse et al., 1974). However, the authors noted that DCA influenced the proportion of active pyruvate dehydrogenase in the perfused rat heart, but TCA was inactive under these circumstances. Although these data were obtained from mitochondria from different sources, they suggest that there may be some differences in effects of DCA and TCA on intermediary metabolism related to their transport into various cellular compartments.

Bhat et al. (1991) administered TCA to male Sprague-Dawley rats at a concentration of 45.8 mmol/litre (7.5 g/litre) in their drinking-water for 90 days to provide an approximate intake of 785 mg/kg of body weight per day. These levels produced minimal evidence of liver toxicity by histopathological examination. However, lower concentrations in drinking-water have been shown to seriously impair water and food consumption in experimental animals (Bull et al., 1990; Davis, 1990; Mather et al., 1990; DeAngelo et al., 1991). Consequently, it is difficult to determine how these data relate to the potential effects of the low concentrations of TCA that are found in chlorinated drinking-water (e.g., in the 10–100 µg/litre range).

The most obvious target organ for TCA is the liver. This effect is marked by a hepatomegaly (Goldsworthy & Popp, 1987; Bull et al., 1990; Mather et al., 1990; Sanchez & Bull, 1990), which is presumably related to the ability of TCA to act as a peroxisome proliferator (DeAngelo et al., 1989), since that is a common finding with this class of rodent carcinogens. It could also be related to the metabolism of TCA to DCA (Larson & Bull, 1992). However, more recent data suggest that the apparent conversion of TCA to DCA has largely been the result of artefactual conversion when fresh oxygenated blood is acidified prior to derivatization (Merdink et al., 1998). TCA is clearly without substantive cytotoxic effects at doses of less than 300 mg/kg of body weight *in vivo* (Bull et al., 1990; Sanchez & Bull, 1990; Acharya et al., 1995) or concentrations of up to 5 mmol/litre *in vitro* (Bruschi & Bull, 1993).

4.2.2.2   Reproductive effects

There have been limited studies of TCA's effects on reproductive performance. TCA was found to inhibit *in vitro* fertilization of gametes from B6D2F$_1$ mice at a concentration of 1000 mg/litre, but was without effect at 100 mg/litre (Cosby & Dukelow, 1992). It is unlikely that these effects at very high doses relative to those that might be expected from human consumption of TCA at concentrations less than 0.1% of the NOEL are of relevance in assessing risks from exposure to TCA in drinking-water.

4.2.2.3   Developmental effects

Treatment of pregnant rats with TCA at 0, 330, 800, 1200 or 1800 mg/kg of body weight per day by gavage in a water vehicle on gestation days 6–15 produced dose-dependent reductions in body weight and length of rat pups from dams administered doses of 800 mg/kg of body weight per day and above. No effects were observed at 330 mg/kg of body weight per day. However, there was a significant and dose-related increase in soft tissue malformations at all doses studied. The mean frequency of soft tissue malformations was 3.5 ± 8.7% (SD), 9.06 ± 12.9%, 30.4 ± 28.1%, 55.4 ± 36.1% and 96.9 ± 8.8% at 0, 330, 800, 1200 and 1800 mg/kg of body weight, respectively. Most of the increased soft tissue abnormalities were accounted for by defects in the cardiovascular system. The major malformation seen was laevocardia. However, at doses of 800 mg/kg of body weight and above, a significant incidence of an interventricular septal defect was observed (Smith et al., 1989a).

Saillenfait et al. (1995) found that TCA, administered to rats in embryo culture, began to produce consistent increases in defects at concentrations of 2.5 mmol/litre and above, with few or no effects observed at 1 mmol/litre. These defects included brain and eye defects, reduction in the branchial arch and otic system defects. At concentrations of 3.5 mmol/litre, some evidence of skeletal defects was observed (i.e., absence of hindlimb bud). As is discussed below, these concentrations can be achieved in the blood of rats administered high doses of TCA (≥ 100 mg/kg of body weight) (Larson & Bull, 1992). However, there is considerable doubt about whether these effects would be induced by the doses of less than 1 µg/kg of body weight experienced by humans consuming chlorinated drinking-water.

4.2.2.4 *Neurotoxicity*

No reports of neurotoxic effects of TCA were located.

4.2.2.5 *Toxicity in humans*

TCA is a strong acid. It is widely recognized that contact of TCA with the skin has the potential to produce acid burns, and ingestion of TCA has the potential to damage tissues of the gastrointestinal tract or produce systemic acidosis, even though specific studies of these effects do not appear in the literature. Such effects would occur from contact with the crystal or strong solutions of the free acid. However, such effects have little relevance to the production of low levels of TCA, as the salt, as a by-product of the chlorination of drinking-water.

Indirectly, it may be presumed that TCA presents little overt hazard to human health because it is a major metabolite of commonly used solvents such as trichloroethylene and tetrachloroethylene. Occupational exposures to these solvents have been quite high in the past, but few, if any, effects of the solvents in humans have been attributed to TCA. Therefore, one would surmise that TCA is relatively non-toxic to humans under circumstances of low exposures such as those encountered in chlorinated drinking-water. However, these largely negative data do not insure against chronic hazards such as cancer or adverse reproductive outcomes or teratogenicity. The only reasonable evidence of carcinogenicity due to TCA in animals relates very specifically to the induction of liver tumours. If TCA's apparent mode of action is taken into consideration, it is difficult to identify other tumours that would be attributable to TCA from animal studies. Recent studies of workers in degreasing operations provide little evidence of hepato-cellular tumours (Spirtas et al., 1991; Weiss, 1996).

4.2.2.6   Carcinogenicity and mutagenicity

IARC has evaluated the carcinogenicity of TCA and concluded that there is inadequate evidence for its carcinogenicity in humans and limited evidence for its carcinogenicity in experimental animals. The compound was assigned to Group 3: not classifiable as to its carcino-genicity to humans (IARC, 1995).

TCA induces hepatocellular carcinomas when administered in drinking-water to male B6C3F$_1$ mice (Herren-Freund et al., 1987; Bull et al., 1990; Daniel et al., 1993a). Although some of the data in the literature are of a preliminary nature, consistent results were obtained in three independent studies (Table 17). In two of these studies, dose-related increases in the incidence of malignant tumours and pre-cancerous lesions were obtained in B6C3F$_1$ mice at concentrations in water of between 1 and 5 g/litre and with as little as 12 months of treatment (Bull et al., 1990; Daniel et al., 1993a). Under similar conditions of treatment, TCA did not induce hepatic tumours in F344 rats (DeAngelo et al., 1997).

In the study in mice by Pereira (1996) reported in Table 17, a NOAEL of 0.35 g of TCA per litre can be identified. Drinking-water consumption and body weight were reported only during the first 4 weeks of the study. These data were not used; instead, it was assumed that the average daily water consumption was about 10% of the animal body weight. On this basis, 0.35 g of TCA per litre is equivalent to approximately 40 mg/kg of body weight per day.

The available data suggest that TCA has some tumour-promoting activity. Pereira (1995) and Pereira & Phelps (1996) reported that TCA increased the yield of both hepatocellular adenomas and hepatocellular carcinomas in MSU-initiated mice (Figure 4). This effect appears to be evident at the lowest concentration tested, 0.35 g/litre of drinking-water. Unlike the circumstance described above with DCA, TCA signi-ficantly increased the yield of hepatocellular carcinomas as well as hepatocellular adenomas after 362 days of treatment. An earlier study by Parnell et al. (1986) suggested that TCA was capable of promoting tumours initiated by diethylnitrosamine. However, this study employed

Table 17. Carcinogenic effects of trichloroacetate in rodents

Species (sex)	Dose (g/litre)	Duration (weeks)	Tumour site	HN & HA[a]		HC[b]		Reference
				Incidence	Tumour/n (multiplicity)	Incidence	Tumour/n (multiplicity)	
Mice								
B6C3F$_1$ (M)	0	61	Liver	2/22	(0.09)	0/22	(0)	Herren-Freund et al. (1987)
	5	61	Liver	8/22	(0.5)	7/22	(0.5)	
B6C3F$_1$ (M)	0	52	Liver	1/35	0.03	0/35	0	Bull et al. (1990)
	1	52	Liver	5/11	0.45	2/11	0.18	
	2	52	Liver	15/24	0.63	4/24	0.17	
	2	37	Liver	2/11	0.18	3/11	0.27	
B6C3F$_1$ (M)	0	60–95	Liver	NR[c]	NR	6.7–10%	0.07–0.15	Daniel et al. (1993a)
	0.05	60	Liver	NR	NR	22%	0.31	
	0.5	60	Liver	NR	NR	38%	0.55	
	4.5	95	Liver	NR	NR	87%	2.2	
	5	60	Liver	NR	NR	55%	0.97	

Table 17 (Contd).

B6C3F₁ (F)							
0	52	Liver	1/40	0.03	0/40	0	Pereira (1996)
0.35	52	Liver	6/40	0.15	0/40	0	
1.2	52	Liver	3/19	0.16	0/19	0	
3.5	52	Liver	2/20	0.10	5/20	0.25	
0	81	Liver	2/90	0.02	2/90	0.02	
0.35	81	Liver	14/53	0.26	0/53	0	
1.2	81	Liver	12/27	0.44	5/27	0.19	
3.5	81	Liver	18/18	1.0	5/18	0.28	
Rats							
F344 (M)							
0	104	Liver	2/23	0.09	0/23	0	DeAngelo et al. (1997)
0.05	104	Liver	2/24	0.08	0/24	0	
0.5	104	Liver	5/20	0.25	0/20	0	
5.0	104	Liver	1/22	0.045	1/22	0.045	

a Combined hyperplastic nodule and hepatocellular adenoma.
b Hepatocellular carcinoma.
c NR = not reported.

190

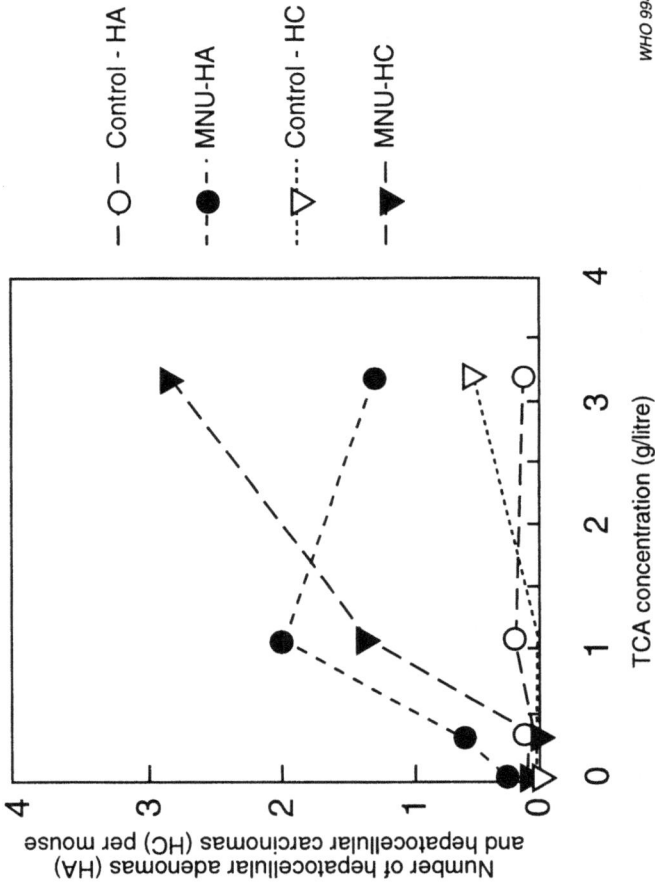

Fig. 4. Tumour-promoting activity of TCA in the liver of B6C3F$_1$ mice that have been previously exposed to methylnitrosourea as an initiator (adapted from the results of Pereira & Phelps, 1996).

WHO 99407

γ-glutamyl transpeptidase (GGT) as a marker for preneoplastic foci and was extended for only 6 months. As a consequence, no increase in tumour yield was noted, although there was a significant increase in GGT-positive foci that appeared dose-related. GGT is a poor marker for foci induced by peroxisome proliferators (Sakai et al., 1995). Therefore, this study may have underestimated the promoting activity of TCA.

The mechanisms by which TCA induces tumours are not clear. TCA induces peroxisome proliferation in male B6C3F$_1$ mice over the same dose range at which it induces hepatic tumours (DeAngelo et al., 1989). Unlike the situation with DCA, the induction of peroxisome synthesis by TCA appears to be sustained over time. Despite a large number of data that strongly link peroxisome proliferation with carcinogenesis, the actual mechanism by which such chemicals actually produce cancer may be only loosely associated with peroxisome proliferation *per se* (discussed further in section 4.2.2.8).

As noted in Table 16, the mutation spectra of mouse liver tumours obtained from mice treated with TCA appear to be different from those observed with DCA (Ferreria-Gonzalez et al., 1995). However, it is important to note that this result was obtained from a very limited number of animals (11), only five of which had hepatic tumours. Although none of the tumours carried the mutation that is apparently selected by DCA treatment, the sparseness of these data prevents a clear conclusion.

Numerous mutagenicity tests have been conducted on TCA (IARC, 1995). TCA did not induce λ prophage in *Escherichia coli* and was not mutagenic to *Salmonella typhimurium* strains in the presence or absence of metabolic activation. TCA, however, reacts with dimethyl sulfoxide (a solvent used commonly in this assay) to form unstable mutagenic substances, which have not been identified (Nestmann et al., 1980). TCA did not induce DNA strand breaks in mammalian cells *in vitro*. Chromosomal aberrations were not induced in human lymphocytes exposed *in vitro* to TCA neutralized to avoid the effects of low pH seen in cultured mammalian cells.

DNA strand breaks were reported in one laboratory in the livers of mice and rats treated 4 h previously with TCA; none was observed

24 h after repeated daily dosing with 500 mg/kg of body weight (Nelson & Bull, 1988; Nelson et al., 1989). Peroxisome proliferation, as indicated by β-oxidation of palmitoyl CoA, was observed only after induction of DNA damage (Nelson et al., 1989). DNA strand breakage was not observed in the livers of mice or rats (Chang et al., 1992). The reasons for the contrasting results obtained using similar techniques are unclear (IARC, 1995).

Giller et al. (1997) examined the effects of TCA in the SOS chromotest in *Escherichia coli* Pq37, the Ames fluctuation assay and the newt micronucleus assay. TCA was negative in the SOS chromotest but exhibited weak activity in the Ames fluctuation assay. Effects were observed at the lowest concentration, 1750 μg/ml, in the absence of S9 fraction. This corresponds to TCA concentrations of approximately 10 mmol/litre in the medium. Newt larvae were found to have an increased frequency of micronuclei at TCA concentrations of 80 μg/ml. As with some previous studies, these tests appear to have been conducted with the free acid, raising issues of potential artefacts in the results.

Harrington-Brock et al. (1998) studied the mutagenic activity of TCA in the mouse lymphoma system. A very weak positive result was obtained at concentrations in excess of 20 mmol/litre. Concentrations of TCA reached in the blood of mice treated with carcinogenic doses can approach the mmol/litre range, so it is possible that these results could be relevant to bioassay data. However, concentrations anticipated in drinking-water would clearly be much lower (in the low μmol/litre range).

In one study, TCA induced micronuclei and chromosomal aberrations in bone marrow cells and abnormal sperm morphology after injection into Swiss mice *in vivo* at doses of 125–500 mg/kg of body weight (Bhunya & Behera, 1987). However, Mackay et al. (1995) could not replicate this finding, even at doses 10-fold higher.

4.2.2.7 Comparative pharmacokinetics and metabolism

TCA is readily absorbed from the gastrointestinal tract in experimental animals and humans (Muller et al., 1974; Larson & Bull, 1992). However, the major determinant of its blood concentrations at a given dose is its relatively slow clearance from blood relative to other HAAs. There are substantial differences in this clearance by different species. The half-life is 5.8 h in mice (Larson & Bull, 1992), 9.3 h in rats (Merdink et al., 1999), 50 h in humans (Muller et al., 1974) and approximately 200 h in dogs (Muller et al., 1974).

TCA is much less extensively metabolized than other HAAs found in drinking-water. However, one metabolite is DCA (Larson & Bull, 1992), which is subsequently converted to glyoxylate, glycolate and oxalate, as outlined in Figure 5. This in turn explains the extensive incorporation of radiolabel from ^{14}C-TCA into blood (Stevens et al., 1992) and tissues (Eyre et al., 1995), as glyoxylate is rapidly trans-aminated and converted to glycine.

In mice, some of TCA's metabolism is independent of the formation of DCA as an intermediate. There is evidence that a signi-ficant amount of oxalate is formed independently of DCA formation and that some direct decarboxylation of trihaloacetates also occurs. The evidence for these pathways comes largely from studies of the metab-olism of bromodichloroacetate (BDCA) (Xu et al., 1995). The conversion of TCA is, however, much slower than that of BDCA. The basis for the overall scheme is discussed more fully in the following section on brominated HAAs. The reader is also referred to Figure 5 and the accompanying text for explanation of the further metabolism of DCA.

4.2.2.8   Mode of action

The tumorigenic effects of TCA in the liver of B6C3F$_1$ mice appear to be closely related to its ability to induce synthesis of peroxi-somes and associated proteins (DeAngelo et al., 1989; Bull et al., 1990; Pereira, 1996). Along with a number of other peroxisome pro-liferators, TCA was shown to be capable of activating the PPAR *in vitro* at concentrations consistent with the levels that are achieved *in vivo* (Issemann & Green, 1990). The cause-and-effect relationships between the activation of this receptor and the induction of cancer are yet to be established. Based upon marked increases in the numbers of peroxisomes that are observed in rodent species that are susceptible to this class of carcinogen and the lack of such responses in other mammalian species, it has been argued that humans are minimally sensitive to the tumorigenic effects of these compounds (Lake, 1995).

194

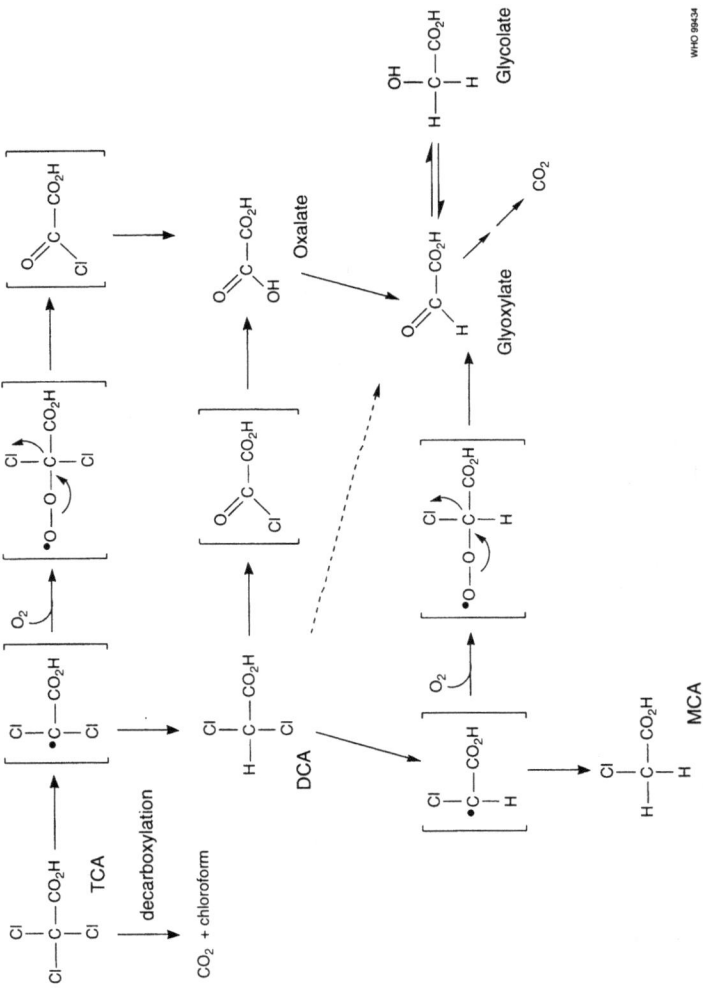

Fig. 5. Scheme for the metabolism of TCA (from Austin & Bull, 1997).

Peroxisome proliferators are also known to variably affect reproduction and development. Considering the types of interactions in which the PPAR is involved, these observations are not too surprising. However, it is not clear whether a consistent pattern of developmental anomalies can be associated with activation of this receptor.

A mouse that was genetically engineered with a targeted disruption PPAR-α gene failed to respond to the pleiotropic effects of peroxisome proliferators (Lee et al., 1995).

Non-rodent species, including humans, express the PPARs, and peroxisome proliferator responsive elements (PPREs) have been identified in the promoter regions of the genes that are analogous to those that are induced in rodents (Varanasi et al., 1996). This suggests that the responsiveness to peroxisome proliferators is in some way modified by other factors. However, the expression of PPARs in humans is low.

It is important to recognize that other mechanisms may be involved in TCA-induced effects. Clearly, the production of DCA as a metabolite could be involved in inducing effects associated with this metabolite. The very high rate of DCA metabolism relative to the rate of TCA metabolism has made it difficult to detect significant amounts of DCA in the blood (Merdink et al., 1998). There is little doubt that some DCA is formed in all species. In addition to DCA, there are a number of reactive and stable metabolites that could contribute to toxicity. At this time, there is no evidence that the acid chloride intermediate postulated between DCA and oxalate contributes anything to the toxic effects of TCA. Chronic TCA administration results in the deposition of lipofuscin, a sign of increased oxidative stress. Moreover, Austin et al. (1995, 1996) obtained evidence of increased lipid peroxidation and increased levels of 8-OH-dG in nuclear DNA of the liver of mice treated with single doses of TCA. Therefore, the accumulation of lipofuscin could be associated with mechanisms unrelated to peroxisome proliferation. The most likely radical-generating sources for lipid peroxidation and oxidative damage to DNA would be through the formation of the radical species (carbon-centred radicals and the peroxy radicals that would be derived from the reaction of molecular oxygen with the carbon-centred radicals). Again, there is no direct evidence to indicate that these processes are important to any toxicological response associated with TCA treatment or exposure.

It is beyond the scope of the present review to resolve risk assessment issues associated with peroxisome proliferators. However, several points should be made specific to TCA. First, peroxisome proliferative responses are not genotoxic responses. Second, TCA is one of the weakest activators of the PPAR known (Issemann & Green, 1990). Finally, TCA appears to be only marginally active as a peroxisome proliferator, even in rats (DeAngelo et al., 1989). Furthermore, treatment of rats with high levels of TCA in drinking-water does not induce liver tumours (DeAngelo et al., 1997). These data strongly suggest that TCA presents little carcinogenic hazard to humans at the low concentrations found in drinking-water.

The key question is whether the carcinogenic and teratogenic effects of TCA observed at very high doses have any relevance at the exposures that are obtained even under extreme conditions in drinking-water. However, the application of conventional uncertainty factors would suggest that TCA in drinking-water represents little hazard to humans at the concentrations normally encountered in chlorinated drinking-water.

4.2.3 Brominated haloacetic acids

Brominated HAAs are formed in waters that contain bromide, which strong oxidants like chlorine and ozone are capable of oxidizing to hypobromous acid. There are very limited data available on the toxicity of these chemicals. Therefore, they will be considered as a group. The discussion below focuses on similarities and differences between brominated and chlorinated HAAs.

4.2.3.1 General toxicological properties and information on dose–response in animals

Linder et al. (1994a) found that the oral LD_{50} for MBA was 177 mg/kg of body weight in adult male Sprague-Dawley rats. DBA was much less toxic, with an LD_{50} of 1737 mg/kg of body weight. The acute toxicities of the bromochloroacetates have not been determined.

No studies have been published on the brominated haloacetates. Some of the information is available in abstract form and will be touched on briefly.

Bull and co-workers (Bull & DeAngelo, 1995; Stauber et al., 1998) conducted a series of experiments with DBA, bromochloro-acetate (BCA) and BDCA administered to male B6C3F$_1$ mice at concentrations ranging from 0.2 to 3 g/litre in their drinking-water. The data obtained from these studies suggest that toxicological effects are observed in approximately the same concentration ranges as for DCA- and TCA-induced toxic effects.

The principal target organ in mice was identified as the liver for all three brominated HAAs, but the nature of the effects on the liver appears to be somewhat different for each compound. All the bro-minated HAAs produce hepatomegaly, but glycogen accumulation and cytomegaly are more prominent with BCA and BDCA than with DBA. Conversely, DBA was reported to produce increases in cyanide-insensitive acyl CoA activity in the liver. BCA and BDCA produced only small and inconsistent effects on this marker of peroxisome proliferation. Thus, it appears that DBA shares TCA's ability to induce peroxisome proliferation, whereas BCA and BDCA appear to produce effects much more like those induced by DCA. Consistent with this, the severity of the hepatomegaly was BCA > BDCA > DBA.

Administration of single doses of BDCA, BCA and DBA by gavage in water as the vehicle induced increases in thiobarbituric acid reactive substances (TBARS) and increased the 8-OH-dG content of nuclear DNA in the liver of male B6C3F$_1$ mice at doses as low as 30 mg/kg of body weight (Austin et al., 1996). These effects were significantly greater than those observed with TCA and DCA and tended to increase as the bromine substitution increased within each series. The order of potency was DBA = BCA > BDCA > DCA > TCA. Increases in 8-OH-dG content were more rapid and more sustained with the brominated HAAs. This indicates that brominated HAAs do induce oxidative stress.

Dose-related increases in the 8-OH-dG content of nuclear DNA of the liver were observed when DBA and BCA were administered in drinking-water to male B6C3F$_1$ mice for periods from 3 to 10 weeks at concentrations of 0.5 g/litre and above (Parrish et al., 1996). The effect of BDCA in drinking-water was not evaluated. It is noted that these effects were observed in the same range in which liver tumours are induced in mice (discussed further below).

4.2.3.2 Reproductive effects

MBA and DBA have been examined for spermatotoxic effects in rats. MBA did not affect parameters related to male reproductive function (Linder et al., 1994a) when administered to rats as a single dose of 100 mg/kg of body weight or at 25 mg/kg of body weight per day administered repeatedly for 14 consecutive days. In contrast, DBA produced degenerating, misshapen epididymal sperm and abnormal retention of step 19 spermatids following single doses of DBA in the range 1000–2000 mg/kg of body weight. Caput sperm counts were significantly reduced on the second day, and substantial reductions of cauda sperm counts were observed at 14 and 28 days after treatment. Serum testosterone levels were significantly depressed on day 2 but returned to control levels by day 14. Sperm displayed defects in development of the shape of sperm heads. Progressive motility of sperm was significantly reduced at 14 and 28 days after treatment.

A subsequent paper by the same group described a study in which doses of 0, 10, 30, 90 or 270 mg of DBA per kg of body weight were administered to rats for 14 consecutive days (Linder et al., 1994b). Marked effects on epididymal sperm counts and sperm morphology effects were observed at the highest dose. Approximately 5% of the caput sperm were fused. In contrast to the single-dose studies, serum testosterone levels appeared to be unaffected. Spermiation also appeared to be mildly affected, with step 19 spermatids being retained beyond stage VIII in animals dosed with as little as 10 mg/kg of body weight per day.

DBA was administered to rats for up to 79 days at 0, 2, 10, 50 or 250 mg/kg of body weight per day by gavage in water. Male fertility was compromised during the second week of treatment at the high dose. This effect appeared to result from behavioural changes, because artificial insemination with sperm collected on day 9 of treatment produced offspring. By day 15, however, no offspring were produced with either biological or artificial insemination, indicating that significant qualitative alterations had occurred in the sperm. Indeed, the 50 mg/kg of body weight per day dose produced abnormal morphology, decreased motility and decreases in epididymal sperm counts. However, rats treated at this dose remained fertile. While no effects on sperm quality were observed at lower doses, reproductive performance appeared depressed at doses as low as 10 mg/kg of body weight per day, suggesting that these lower doses modified behaviour (Linder et al., 1995).

Histopathological changes were observed in the testis and epididymis of rats gavaged daily for 2–79 days with DBA. On treatment day 2, abnormal retention of step 19 spermatids was observed in animals given the highest dose of 250 mg/kg of body weight per day. Additional changes on day 5 included the fusion of mature spermatids and the presence of atypical residual bodies (ARB) in the epithelium and lumen of stage X–XII seminiferous tubules. By day 9, ARB were seen in most stages of the seminiferous epithelial cycle and in the caput epididymis. On day 16, distorted sperm heads were recognized in step 12 and older spermatids, and luminal cytoplasmic debris was found throughout the epididymis. On day 31, there was vacuolation of the Sertoli cell cytoplasm, extensive retention of step 19 spermatids near the lumen of stage IX and X tubules, and vesiculation of the acrosomes of late spermatids. Marked atrophy of the seminiferous tubules was present 6 months after 42 doses of 250 mg/kg of body weight per day. ARB and retention of step 19 spermatids were observed after 31 and 79 doses of 50 mg/kg of body weight per day, and increased retention of step 19 spermatids was seen in several rats dosed with 10 mg/kg of body weight per day. No abnormalities were detected at 2 mg/kg of body weight per day. The changes suggest that the testicular effects of DBA are sequelae to structural or functional changes in the Sertoli cell (Linder et al., 1997b).

4.2.3.3   Neurotoxicity

Reference was made to neurotoxic effects in male Sprague-Dawley rats treated with DBA in reproductive studies (Linder et al., 1994a,b, 1995). However, no specific investigations of the neurotoxic effects of brominated HAAs appear to be available.

4.2.3.4   Toxicity in humans

There are no studies on the health effects of brominated HAAs in humans.

4.2.3.5   Carcinogenicity and mutagenicity

No formal reports have been made of carcinogenic or mutagenic effects of brominated HAAs. Indications that DBA, BCA and BDCA share the hepatocarcinogenic effects of TCA and DCA in B6C3F$_1$ mice have been referred to in an abstract (Bull & DeAngelo, 1995).

Giller et al. (1997) examined the genotoxicity of MBA, DBA, and tribromoacetic acid (TBA) in the SOS chromotest in *Escherichia coli* PQ37, the Ames fluctuation assay utilizing *Salmonella typhimurium* strain TA100 and the newt micronucleus assay in larvae at stage 53 of the developmental table. MBA was negative in the SOS chromotest at levels as high as 1000 µg/ml and in the newt micronucleus assay. However, it was active at concentrations as low as 20 µg/ml in the Ames fluctuation assay with S9 fraction added to the incubation medium. DBA was positive with and without S9 fraction in the SOS chromotest, requiring 100 µg/ml in the former case and 200 µg/ml in the latter. Thus, it is about 5 times as potent as DCA in this test. In the Ames fluctuation assay, DBA was active at 10 µg/ml without S9 and at 30 µg/ml with S9. TBA was active in the SOS chromotest at 100 µg/ml with S9 but required 2000 µg/ml for activity in the Ames fluctuation assay without S9.

4.2.3.6   Comparative pharmacokinetics and metabolism

Metabolism of brominated HAAs has received little attention. Xu et al. (1995) studied the metabolism of BDCA in male B6C3F$_1$ mice. As predicted, substitution of a bromine for a chlorine in TCA resulted in a substantially greater extent of trihaloacetate metabolism. Whereas 45% of a 100 mg/kg of body weight dose of TCA was eliminated unchanged in the urine of mice within 24 h, less than 4% of the same dose of BDCA was found in the urine. At lower doses, only a fraction of a percent of the BDCA was eliminated unchanged.

There is evidence for substantial conversion of BDCA to DCA in both rats and mice (Xu et al., 1995; Schultz et al., 1999). Because of the established ability of DCA to induce hepatic tumours in both mice and rats (discussed above), this may have implications for assessing the risk associated with this compound (see Figures 3 and 5 for a general description of dihaloacetate and trihaloacetate metabolism, respectively).

The metabolism of BDCA is differentially modified in mice and rats as doses are increased. Xu et al. (1995) found that the kinetics of carbon dioxide production from 1-^{14}C-BDCA suggested an efficient conversion of BDCA to carbon dioxide through DCA at low doses, but a direct decarboxylation reaction became important as doses approached 100 mg/kg of body weight (Xu et al., 1995; Austin & Bull, 1997). This complex activity was not observed in rats (Schultz et al., 1999), in that a progressively smaller fraction of the dose is converted to carbon dioxide as dose is increased. This suggests that direct decarboxylation plays a less important role in the metabolism of BDCA in rats than in mice.

The ratios of urinary metabolites produced by mice and rats suggest that there are some substantive differences in the metabolism of BDCA in the two species. Mice (Xu et al., 1995) produce much higher amounts of oxalate (about 30% of the orally administered dose) than do rats (about 20%) (Schultz et al., 1999). The much greater conversion of BDCA to oxalate than for equivalent doses of DCA suggests that much of the extra oxalate seen in mouse urine arises from reductive dehalogenation of BDCA, followed by peroxy radical formation and decomposition to oxalate (Xu et al., 1995).

As the BDCA dose is increased from 20 to 100 mg/kg of body weight in the rat, the fraction of the dose that is eliminated in the urine as DCA increases from about 2% to 13% (Schultz et al., 1999), whereas in mice the increase is from 0.2% to approximately 3%. In the rat, increasing the dose from 5 mg/kg of body weight to 20 or 100 mg/kg of body weight was associated with a significantly extended half-life of both BDCA and DCA (from 0.9 to 3.7 h). The increased half-life appears to be attributed to saturation of the conversion of BDCA to DCA. Despite this inhibition of DCA formation, the blood levels of DCA observed are actually higher than those observed when equivalent doses of DCA itself are administered. Thus, high doses of BDCA would appear to inhibit the metabolic clearance of DCA as well. Consequently, the toxicology of BDCA should share many of the attributes of DCA toxicology in the rat. Comparable data do not exist on the blood levels of DCA achieved by BDCA administration in mice, but the urinary levels of DCA metabolites appear to be largely offset by the conversion of BDCA to oxalate, suggesting that the blood levels of DCA would be significantly lower in mice than in rats.

In animals previously treated with 1 g of DCA per litre in drinking-water, metabolism of BDCA to carbon dioxide is significantly increased in mice (Austin & Bull, 1997). This appears to be associated with an increase in the capacity for the direct decarboxylation of BDCA to form BDCM and carbon dioxide. Therefore, some effects of BDCA in mice may be attributed to the formation of BDCM.

These data and data indicating that pretreatment with DCA also affects its own metabolism suggest that there may be significant interactions in the toxicity of these chemicals at high doses. It remains to be seen if such interactions occur at treatment concentrations that more closely approximate those observed in drinking-water.

4.2.3.7   Mode of action

It is premature to attempt a definitive discussion of the mechanisms by which brominated HAAs induce tumours. There are suggestions of mechanisms that need to be pursued with this class, but there are really no data that demonstrate how they contribute to the induction of cancer, nor is there a firm basis for considering whether these mechanisms are relevant at the low concentrations of these chemicals found in drinking-water.

The mechanisms associated with the carcinogenic effects of HAAs include those identified for DCA and TCA. It is apparent that more than one mechanism is responsible for the effects of this class and that the importance of these mechanisms to the activity of individual members of the class varies. In part, these differences in mechanism can be related to the differences in tumour phenotypes that are induced. One phenotype seems to be associated with prior characterizations of tumours induced by peroxisome proliferators and is induced by TCA (DeAngelo et al., 1989; Stauber et al., 1998). The second phenotype involves glycogen-poor tumours that stain heavily with antibodies to c-Jun and c-Fos. This phenotype is produced by DCA. These effects are probably produced by selection of lesions with differing defects in cell signalling pathways that control the processes of cell division and cell death.

Based upon the data of Giller at al. (1997), the brominated HAAs are about 10-fold more potent than their chlorinated analogues in their ability to induce point mutations. This does not establish that they are inducing cancer by mutagenic mechanisms *in vivo*, but this activity will have to be taken into account as data on their carcinogenic activity become more complete.

The HAAs vary widely in their ability to induce oxidative stress and to elevate the 8-OH-dG content of nuclear DNA of the liver. This property becomes increasingly apparent with the brominated compounds (Austin et al., 1996; Parrish et al., 1996). It is notable that the brominated analogues are not more potent inducers of hepatic tumours than the corresponding chlorinated HAAs. Therefore, it is doubtful that this mechanism is the most important determinant of this effect.

No specific mechanisms have been associated with the effects of DBA on male reproduction or as a developmental toxin. However, it would be surprising if the effects on cell signalling systems that appear to be involved in the carcinogenic responses do not also contribute to these effects.

4.2.4 *Higher molecular weight halogenated acids*

Studies of by-product formation from humic and fulvic acids in the 1970s and early 1980s demonstrated that there is a complex array of halogenated carboxylic acids in addition to the HAAs (Christman et al., 1983). Some of these acids have been identified in drinking-water as well, but, as discussed elsewhere in this document, both the scope and quantitative nature of the data that are available for drinking-water itself are limited. Little attention has been paid to these higher molecular weight acids in either the toxicological or epidemiological literature. However, it is important to recognize that they make up the bulk of the total organic halogen that is present in drinking-water.

Beyond the HAAs, the most studied group of halogenated acids are the chloropropionic acids. As with DCA, the major impetus for these studies has been potential therapeutic applications rather than concerns over exposure to the compounds as contaminants of drinking-water. Therefore, there are few data that have been developed for hazard identification purposes, and even less information is available on dose–response on effects other than those being explored for therapeutic purposes.

By far the most data on chloropropionic acids exist for 2-chloropropionate (2-CP). This compound shares the hypoglycaemic effects of DCA. It was first used as an experimental tool to segregate direct effects of DCA from those of its metabolites. Oxalate and glyoxylate are two metabolites of DCA that seem to be responsible for its effects on gluconeogenesis from lactate (Crabb & Harris, 1979). Since 2-CP is not metabolized to these compounds and failed to inhibit gluconeogenesis, these data effectively argue that this effect of DCA is largely attributable to these two metabolites. In contrast, 2-CP still decreased blood glucose in rats when infused intravenously at a rate of 300 mg/kg of body weight per hour. As with DCA, 2-CP increased concentrations of circulating ketone bodies but significantly reduced blood concentrations of lactate. As had been previously demonstrated with DCA, concentrations of 1 and 5 mmol of 2-CP per litre significantly enhanced the activity of pyruvate dehydrogenase.

Yount et al. (1982) compared the effects of DCA and 2-CP in mice and rats. They extended these investigations into the area of comparative toxicities of the two compounds as well. The acute oral LD_{50} for 2-CP in fasted ICR mice was 15.4 ± 0.1 mmol/kg of body weight, making it approximately twice as toxic as DCA on a molar basis. However, neither compound is really very toxic acutely (2-CP = 1671 mg/kg of body weight; DCA = 4100 mg/kg of body weight).

Male Wistar rats were administered the sodium salts of 2-CP and DCA at 0.04 mol/kg of feed for 12 weeks. These concentrations correspond to about 4.3 and 5.1 g of 2-CP and DCA per kg of feed, respectively. Actual doses to the animals are difficult to calculate accurately because the body weights were not provided and because significant effects of both compounds on body weight gain were noted. If an average weight of 300 g is assumed for rats for the duration of the experiment (i.e., study was started with weanling rats), the doses can be estimated to be roughly 300 mg/kg of body weight per day for DCA and 250 mg/kg of body weight per day for 2-CP.

Both DCA and 2-CP decreased the growth rate and food consumption of treated rats and caused neurotoxic effects (e.g., hind limb weakness). 2-CP treatment caused testicular abnormalities and significantly lowered plasma triacylglycerol levels compared with control or DCA-treated rats. In mature rats, total serum ketone bodies were increased by DCA but not by 2-CP (Yount et al., 1982).

2-CP, as either the L- or D-isomer, is rapidly and extensively metabolized in the liver cytosol by a mechanism that depletes GSH (Wyatt et al., 1996). Significant depletion of non-protein sulfhydryl content (primarily GSH) was observed with single acute oral doses of 62.5 mg/kg of body weight and above in male Alderley Park Wistar-derived rats. This effect was observed to be maximal at 4 h and returned to control values in approximately 48 h. A slower depletion of non-protein sulfhydryl content was observed in the cerebellum and forebrain with doses of 750 mg/kg of body weight. The depletion was observed to be maximal about 24 h after administration in the cerebellum and between 12 and 24 h in the forebrain. The depletion in the cerebellum occurred with doses that also resulted in the induction of granule cell necrosis in the cerebellum. Although depletion of non-protein sulfhydryl groups tended to recover in the liver, the effect in the cerebellum appeared to be partially cumulative with each daily dose.

As with DCA, the largest capacity for 2-CP metabolism appears to be in the cytosolic fraction of the hepatocyte, whereas metabolism in microsomes is quite small. L-CP appears to be slightly more active in depleting cytosolic fractions of GSH. In the process, the metabolite 2-*S*-glutathionylpropanic acid is formed. On the basis of the stoichiometry between GSH depletion and formation of this product and prior observations of Polhuijs et al. (1989, 1991) with 2-bromocarboxylic acids, it was concluded that 2-CP was a substrate for a θ-class GST.

4.3 Haloaldehydes and haloketones

A diverse set of halogenated aldehydes and ketones are formed in the disinfection of drinking-water. The most important in terms of having been identified in drinking-water is trichloroacetaldehyde or chloral hydrate, which is discussed separately. The remainder of the group is discussed collectively. From the perspective of drinking-water problems, the class has received very little attention, but its members have been identified as key metabolites of chemicals such as trichloroethylene, vinyl chloride and dibromochloropropane (Omichinski et al., 1988; Spengler & Singer, 1988). The principal evidence that they are formed comes from studies of chlorinated humic and fulvic acids (Meier et al., 1983, 1985a) and of kraft pulp chlorination (Kringstad et al., 1981). However, when specifically looked for in drinking-water using techniques with adequate analytical sensitivity, selected members of the group have been found in concentrations that are somewhere between those of the HANs and HAAs (Coleman et al., 1984).

These two classes of chemicals played an important role in the initial studies of chemicals formed in the chlorination of drinking-water. The interest in them was sparked by the fact that they were among the first by-products to be identified that contributed to the mutagenic activity produced in chlorinated water (Cheh et al., 1980). Attention faded from this group when MX was identified, because this compound contributed the major proportion of the mutagenic activity produced by chlorine (Meier, 1988). Because these chemicals represent an additional group of mutagenic chemicals, some of which are capable of initiating skin tumours, it is important to acknowledge their presence. However, because of the lack of data that can be used to assess the degree of hazard, the present review will not be comprehensive.

4.3.1 Chloral hydrate (trichloroacetaldehyde, chloral)

Trichloroacetaldehyde (chloral) is hydrated in water and in the body to form the well-known sedative-hypnotic, chloral hydrate. Most toxicological and metabolic studies have been conducted with chloral hydrate rather than trying to deal with maintaining the aldehyde in the dehydrated state.

It should be recognized that where there are significant amounts of bromide in treated drinking-water, the use of oxidants will also produce brominated analogues of chloral hydrate. This has been poorly documented with the trihaloacetaldehydes, but the brominated analogues have been observed in a system where chlorination reactions with fulvic acid are conducted in the presence of high bromide concentrations (Xie & Reckhow, 1993). The lack of data from actual water supplies is in large part due to the lack of appropriate analytical standards. In a broad sense, however, the ratios of chloral hydrate, bromodichloroacetaldehyde, dibromochloroacetaldehyde and tribromo-acetaldehyde should more or less parallel those seen with the analogous trihaloacetates. A second problem is that there is not a significant body of toxicological literature available for these analogues because they are not utilized in commerce. This represents a significant data gap because bromine substitution can be anticipated to result in greater metabolism of the trihaloacetaldehydes, as has been demonstrated for the trihaloacetates (Xu et al., 1995). As a consequence, an exaggeration of those effects of chloral hydrate that are secondary to metabolism through reactive intermediates might be expected (Hoz et al., 1991). Owing to the lack of data, however, it is inappropriate to speculate much further. Therefore, the remainder of this section will specifically address the data that are available for chloral hydrate.

4.3.1.1   *General toxicological properties and information on dose–response in animals*

Chloral hydrate is primarily known for its depressant effects on the central nervous system (Gilman et al., 1991). The usual doses required to produce central nervous system depression in humans range from about 500 to 2000 mg in adults. These effects do not appear to have been extensively studied in experimental animals.

Chloral hydrate was administered for 90 days in drinking-water to male and female Sprague-Dawley rats at concentrations of 300, 600, 1200 or 2400 mg/litre. Hepatocellular necrosis was observed in 2 of 10 male rats treated with concentrations of either 1200 or 2400 mg of chloral hydrate per litre (Daniel et al., 1992b). No liver damage was seen in female rats. The necrosis observed at the highest dose was indicated as being more severe than that observed at 1200 mg/litre, providing some indication of a dose–response. It is of interest that there was no sign of hepatomegaly produced by chloral hydrate at either this dose or any lower dose. If it is assumed that rats drink about 10% of their body weight per day, the level of 1200 mg/litre corresponds to approximately 120 mg/kg of body weight per day, or about 8 g for a 70-kg human, close to the estimated doses in the study by van Heijst et al. (1977).

In contrast to findings in rats, male CD-1 mice displayed hepatomegaly when doses of 144 mg of chloral hydrate per kg of body weight per day were administered by gavage for a period of 14 days (Sanders et al., 1982). No effect was observed at 14.4 mg/kg of body weight per day. Other organs remained normal at gross necropsy, and there were no signs of altered serum enzyme levels (e.g., LDH or serum glutamate–pyruvate transaminase [SGPT]) or altered BUN. These data suggest that chloral hydrate is not cytotoxic at these doses. This short-term experiment was followed by a second experiment in which mice (140 per sex per group) were administered 70 or 700 mg of chloral hydrate per litre in drinking-water for up to 90 days. These levels were estimated to yield the same doses as those used in the 14-day range-finding study and averaged 18 or 173 mg/kg of body weight per day for female mice and 16 or 160 mg/kg of body weight per day for male mice. Male mice displayed hepatomegaly after 90 days of treatment at both the low and high doses (Sanders et al., 1982). Small, but statistically significant, increases in LDH and serum glutamate–oxaloacetate transaminase (SGOT) were observed at the high dose, but not at 70 mg/litre. The female mice did not demonstrate the hepatomegaly observed in males, but they did show alterations in hepatic microsomal parameters. These data are of potential significance in considering the greater sensitivity of mice (albeit of another strain) to the hepato-carcinogenic effects of chloral hydrate as compared with rats.

Chloral hydrate has the potential of interacting with other drugs by direct and indirect means. Most commonly cited is a potentiation with alcohol that has been associated with the so-called "Mickey Finn" (Gilman et al., 1991). This is attributed to interactions with common steps in the metabolism of both chloral hydrate and alcohol (Gessner & Cabana, 1970; Sellers et al., 1972). Combined exposure appears to interfere with glucuronidation of the metabolite trichloroethanol and with its conversion to TCA (Kaplan et al., 1967; Sellers et al., 1972). Moreover, trichloroethanol is probably the metabolite of chloral hydrate that is primarily responsible for its central nervous system depressant effects (Gilman et al., 1991); thus, there is undoubtedly somewhat of a pharmacological interaction as well. Increased sensitivity to the hypnotic activity of chloral hydrate in paraoxon-treated animals has been suggested to result from an increased sensitivity of the brain to hypoxia (Koepke et al., 1974). The other major interaction associated with chloral hydrate is the ability of its metabolites, particularly TCA, to compete for binding sites on plasma proteins. This type of interaction has been held responsible for increased pharmacological and toxicological reactions to warfarin (Sellers & Koch-Weser, 1970; Koch-Weser et al., 1971) and bis-hydroxycoumarin (Cucinell et al., 1966).

4.3.1.2   Toxicity in humans

The primary effect seen with ingestion of chloral hydrate is central nervous system depression, the basis of its use in therapeutics. The usual dose recommended for sedation is 250 mg 3 times daily. The hypnotic dose is generally given as 500–1000 mg, but 2000 mg is required to be effective in many adults (Gilman et al., 1991). Neonates are frequently treated with doses of chloral hydrate in the range of 30–40 mg/kg of body weight (Lambert et al., 1990). In recent years, chloral hydrate has become popular for sedating subjects, particularly children, to aid in performing diagnostic procedures such as CT scans, electroencephalograms (EEG) and electrocardiograms (ECG), where relatively higher doses have been utilized (32–80 mg/kg of body weight, Silver & Steir, 1971; 100 mg/kg of body weight, Farber & Abramow, 1985).

The most important acute toxic effect is the production of cardiac arrhythmias. Where doses in adults have been estimated, they are considerably above those commonly used for therapeutic purposes, most often in excess of 8 g. Most of the available studies involved poisoning or overdose situations. However, one study closely examined the induction of arrhythmias in paediatric cases undergoing EEGs (Silver & Steir, 1971). The dose range was 32–80 mg/kg of body weight, and in only 2 of 12 subjects was a sinus arrhythmia associated with the administration of chloral hydrate. This suggests that doses at the lower end of this range may approximate a threshold. Doses in the range of 96 mg/kg of body weight and above have consistently been shown to produce arrhythmias in children (Nordenberg et al., 1971; Farber & Abramow, 1985; Hirsch & Zauder, 1986). In a 70-kg adult, 32 mg/kg of body weight would equal a dose of 2240 mg.

Lower doses of chloral hydrate have been associated with some adverse side-effects. A study of newborns administered chloral hydrate indicated a high incidence of direct hyperbilirubinaemia (Lambert et al., 1990). This effect was associated more with continuous use than with an acute dose, however. The dose rate to affected (40 mg/kg of body weight) and unaffected (33 mg/kg of body weight) neonates was not significantly different. The total dose in affected children was 1035 mg relative to 135 mg in the unaffected children. Thus, a more protracted use of chloral hydrate in the affected group was apparently responsible for the hyperbilirubinaemia observed. These data suggest that there is little concern over this effect with single doses of chloral hydrate. Because neonates are generally thought to be more sensitive to hyperbilirubinaemia, this effect is probably of less concern for adults.

There have been occasional reports of liver damage induced by high doses of chloral hydrate by ingestion (van Heijst et al., 1977; Gilman et al., 1991). The short-term data from mice, discussed previously, support the conclusion that an effect on the liver is unlikely to be observed in humans until very high doses are reached. Longer-term exposures (e.g., months) lead to some enlargement of the liver, if humans are as sensitive as mice in this regard, but the doses remain considerably above the fraction of a μg/kg of body weight that would be expected from most chlorinated drinking-waters. The clinical literature suggests that humans are closer to rats in the sensitivity of their livers to chloral hydrate.

A single modern case of fixed cutaneous eruptions was noted in the literature (Miller et al., 1966). This was associated with a thera-peutic dose of chloral hydrate (500 mg) in a 57-year-old man. These lesions are termed "fixed" because they tend to occur at the same locations on the body with repeated exposures. An earlier case was reported in 1878. This seems to be a rare side-effect of chloral hydrate that is completely reversible. There have been other reported skin reac-tions to chloral hydrate ingestion, but these appear to be relatively rare as well (Almeyda & Levantine, 1972).

4.3.1.3 Carcinogenicity and mutagenicity

IARC has evaluated the carcinogenicity of chloral and chloral hydrate and concluded that there is inadequate evidence for their carcinogenicity in humans, limited evidence for the carcinogenicity of chloral hydrate in experimental animals and inadequate evidence for the carcinogenicity of chloral in experimental animals. Both chloral and chloral hydrate were assigned to Group 3: the compounds are not classifiable as to their carcinogenicity to humans (IARC, 1995).

A more recent concern with chloral hydrate has been findings that it has some genotoxic and carcinogenic effects in animals and *in vitro* test systems (Table 18). Interpretation of some of these data is difficult, as many investigators failed to document the purity of the chemical

Table 18. Results of genotoxicity assays of chloral hydrate

Dose [conc.]*	Test system	Result	Reference
10 mg/plate	*Salmonella* TA100 TA98	Chloral hydrate purified before use Positive, S9 enhanced slightly Negative	Waskell (1978)
1–5 mg/plate	*Salmonella* TA1535 TA100	 Negative Positive; decreased with S9	Bignami et al. (1980)
2–10 mg/plate	*Streptomyces coelicolor*	Positive	Bignami et al. (1980)
1–10 mg/plate	*Aspergillus nidulans*	Positive	Bignami et al. (1980)
82.7– 413.5 mg/kg bw, i.p.	Mouse spermatocytes	Produces non-disjunction Increases hyperhaploidy at all doses tested	Russo et al. (1984)
[5–20 mmol/ litre]	*Saccharomyces cerevisiae*	Increased mitotic gene conversion at trp+ locus in presence of S9; ilv+ revertants not affected	Bronzetti et al. (1984)
[5–10 mmol/ litre]	*Aspergillus nidulans*	Increased mitotic segregation at both doses, purity stated 99%	Crebelli et al. (1985)
[1–25 mmol/ litre]	*Saccharomyces cerevisiae*	Inhibits sporulation and increased diploid and disomic clones	Sora & Carbone (1987)
[25–250 mmol/ litre]	DNA–protein cross-links in isolated rat liver nuclei	Negative	Keller & Heck (1988)
[0.001– 0.003%]	Chinese hamster embryonic diploid cells	Increased number of aneuploid cells at all doses; other chromosomal aberrations produced at two higher concentrations	Furnus et al. (1990)
0.008–5 mg/plate	*Salmonella* TA98 TA100 TA1535 TA1537 TA1538	All negative, purity of compound specified	Leuschner & Leuschner (1991)

Table 18 (contd).

Dose [conc.][a]	Test system	Result	Reference
500 mg/kg bw, i.p.	Mouse micronucleus	Negative	Leuschner & Leuschner (1991)
100– 1000 mg/kg bw, p.o.	Chromosome, rat bone marrow	Negative at 6 and 24 h	Leuschner & Leuschner (1991)
250–750 µg/ml	Human peripheral blood lymphocytes	Increased hyperdiploid nuclei, and percentage of aneuploid mitosis; purity specified at 99%	Vagnarelli et al. (1990)
300 µg/ml	Ames fluctuation assay	Metabolism-dependent positive response in TA100; negative at 100 µg/ml	Giller et al. (1995)
200 µg/ml	Newt larvae micronucleus assay	Micronuclei in peripheral blood erythrocytes *in vivo*; negative at 100 µg/ml	Giller et al. (1995)

[a] Abbreviations used: conc. = concentration; bw = body weight; i.p. = intraperitoneal; p.o. = per os.

tested. Nevertheless, chloral hydrate tends to be positive in *Salmonella typhimurium* strain TA100, but not in TA98 (Waskell, 1978) or TA1535 (Bignami et al., 1980). The activity towards TA100 was very weak in one assay (Waskell, 1978) and substantially greater in another (Bignami et al., 1980). It was notable that Waskell (1978) recrys-tallized chloral hydrate from alcohol 6 times before subjecting it to test. Bignami et al. (1980) also found that chloral hydrate was capable of inducing point mutations in other test systems. A third group found chloral hydrate to be negative in TA98, TA100, TA1535, TA1537 and TA1538 (Leuschner & Leuschner, 1991), and the purity of the chloral hydrate was specified. Keller & Heck (1988) could find no evidence of DNA–protein cross-links with chloral hydrate treatment of isolated rat liver nuclei. A number of laboratories have shown that chloral hydrate is capable of producing chromosomal aberrations *in vitro* (Bronzetti et al., 1984; Crebelli et al., 1985; Sora & Carbone, 1987; Furnus et al., 1990; Vagnarelli et al., 1990), including aneuploid cells. Chromosomal effects appear to be more consistently observed, and, thus, these results are more convincing. Even in these cases, however, the purity of the compound tested was generally not determined.

Chloral hydrate has been extensively studied as a potentially genotoxic agent. It has been evaluated in the recommended screening battery and several other assays, including genetic alterations in rodent germ cells. Chloral hydrate is positive in bacterial mutation tests, indicating that it is capable of inducing point mutations (Waskell, 1978; Haworth et al., 1983; Giller et al., 1995). It is positive in the mouse lymphoma assay for mutations at the *Tk* locus (Harrington-Brock et al., 1998). Chloral hydrate is also positive in several other *in vitro* assays for genetic damage. It induces anueploidy in Chinese hamster embryonic fibroblasts (Natarajan, 1993), Chinese hamster pulmonary lines LUC2 and Don.Wq.3H (Warr et al., 1993) and human peripheral blood lymphocytes (Sbrana et al., 1993). Positive micronuclei induction was observed in Chinese hamster cells (Lynch & Parry, 1993) and human peripheral blood lymphocytes (Ferguson et al., 1993), and chromosomal aberrations were found in Chinese hamster embryonic diploid cells (Furnus et al., 1990). It is not clear whether chloral hydrate is capable of inducing genetic damage *in vivo*. There is a mixture of positive and negative *in vivo* data. Russo & Levis (1992) found chloral hydrate to be capable of inducing aneuploidy in mouse spermatocytes. Two different groups observed an increase in micronuclei in mouse spermatids when treatment involved exposure of spermatogonia stem cells (Allen et al., 1994; Nutley et al., 1996). Russo et al. (1992) found chloral hydrate to induce micronuclei in mouse bone marrow erythrocytes. Other laboratories have found chloral hydrate to be negative in *in vivo* experiments (Xu & Adler, 1990; Adler, 1993). So far, chloral hydrate has been found to give negative test results in studies with mouse oocytes (Mailhes et al., 1993). Although chloral hydrate can induce a variety of genetic events (mutation, aneuploidy, structural chromosomal aberrations), it does so with a very low potency.

Chloral hydrate has been reported to produce hepatic tumours in male B6C3F₁ mice in two studies. One study administered by gavage a single dose of 5 or 10 mg of chloral hydrate per kg of body weight to groups of 25 and 20 male mice at 15 days of age (Rijhsinghani et al., 1986). The response to the 10 mg/kg of body weight dose led to statistically elevated levels of tumours between 48 and 92 weeks, but the results are based on the appearance of three adenomas and three carcinomas among eight animals. Moreover, the historical control incidence of hepatic tumours in the male of this hybrid is generally about 25% and has been reported to be in excess of 40% in individual studies. Thus, the small numbers of animals make it difficult to give much credence to the results of this study. A second study (Daniel et al., 1992a), however, showed that chloral hydrate administered in drinking-water to a group of 40 male B6C3F$_1$ mice for 104 weeks at 1 g/litre (166 mg/kg of body weight per day) resulted in a 71% incidence of hepatic tumours (combined adenomas and carcinomas). The fact that much higher doses were required to induce tumours in the same hybrid mouse in this study raises further questions about the Rijhsinghani et al. (1986) study; however, mice of this age are known to be very sensitive to tumour initiators (Vesselinovich et al., 1974). However, the Daniel et al. (1992a) study does clearly indicate that chloral hydrate is capable of inducing tumours in B6C3F$_1$ mice when the mice are subjected to a lifetime exposure.[a]

The question of whether chloral hydrate itself contributes to its carcinogenic effects is critical because at least two of its metabolites, TCA and DCA, are comparatively potent inducers of hepatic tumours in B6C3F$_1$ mice. This question can be resolved only by demonstrating (i) that the clastogenic effects of chloral hydrate play a role in the development of tumours or (ii) that TCA, DCA or a combination of both chemicals are produced in sufficient quantities to completely

---

[a] After the Task Group meeting, three new studies in B6C3F$_1$ mice on the carcinogenicity of chloral hydrate appeared (NTP, 2000a,b; George et al., in press). In the first (NTP, 2000a), no carcinogenic effect was observed following the administration of a single dose of chloral hydrate (the dose was up to 5 times higher than that used in the study of Rijhsinghai et al., 1986), while in the two other studies, males had an increased incidence of hepatic tumours after life-time exposure (NTP, 2000b; George et al., in press). In the NTP life-time study (NTP, 2000b), a slightly elevated incidence of pituitary adenomas, of borderline statistical significance, was observed in female mice.

References:

NTP (2000a) Toxicology and carcinogenesis studies of chloral hydrate in B6C3F$_1$ mice (gavage studies). Research Triangle Park, North Carolina, US department of Health and Human Services, National Toxicology Program (NTP-TR-502).

NTP (2000b) Toxicology and carcinogenesis studies of chloral hydrate (ad libitum and dietary controlled) in male B6C3F1 mice (gavage study). Research Triangle Park, North Carolina, US department of Health and Human Services, National Toxicology Program (NTP-TR-503).

George MH, Kilburn S, Moore T & DeAngelo AB (in press) The carcinogenicity of chloral hydrate administered in the drinking water to the male B6C3F$_1$ mouse and F344/N rat. Toxicol Pathol.

account for the induction of liver tumours without significant contribution from earlier, more reactive metabolites. This question is more critically assessed in the next section.

4.3.1.4   Comparative metabolism and pharmacokinetics

The metabolism of chloral hydrate has received considerable attention over the years because of its extensive use as a sedative-hypnotic (Marshall & Owens, 1954; Kaplan et al., 1967; Gessner & Cabana, 1970; Cabana & Gessner, 1970; Sellers et al., 1972; Garrett & Lambert, 1973; Mayers et al., 1991). A series of older studies provide a still valid general picture of the conversion of chloral hydrate to its two major metabolites, trichloroethanol and TCA. More recent studies have focused more specifically on species differences in this metabolism and have begun to focus on minor metabolic pathways.

Figure 6 provides a simplified scheme of chloral hydrate metabolism. The reader is referred to the appropriate sections of this document to evaluate the further metabolism of the products TCA and DCA.

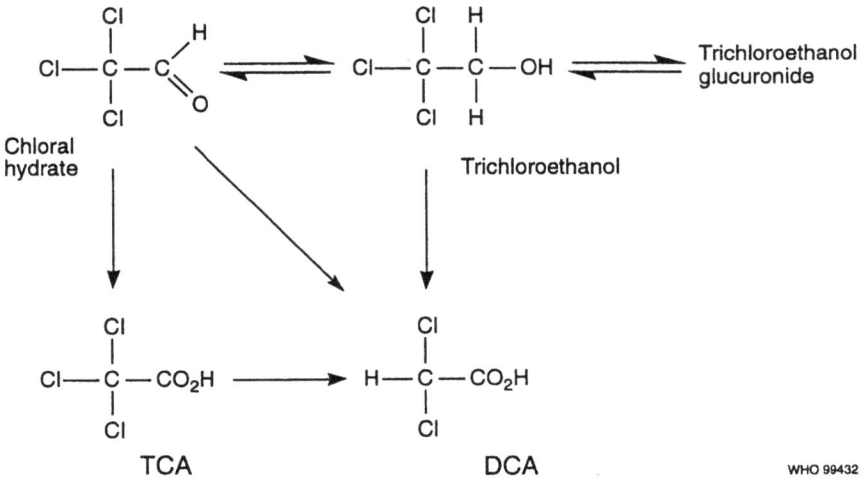

Fig. 6. Metabolism of chloral hydrate in mammalian systems (adapted from Marshall & Owens, 1954; Kaplan et al., 1967).

The major fate of chloral hydrate is to undergo reduction to trichloroethanol, with a smaller, but significant, fraction being oxidized to TCA. Initially, formation of trichloroethanol is favoured because the redox potential within cells *in vivo* favours reduction (Kawamoto et al., 1987). This initial tendency is accentuated by a rapid glucuronidation of the trichloroethanol that is formed (Marshall & Owens, 1954). As is pointed out below, this may be a key feature in the interspecies differences in chloral hydrate metabolism. With time, however, more TCA is formed as a result of enterohepatic circulation of the trichloroethanol glucuronide (Stenner et al., 1996). The glucuronide is hydrolysed to trichloroethanol, which can be oxidized to TCA, with chloral hydrate as an intermediate. Under physiological conditions, the formation of TCA is for all practical purposes irreversible, and the net conversion of chloral hydrate to TCA will continue as long as there are significant amounts of trichloroethanol entrained in the enterohepatic circulation.

The production of these major products of chloral hydrate metabolism is relatively well understood. However, the exact source of a number of minor metabolites is less well understood. The reaction rates and mechanisms involved are just beginning to be studied. Understanding these mechanisms will be key to understanding whether the effects of chloral hydrate can be attributed primarily to its conversion to chemicals of established toxicological properties, such as trichloroethanol, DCA and TCA, or whether the activities of reactive intermediates must also be considered. Formation of DCA probably requires radical formation, but it is not clear whether the radical would be formed from trichloroethanol, chloral hydrate or TCA. If DCA is derived from the first two compounds, the dichloroacetaldehyde that would result as an intermediate could pose some toxicological problems as well. Moreover, Ni et al. (1996) suggested from their ESR data that a trichloromethyl radical is formed from chloral hydrate. Such an intermediate could contribute to the toxicological effects of chloral hydrate as well.

Available pharmacokinetic data have focused upon the relative role of trichloroethanol as the metabolite of chloral hydrate that is responsible for its central nervous system-depressant activity (Butler, 1948, 1949; Marshall & Owens, 1954; Garrett & Lambert, 1973). Conversely, a variety of metabolites have been suggested as responsible for the toxic effects of chloral hydrate and its ability to induce liver cancer in mice, in particular (Daniel et al., 1992a). The critical question is whether an early reactive metabolite — e.g., the free radicals identified by Ni et al. (1996) — induces clastogenic effects that are important to tumour development. The competing, but not necessarily exclusive, hypothesis is that the clearly hepatocarcinogenic metabolites TCA and DCA are produced in sufficient quantity to account for some or all of the liver cancer that results from chloral hydrate treatment.

While TCA and trichloroethanol are well established metabolites of chloral hydrate, DCA has been only recently recognized as a potentially important metabolite with respect to liver tumour induction. Part of the difficulty is that DCA is much more rapidly metabolized than either TCA or trichloroethanol, and peak concentrations would be expected to be significantly lower. This first became apparent when DCA appeared to be produced in significant quantities from trichloro-ethylene administered to B6C3F$_1$ mice (Templin et al., 1993). Chloral hydrate is the first stable metabolite of trichloroethylene metabolism (Cole et al., 1975); thus, these data prompt an examination of the role that chloral hydrate plays in the formation of DCA. In contrast with these results in mice, DCA was not detectable in rats and dogs administered similar doses (Templin et al., 1995). It became apparent that some of the DCA that was measured in these studies may have arisen artefactually through dehalogenation of TCA under acid con-ditions in fresh blood (Ketcha et al., 1996). As a consequence of this series of findings, newer studies have examined whether DCA is produced from chloral hydrate in a number of species.

Recent results of Abbas et al. (1996) showed that doses of 10 and 100 mg of chloral hydrate per kg of body weight result in approxi-mately 2.4 and 10 µg of DCA per ml of blood. However, it must be noted that a variety of artefacts of DCA formation from TCA in blood suggest that these results need to be viewed with caution (Ketcha et al., 1996). Indeed, Merdink et al. (1998) found that DCA was not measur-able in mice dosed with 50 mg of chloral hydrate per kg of body weight.

4.3.1.5   Mode of action

The mechanism of action involved in chloral hydrate-induced liver tumours in mice remains to be established. Clearly, chloral hydrate is converted to at least one metabolite, TCA, that appears to act as a peroxisome proliferator. There is some possibility that it is converted to DCA, a compound that acts primarily as a tumour promoter (Stauber & Bull, 1997). On the other hand, chloral hydrate is distinct from these other two compounds in that it appears to be clastogenic *in vivo*, but at very high doses. The question is, does this clastogenic activity play a role in tumorigenesis? The fact that chloral hydrate appears to produce only hepatic tumours in mice parallels the species specificity of TCA and suggests that other activities are perhaps not involved.

4.3.2 Halogenated aldehydes and ketones other than chloral hydrate

4.3.2.1 General toxicological properties and information on dose–response in animals

1) Haloaldehydes

Relatively few data are available to describe acute, short-term or chronic toxicities for the haloacetaldehydes. In general, aldehydes are irritant chemicals, and substitution of chlorine generally increases this irritancy. However, it is unlikely that irritant effects will occur at concentrations that are encountered in drinking-water. Chloroacetaldehyde is an example of a haloaldehyde for which some data exist, although it has not been commonly found in drinking-water. Concentrations of chloroacetaldehyde as low as 0.02% produced intradermal irritation, 7.5% produced rather severe dermal irritation and 0.03% irritated the eyes of rabbits (Lawrence et al., 1972).

When administered systemically, halogenated aldehydes are quite toxic. Again because of a lack of appropriate data, chloroacetaldehyde will be used for illustrative purposes. Lawrence et al. (1972) reported the oral LD_{50} in Sprague-Dawley rats to be 89 and 103 mg/kg of body weight in males and females, respectively. In male ICR mice, the oral LD_{50} was found to be 82 mg/kg of body weight. In longer-term investigations, Lawrence and co-workers (1972) utilized intraperitoneal injections or inhalation as the method of administration. Intraperitoneal injections of 2.2 or 4.4 mg/kg of body weight per day for 30 days in male Sprague-Dawley rats produced significant decreases in haemoglobin, haematocrit and erythrocytes at the highest dose. This was consistent with its ability to induce haemolysis of erythrocytes at concentrations of 0.2 mol of chloroacetaldehyde per litre and above.

However, the validity of this *in vitro* observation as a dependable indicator of *in vivo* effects is suspect because of the extremely high concentrations that were utilized. The 4.4 mg/kg of body weight dose produced reductions in body weight and induced significant increases in the organ to body weight ratios for the brain, gonads, heart, kidneys, lungs and spleen. These effects appeared to be largely the result of reduced body weight rather than changes in absolute organ weights.

Lawrence et al. (1972) pointed out the importance of route of administration to the toxicity of chloroacetaldehyde. If administered intraperitoneally, it is 10–30 times as potent as its metabolite 2-chloroethanol. However, the toxicity of the two compounds is more or less equivalent when they are administered orally, and 2-chloroethanol is about 4 times as toxic as chloroacetaldehyde when applied topically. These differences are most likely attributed to relative rates of absorption versus metabolic conversion and the many non-specific reactions in which chloroacetaldehyde would be expected to be involved in the gastrointestinal tract and on the skin. This issue should be reflected in the systemic toxicities of halogenated aldehydes, in general.

A 104-week study of chloroacetaldehyde utilizing drinking-water as the mode of administration was conducted in male B6C3F$_1$ mice (Daniel et al., 1992a). Only a single concentration was used (100 mg/litre), which yielded an average dose of 17 mg/kg of body weight (i.e., larger than administered to rats intraperitoneally). This dose did not lead to excessive mortality or depress body weight gains. It did not affect weights of the liver, kidneys, testes or spleen. There was no remarkable non-tumour pathology in 40 tissues that were sampled and examined microscopically in five of the animals that were serially sacrificed during the course of the experiment. An apparent increase in the incidence of liver histopathological change was described as hepatocellular necrosis, hyperplasia and cytomegaly. However, these effects were very mild and of doubtful significance as compared with the same types of pathology in control mice.

Sood & O'Brien (1993) examined the effects of chloroacetaldehyde in isolated rat hepatocytes. A concentration of 0.5 mmol/litre was found to be cytotoxic, whereas 0.2 mmol/litre was without apparent effect. The cytotoxicity could be essentially abolished by dithiothreitol in the incubation media. The requirement for high concentrations in this *in vitro* experiment and the apparent lack of effect (albeit administered to a different species) at relatively high concentrations in the animals' drinking-water (100 mg/litre) suggest that there is little concern about hepatotoxicity at the very low concentrations that might be expected to be found in chlorinated drinking-water.

2)   Haloketones

Toxicological data in experimental animals for the haloketones are extremely limited. The halopropanones are the most commonly studied group of this class, but most of the work has been directed at mutagenic effects of the chemicals.

Laurie et al. (1986) studied the effects of 1,1- and 1,3-DCPN in CD-1 mice. 1,1-DCPN was administered in paraffin, and 1,3-DCPN was administered as an aqueous solution. 1,1-DCPN significantly increased the levels of ASAT, ALAT and LDH at doses of 325 mg/kg of body weight. 1,3-DCPN was evaluated to a maximum dose of 20 mg/kg of body weight and appeared to be without effect on the serum enzymes. However, the LD_{50} for 1,3-DCPN was stated to be 25 mg/kg of body weight, indicating that the liver was probably not the critical target organ for this compound, at least with acute treatment. At doses of 130 mg/kg of body weight and greater, 1,1-DCPN significantly depressed hepatic GSH levels. Again, 1,3-DCPN was without effect at the dose of 20 mg/kg of body weight. Most of the decrease in GSH produced by 1,1-DCPN was observed in the post-mitochondrial cellular fraction as opposed to the mitochondrial fraction.

A major thrust of the Laurie et al. (1986) paper was to determine the extent to which 1,1- and 1,3-DCPN modified the toxicity of carbon tetrachloride. Carbon tetrachloride was administered at doses ranging from 0.02 to 1.0 ml/kg of body weight. The 0.02 ml/kg of body weight dose produced an elevation of serum enzymes on its own. However, when carbon tetrachloride was administered 4 h after 1,1-DCPN, the dose of 1,1-DCPN that was required to significantly increase serum enzyme levels was decreased from 325 to 130 mg/kg of body weight. Since a doubling of the dose of 1,1-DCPN would have produced a similar response and the dose of carbon tetrachloride was above a threshold response level, the interaction between carbon tetrachloride and 1,1-DCPN would seem to be no more than additive. Inhibition of the toxicological effects of carbon tetrachloride in a dose-related manner was observed when 1,3-DCPN was administered prior to carbon tetrachloride.

Merrick et al. (1987) studied the cytotoxic effects of chloro-propanone (CPN), 1,1-DCPN and 1,3-DCPN on isolated hepatocytes of male Sprague-Dawley rats. The chloropropanones were all shown to react with GSH in solution. At concentrations of 10 mmol/litre, the rate of GSH reaction was most rapid with 1,3-DCPN, followed by CPN and then 1,1-DCPN. This reactivity paralleled the ability of the com-pounds to induce cytotoxicity in isolated hepatocytes. Significant increases in ASAT release were observed with 1,3-DCPN at 0.5 mmol/litre, CPN at 1 mmol/litre and 1,1-DCPN at 5 mmol/litre. As would be expected, GSH depletion was observed at concentrations of 1,3-DCPN as low as 0.1 mmol/litre. The other two compounds were significantly less active in depleting GSH, but were of approximately equivalent potency with one another.

A study of 1,1,1-TCPN was conducted in Sprague-Dawley rats by Daniel et al. (1993b). Acute, 10-day and 90-day experiments were performed. 1,1,1-TCPN was administered in corn oil by gavage. Doses in the 10-day study were 0, 16, 48, 161 or 483 mg/kg of body weight per day. In the 90-day study, doses of 30, 90 or 270 mg/kg of body weight per day were administered. In the 10-day study, 8 out of 10 male and 7 out of 10 female rats died at 483 mg/kg of body weight per day before the conclusion of the treatments. Two male rats also died at 161 mg/kg of body weight per day. Although there was not a significant effect on body weight in the survivors, there was a 10% increase in liver to body weight ratios at 161 mg/kg of body weight per day in both male and female rats. Evidence of hyperkeratosis was found in the forestomach of both male and female rats treated at doses of 48 mg/kg of body weight per day and greater. No adverse effect was observed at 16 mg/kg of body weight per day.

Increases in relative liver weight were observed in the 90-day experiment at 270 mg/kg of body weight per day in male rats, but not at 90 mg/kg of body weight per day. Ataxia was reported in both sexes at the 270 mg/kg of body weight per day dose level. Increases in the incidence of forestomach lesions were observed in both sexes at 90 and 270 mg/kg of body weight per day, with the most frequent observation being hyperkeratosis followed by acanthosis. The overall NOAEL in the 10-day and 90-day studies is 30 mg/kg of body weight per day.

In summary, the toxicological effects of the halopropanones provide evidence that some of the representatives of this class are highly toxic, with acute lethal doses being as low as 25 mg/kg of body weight. The gastrointestinal tract and liver appear to be key target organs for some members of the class. However, no target organ was identified for the most acutely toxic of the group, 1,3-DCPN.

4.3.2.2   Toxicity in humans

No data on the effects of either halogenated aldehydes or halogenated ketones on human subjects were identified.

4.3.2.3   Carcinogenicity and mutagenicity

There are considerable data on the mutagenic properties of various halogenated aldehydes and ketones. A comparison of the mutagenic activity, measured in *Salmonella typhimurium* tester strains, of the halogenated aldehydes found in drinking-water with that of chloroacetaldehyde is summarized (not comprehensively) in Table 19. Table 20 provides a similar summary of results with halogenated ketones. These data are presented to demonstrate that the activity of these compounds is not dissimilar from that observed with chloroacetaldehyde, a metabolite of a large number of carcinogenic chemicals, including vinyl chloride. Therefore, it will be used as a prototype for the class. This is not to suggest that this is an adequate substitute for appropriate data for the other compounds. It must be recognized that the data available for this class are completely inadequate for making substantive estimates of the impact of these chemicals on human health; in particular, mutagenicity data in bacterial systems do not necessarily reflect activity *in vivo*.

1)   Haloaldehydes

Chloroacetaldehyde has been extensively studied with respect to the types of interactions that it has with DNA. The adducts formed in animals treated with vinyl chloride are the same as those produced with chloroacetaldehyde (Green & Hathway, 1978). The cyclic etheno adducts formed with cytosine and adenine seem particularly important in mutagenic responses observed with chloroacetaldehyde (Spengler & Singer, 1988; Jacobsen et al., 1989).

Table 19. Mutagenic activity of halogenated aldehydes produced by chlorination in the *Salmonella*/microsome assay

Compound	Strain	Net revertants/ plate		Reference
		−S9	+S9	
Chloroacetaldehyde	TA100	440	~330	Bignami et al. (1980)
2-Chloropropenal	TA100	135	49	Segall et al. (1985)
2-Bromopropenal	TA100	1140	108	Segall et al. (1985)
2-Bromopropenal	TA100	400		Gordon et al. (1985)
2,3-Dibromopropanal	TA100	300		Gordon et al. (1985)
2,3-Dichloropropenal	TA100	91	5	Segall et al. (1985)
3,3-Dichloropropenal	TA100	0.7		Meier et al. (1985a,b)
2,3,3-Trichloropropenal	TA100	224		Rosen et al. (1980)
3-Chloro-2-butenal	TA100	68	42	Segall et al. (1985)
3-Bromo-2-butenal	TA100	108	39	Segall et al. (1985)
2-Bromo-3-methyl-2-butenal	TA100	<0.5	<0.5	Segall et al. (1985)

Table 20. Mutagenic activity of halogenated ketones produced by chlorination in the *Salmonella*/microsome assay

Compound	Strain	Net revertants/ plate		Reference
		−S9	+S9	
CPN	TA100	NM[a]	NM	Merrick et al. (1987)
1,1-DCPN	TA100	0.04		Meier et al. (1985a)
1,3-DCPN	TA100	25.2		Meier et al. (1985a)
1,1,1-TCPN	TA100	0.12		Meier et al. (1985a)
1,1,3-TCPN	TA100	3.9		Douglas et al. (1985)
1,1,3,3-Tetrachloro-propanone	TA100	1.5		Meier et al. (1985a)
Pentachloropropanone	TA100	0.86		Meier et al. (1985a)

[a] NM = non-mutagenic.

There are a limited number of studies that have examined the carcinogenic properties of chloroacetaldehyde in rather specialized test systems. Van Duuren et al. (1979) examined the carcinogenic activity of chloroacetaldehyde in mouse skin initiation/promotion studies, with subcutaneous injection and by stomach tube. In the initiation/promotion assay, chloroacetaldehyde was applied to the skin of 30 female Ha:ICR Swiss mice, at a dose of 1.0 mg per application per mouse, 3 times weekly for up to 581 days, or as a single dose followed by 2.5 µg of TPA 3 times weekly for 576 days. No evidence of increased skin tumour yield was found. The intragastric treatments involved administration of 0.25 mg per mouse per week (1.8 mg/kg of body weight per day if a 20-g body weight is assumed). In this case, sections of lung, liver and stomach were taken for histopathological examination. No signs of increased tumour incidence were found. A fourth experiment involved the subcutaneous injection in 30 mice of 0.25 mg per mouse (1.8 mg/kg of body weight per day, assuming a 20-g body weight for the mouse). Microscopic examination of sections of the liver and injection sites revealed no evidence of increased tumour yield.

A second group of mouse skin initiation/promotion experiments with chloroacetaldehyde were conducted by Zajdela et al. (1980). Single doses of 0.05, 0.1, 1.0 or 2.5 mg of chloroacetaldehyde dissolved in acetone were applied to male and female XVIInc/Z mice (20–28 per group). This was followed by application of TPA at 2 µg, 3 times weekly for 42 weeks. There was no significant difference between mice receiving TPA alone and those that had been initiated by chloroacetaldehyde.

There appears to be only one study that examined the carcinogenic activity of halogenated aldehydes administered in drinking-water over a lifetime (Daniel et al., 1992a). Male B6C3F$_1$ mice treated with 0.1 g of chloroacetaldehyde per litre of drinking-water for 104 weeks were found to have an incidence of eight hepatocellular carcinomas in 26 mice examined (31%). In addition, 8% of these mice were diagnosed as having hepatocellular adenoma, and another 8% were found to have hyperplastic nodules. This compared with two carcinomas in 20 control mice examined (10%), one with adenoma (5%) and no hyperplastic nodules (0%). In a comparison with previous studies, the experiment utilized a significantly higher dose (17 mg/kg of body weight per day) as well as a continuous treatment. It is possible that these tumours were induced by the genotoxic properties of the chemical.

Robinson et al. (1989) examined the ability of four other halogenated aldehydes to act as tumour initiators in the skin of Sencar mice: 2-chloropropenal, 2-bromopropenal, 3,3-dichloropropenal and 2,3,3-trichloropropenal. The compounds were administered topically in six divided doses over a 2-week period (total doses were 600–2400 mg/kg of body weight). Two weeks after the final initiating dose, TPA was applied at a dose of 1 μg, 3 times weekly for 20 weeks. Both 2-chloropropenal and 2-bromopropenal significantly increased tumour yield at 24 weeks and significantly increased the yield of squamous cell carcinomas at 52 weeks at total topical doses of 1200 mg/kg of body weight and above. Both the benign tumour and malignant tumour yields were greater with 2-bromopropenal than with 2-chloropropenal. An experiment utilizing oral administration of these compounds during the initiation period was included in this study. Oral administration of 2-chloropropenal did not produce consistent, dose-related responses. However, there appeared to be a substantial increase in skin tumour yield at an oral dose of 300 mg of 2-bromopropenal per kg of body weight (19 tumours in 38 mice [50%] vs. 20 tumours in 110 control mice [18%]).

On the basis of these studies, it must be concluded that there is a potential carcinogenic hazard associated with the halogenated aldehydes. Only a single compound, chloroacetaldehyde, was evaluated as a carcinogen in a lifetime study, and only one dose level was studied. It appears to be more potent as a carcinogen than the corresponding THM and HAA by-products. Many members of the class are mutagenic, and chloroacetaldehyde, at least, appears to produce tumours in the liver at less than cytotoxic doses. Based upon the comparison between 2-chloropropenal and 2-bromopropenal, there is some reason to believe that the brominated by-products are more potent than the corresponding chlorinated by-products. Therefore, concern must be expressed over disinfection processes that activate bromide, as well as those that simply chlorinate. However, the currently available data are not sufficient to allow the hazards associated with these compounds to be estimated.

2)   Haloketones

A number of halopropanones have been tested in mutagenesis assays. To facilitate comparison of their relative potencies, selected results from assays that were conducted in *Salmonella typhimurium* tester strain TA100 were incorporated into Table 20. For the most part, the data selected for this table were abstracted from papers in which more than one haloketone was evaluated, rather than being selected because they were identified as the best value for each individual chemical that exists in the literature. Some of the compounds have been shown to be active in other *Salmonella* tester strains and other mutagenesis and clastogenesis assays. There was little to be gained from an exhaustive review of this literature, so further consideration of the mutagenic activity will be limited to those systems that extended evaluations to other end-points *in vitro* or attempted to confirm *in vitro* observations *in vivo*.

1,3-DCPN was found to induce SCEs in V79 cells at concentrations as low as 0.002 mmol/litre (von der Hude et al., 1987). Blazak et al. (1988) found that 1,1,1-TCPN and 1,1,3-TCPN were able to act as clastogens in CHO cells *in vitro*. Structural aberrations were produced at a 1,1,3-TCPN concentration of 1.5 g/ml, whereas a concentration of 23 µg/ml was required for a similar response to 1,1,1-TCPN. However, the dose–response for 1,1,3-TCPN was limited by cytotoxicity. Experiments were also conducted focusing on the ability of 1,1,1-TCPN and 1,1,3-TCPN to induce micronuclei in polychromatic erythrocytes and to induce sperm head abnormalities in mice *in vivo*. 1,1,1-TCPN was found to be negative in both assays in the dose range 75–300 mg/kg of body weight, whereas 1,1,3-TCPN was negative in the range 3–12 mg/kg of body weight.

Robinson et al. (1989) tested CPN, 1,1-DCPN, 1,3-DCPN, 1,1,1-TCPN and 1,1,3-TCPN as initiators in the skin of Sencar mice. The compounds were administered by topical application in acetone with total doses that ranged from 37.5 to 4800 mg/kg of body weight (doses of 600 mg/kg of body weight and above were administered in six equal doses over a 2-week period to avoid cytotoxic or lethal effects of the compounds). Other groups of animals treated with the chemicals were also administered similar doses by intragastric intubation. The initiating treatments were followed by a promotion schedule that involved the topical application of 1 μg of TPA 3 times weekly for 20 weeks. Tumour counts were reported at 24 weeks; if the incidence was elevated within this time period, the mice were held until 52 weeks on study prior to sacrifice, and histological evaluations of the tumours were made. Among the haloketones, only 1,3-DCPN was found to produce a dose-related increase in tumour incidence. A single topical dose of 37.5 mg/kg of body weight was sufficient to initiate skin tumours, and the response increased progressively as doses were increased to 150 mg/kg of body weight. At higher doses, the response decreased in magnitude. Splitting the 300 mg/kg of body weight dose into six equal doses over a 2-week period increased the tumorigenic response relative to a single dose of 300 mg/kg of body weight. However, this response was also attenuated, as the multiple-dose schedule utilized higher doses. This attenuation of the response was particularly marked in total tumour yields, which included many benign tumours. It was less effective in limiting the yield of squamous cell carcinomas.

In conclusion, the carcinogenic activity of the DBPs in the haloaldehyde and haloketone classes, with the exception of chloro-acetaldehyde, has not been evaluated in lifetime studies in experimental animals. However, other tests confirm that they have carcinogenic properties. 1,3-DCPN was the most potent tumour initiator in both classes of DBPs. A single dose of 75 mg/kg of body weight produces a total tumour yield equivalent to that produced by 1200 mg of 2-bromopropenal, the most potent of the haloaldehydes, per kg of body weight. 2-Bromopropenal is about 40 times as potent as 1,3-DCPN as a mutagen. The other halopropanones do not appear to be capable of acting as tumour initiators in the mouse skin.

4.3.2.4   Comparative pharmacokinetics and metabolism

No information was identified in the available literature.

4.3.2.5   Mode of action

The data available indicate that these two groups of chemicals contain compounds that possess mutagenic activity. As these effects have been identified in *in vitro* or bacterial test systems, there is no assurance that this is the manner in which they contribute to toxicity or carcinogenicity. A few chemicals have been shown to be initiators in the mouse skin, but it is not clear whether that would be a target organ as a result of chronic ingestion of these chemicals. Other chemicals appear to have activities that could contribute less directly to the induction of cancer, particularly as cytotoxic compounds. It is clear from the limited data available that it would be inappropriate to try to generalize data from only a few examples to these two larger classes of DBPs.

4.4 Haloacetonitriles

4.4.1 *General toxicological properties and information on dose–response in animals and humans*

The HANs are discussed in a single section of this document because the toxicological data on them are quite limited. The dihaloacetonitriles (DHAN) — DCAN, BCAN and DBAN — are the most important in terms of concentrations found in chlorinated drinking-water. However, there are limited data on bromoacetonitrile (BAN), chloroacetonitrile (CAN) and trichloroacetonitrile (TCAN) that are included for completeness.

Hayes et al. (1986) examined the general toxicological effects of DCAN and DBAN in male and female ICR mice and CD rats. In mice, the acute oral (by gavage in corn oil) LD_{50} was reported to be 270 (males) and 279 (females) mg/kg of body weight for DCAN and 289 (males) and 303 (females) mg/kg of body weight for DBAN. In rats, the LD_{50} was found to be 339 (males) and 330 (females) mg/kg of body weight for DCAN and 245 (males) and 361 (females) mg/kg of body weight for DBAN. Hussein & Ahmed (1987) found somewhat lower oral LD_{50}s in rats: BAN, 25.8 mg/kg of body weight; DBAN, 98.9 mg/kg of body weight; CAN, 152.8 mg/kg of body weight; and DCAN, 202.4 mg/kg of body weight. These latter data were reported only in abstract form, and the vehicle used was not indicated. As discussed below, some of the toxicological responses to chemicals in this class appear to depend on the nature of the vehicle in which they were administered.

DCAN and DBAN were also studied over 14- and 90-day treatment intervals (Hayes et al., 1986). DCAN dissolved in corn oil was administered to male and female CD rats by gavage at 12, 23, 45 or 90 mg/kg of body weight per day for 14 days and at 8, 33 or

65 mg/kg of body weight per day for 90 days. DBAN was administered to male and female CD rats at daily doses of 23, 45, 90 or 180 mg/kg of body weight per day for 14 days and at 6, 23 or 45 mg/kg of body weight per day for 90 days. Increased mortality was produced at 33 mg of DCAN per kg of body weight per day and at 45 mg of DBAN per kg of body weight per day in the 90-day studies. Body weight was decreased and lower weights and organ to body weight ratios were observed for spleen and gonads with doses of 65 mg of DCAN per kg of body weight per day and above. The NOAELs for DCAN were 45 mg/kg of body weight per day for 14 days and 8 mg/kg of body weight per day for 90 days of exposure. The NOAELs for DBAN were 23 mg/kg of body weight per day at 90 days and 45 mg/kg of body weight per day at 14 days. No serum chemistry changes indicative of adverse effects were seen with either compound at sublethal doses.

4.4.2   *Reproductive and developmental toxicity*

Smith et al. (1987) examined the effect of CAN, DCAN, TCAN, BCAN and DBAN on female reproduction in an *in vivo* teratology screening test in Long-Evans hooded rats. DCAN and TCAN at doses of 55 mg/kg of body weight administered in tricaprylin by gavage from day 7 to day 21 of gestation significantly reduced the percentage of females delivering viable litters, increased resorption rates and reduced maternal weight gain. BCAN and DBAN at the same dose were without effect. All of the HANs reduced the mean birth weight of pups, and the DHANs reduced the postnatal weight gain till the fourth day after birth. Postnatal survival was reduced with DCAN and TCAN but not with BCAN or DBAN. These pups continued to display reduced body weights into puberty. BCAN also resulted in significantly depressed weights at puberty, although the effect was smaller than that observed with DCAN or TCAN.

The hydra assay system for developmental toxicity has also been used to screen some of the HANs (Fu et al., 1990). Both DBAN and TCAN were found to be of the same general order of toxicity to adult and embryonic animals. Based on these findings, the authors predicted that DBAN and TCAN would not be teratogenic at non-maternally toxic doses.

The developmental toxicity of DCAN was followed up in full-scale teratology studies (Smith et al., 1989b). In this case, DCAN dissolved in tricaprylin was administered to Long-Evans rats at doses of 0, 5, 15, 25 or 45 mg/kg of body weight per day from day 6 to day 18 of gestation. Embryolethality and fetal resorptions were statistically significant at 25 and 45 mg/kg of body weight per day. The highest dose was also maternally toxic. Soft tissue anomalies, including an intraventricular septal defect in the heart, hydronephrosis, fused ureters and cryptorchidism, were observed at this dose. Skeletal abnormalities (fused and cervical ribs) were produced in a dose-dependent manner and were significantly increased at 45 mg/kg of body weight per day. A NOAEL was found to be 15 mg/kg of body weight per day.

TCAN was evaluated in two teratology studies by the same laboratory (Smith et al., 1988; Christ et al., 1996). The first of these studies utilized tricaprylin as the vehicle, whereas the second utilized corn oil. In the first study, embryolethality was observed at doses as low as 7.5 mg/kg of body weight per day. Doses of 15 mg/kg of body weight per day and above produced soft tissue abnormalities, including fetal cardiovascular anomalies (Smith et al., 1988). TCAN administered in a corn oil vehicle produced cardiovascular defects at 55 mg/kg of body weight per day (Christ et al., 1996). The effects observed at this dose were found at significantly lower incidence than observed in the 15 mg/kg of body weight per day dose of the previous study. The abnormalities were milder, being simply positional (laevocardia), instead of the interventricular septal defect and a defect between the ascending aorta and right ventricle that were observed with the tricaprylin vehicle. On the other hand, more skeletal defects were observed with the corn oil vehicle. The authors attributed these differences to an interaction between the tricaprylin vehicle and TCAN. However, tricaprylin and corn oil are not representative of drinking-water exposure. It is not possible to determine whether the results obtained with tricaprylin or the results obtained with corn oil provide the most valid test. The results could be just as readily ascribed to an inhibition of the effects of the corn oil vehicle. As a consequence, these data present somewhat of a difficulty in interpreting results for all of the HANs that have been tested, because the only vehicle in which most have been evaluated was tricaprylin.

4.4.3   *Carcinogenicity and mutagenicity*

IARC has evaluated BCAN, CAN, DBAN, DCAN and TCAN and concluded that there is inadequate evidence for their carcinogenicity in experimental animals. No data were available on their carcinogenicity in humans. Consequently, these HANs were assigned to Group 3: the agent is not classifiable as to its carcinogenicity to humans (IARC, 1991, 1999).

Bull et al. (1985) tested the ability of CAN, DCAN, TCAN, BCAN and DBAN to induce point mutations in the *Salmonella*/ microsome assay, to induce SCEs in CHO cells *in vitro*, to produce micronuclei in polychromatic erythrocytes in CD-1 mice and to act as tumour initiators in the skin of Sencar mice.

DCAN produced a clear increase in mutagenic activity in *Salmonella typhimurium* strains TA1535 and TA100. This response was not altered by the inclusion of the S9 system to metabolically activate the compound, if needed. BCAN also produced a positive response at low doses, but the dose–response curve was interrupted at high doses by cytotoxicity. In this case, the inclusion of the S9 fraction appeared to simply allow the bacteria to survive cytotoxic effects. This perhaps arose through a non-specific inactivation of the electrophilic character of the compound. BCAN produced a similar, but less marked, trend in strain TA100. The other HANs were negative in the *Salmonella*/microsome assay.

All of the HANs tested increased the frequency of SCEs in CHO cells. The potencies in the absence of S9 were DBAN > BCAN > DCAN ≈ TCAN > CAN. As in the *Salmonella*/microsome assay, the addition of S9 allowed higher doses to be tested rather than modifying the response to a given concentration. In contrast, none of the HANs was found to induce micronuclei in CD-1 mice *in vivo*.

The HANs were tested for their ability to initiate tumours in the skin of Sencar mice (Bull et al., 1985). In this experiment, the HANs were administered topically to the shaved backs of the mice in six doses over a 2-week period. Two weeks following the last initiation treatment, TPA dissolved in acetone was applied topically at a dose of 1 µg per mouse, 3 times weekly for 20 weeks. The total initiating doses were 1200, 2400 and 4800 mg/kg of body weight. Significant increases in skin tumours were observed with CAN, TCAN, BCAN and DBAN. DBAN produced the greatest response at a dose of 2400 mg/kg of body weight, but the response decreased in magnitude as the dose was increased to 4800 mg/kg of body weight. The shape of this dose–response curve was checked in a repetition of the experiment, and the results were virtually identical. It was postulated that the attenuated response at the higher dose was caused by the cytotoxicity to initiated cells. BCAN also increased the incidence of skin tumours, but no significant increase in tumour incidence was induced by DCAN. The carcinogenicity of the DHANs in mouse skin was seen to progressively increase as bromine was substituted for chlorine in the compound. On the other hand, CAN appeared to be among the more potent of the HANs in initiating skin tumours. TCAN gave inconsistent results.

CAN, TCAN and BCAN produced small, but significant, increases in the incidence of lung tumours in female A/J mice (40 mice per chemical tested) when administered by gavage at doses of 10 mg/kg of body weight, 3 times weekly for 8 weeks (Bull & Robinson, 1985). Mice were started on treatment at 10 weeks of age and sacrificed at 9 months of age. No significant effects were observed with DBAN and DCAN. The differences in tumorigenic response are too small for meaningful rankings of the compounds for potency in this lung tumour-susceptible strain.

DCAN was found to induce aneuploidy in *Drosophila* (Osgood & Sterling, 1991) at a concentration of 8.6 mg/litre. On the other hand, DBAN produced inconsistent results but was tested at much lower concentrations (0.3 mg/litre) because of its higher degree of toxicity. Low levels of sodium cyanide (0.2 mg/litre) were also found to be active in this test system. Since DCAN is metabolized to cyanide, the authors suggested that the cyanide ion (CN^-) was responsible for the response. DCAN is somewhat more efficiently converted to cyanide in rats than is DBAN (Pereira et al., 1984). This difference would be multiplied by the much higher concentration of DCAN that was tested.

Daniel et al. (1986) found that the HANs were direct-acting electrophiles with the following decreasing order of reactivity: DBAN >> BCAN > CAN >> DCAN >> TCAN. The ability to induce DNA strand breakage in human CCRF-CEM cells was found to follow a considerably different order: TCAN >> BCAN > DBAN > DCAN > CAN. It is of interest that tumour-initiating activity paralleled alkylation potential in a cell-free system rather than an ability to induce strand breaks in DNA in intact cells or to induce mutation in *Salmonella* (BCAN > DCAN >> DBAN > TCAN = CAN = 0). If CAN is omitted from the group, mutagenicity parallels the extent to which the HAN is converted to cyanide *in vivo* (Daniel et al., 1986). This discordant set of parallels suggests that some property may be affecting the ability of the test systems to measure the response or that the responses are not mediated through a common mechanism. Clearly, cytotoxic effects limited the responses of *Salmonella* to the brominated HANs. Similar activity appeared to be affecting the mouse skin initiation/promotion studies, but only after a fairly robust response was observed. Some of the other effects may be only loosely associated with a health effect. For example, the induction of SSBs in DNA can arise from cytolethal effects. Moreover, such breaks reflect DNA repair processes as well as damage. Therefore, it is suggested that the carcinogenic potency of this class best parallels alkylation potential.

TCAN was found to covalently bind with macromolecules in liver, kidney and stomach of the F344 rat (Lin et al, 1992). The covalent binding index was found to be the highest in the DNA of the stomach, followed by the liver, and was lowest in the kidney. The binding of ^{14}C was significantly higher when it was in the C_2 position rather than in C_1, indicating that the nitrile carbon is lost. The adducts formed were labile, and no specific adducts were identified. Adducts to blood proteins were also observed with TCAN. Covalent binding of DBAN or DCAN to DNA could not be demonstrated (Lin et al., 1986), but binding to proteins was apparently not investigated with these HANs.

In conclusion, the HANs do possess carcinogenic and mutagenic properties in short-term tests. However, without appropriate long-term animal studies, the carcinogenic risk from HANs cannot be estimated.

4.4.4   *Comparative pharmacokinetics and metabolism*

The metabolism of the HANs has received some preliminary study, but little information exists on the pharmacokinetics of the parent compounds or their products. It is also important to note that some of the HANs inhibit enzymes that are important in the metabolism of other chemicals that are foreign to the body.

Pereira et al. (1984) found the following percentage of the original doses of the HANs eliminated in the urine within 24 h as thiocyanate: CAN, 14%; BCAN, 12.8%; DCAN, 9.3%; DBAN, 7.7%; and TCAN, 2.3%. This was compared with 42% of a dose of propionitrile. On the basis of this limited information and a general scheme for the elimination of cyanide from nitriles, published by Silver et al. (1982), Pereira et al. (1984) proposed that additional products of HAN metabolism would be as follows: CAN, formaldehyde; DHANs, formyl cyanide or formyl halide; and TCAN, phosgene or cyanoformyl chloride. These products would be direct-acting alkylating agents.

Roby et al. (1986) studied the metabolism and excretion of DCAN labelled with ^{14}C in either the C_1 or C_2 position in both male F344 rats and B6C3F$_1$ mice. The metabolic fate of the two carbons was significantly different in both mice and rats: C_2 is metabolized much more efficiently to carbon dioxide, whereas a very much higher proportion of C_1 is found as urinary metabolites, at least in mice. These results are consistent with the proposal of Pereira et al. (1984) suggesting metabolites that would be converted efficiently to carbon dioxide from C_2.

The HANs inhibit enzymes in the liver of the rat that are traditionally associated with the metabolism of foreign compounds. Pereira et al. (1984) demonstrated the inhibition of dimethylnitrosamine demethylase activity. This activity has been traditionally associated with the cytochrome P450 isoform 2E1, although there was no direct confirmation of this in the study. However, two forms of the enzyme activity were identified, one with a K_m of 2×10^{-5} and the other with a K_m of 7×10^{-2}. Based on a plot presented in the paper, DBAN appears to be inhibiting the high-affinity enzyme by either a noncompetitive or uncompetitive mechanism. The kinetics of inhibition were examined *in vitro* and the enzyme : inhibitor dissociation constants (K_is) reported to be as follows: DBAN, 3×10^{-5}; BCAN, 4×10^{-5}; DCAN or TCAN, 2×10^{-4}; and CAN, 9×10^{-2}. Although not commented upon by the authors, the kinetics of inhibition by TCAN were clearly different from those of the DHANs, suggesting some differences in the mechanism or the form of the enzyme that might be affected. The authors examined the effects of DBAN or TCAN administered orally to rats at doses of 0.75 mmol/kg of body weight on the dimethylnitrosamine demethylase activity in the liver at 3 and 10 h after administration. TCAN significantly reduced the activity of the enzyme by about 30% at both time intervals, but DBAN did not, despite the fact that it was the more potent inhibitor *in vitro*. This could represent a difference in the extent to which the two compounds are absorbed systemically, or it could be related to the nature of the inhibition (i.e., reversible vs. irreversible).

Ahmed et al. (1989) demonstrated inhibition of cytosolic GSTs by HANs *in vitro*. Doses (mmol/litre) at which 50% inhibition of the activity of the enzyme GST occurred were as follows: DCAN, 2.49; TCAN, 0.34; DBAN, 0.82; CAN, >10; and BAN, >10. This latter observation has not been established to occur in animals (Gao et al., 1996). Activation and inactivation of various DBPs are catalysed by various isoforms of GST (Pegram et al., 1997; Tong et al., 1998). In this case, toxicity is reduced by inhibition of GST; however, mutagenic activity of brominated THMs appears to depend upon a GSH pathway (Pegram et al., 1997). Similarly, GSTs appear to play an important role in the metabolism of HAAs (Tong et al., 1998).

While these effects on the metabolism of other DBPs could be of importance, there are no data with which to relate these effects to concentrations that would be encountered in drinking-water.

4.4.5   Mode of action

The induction of skin tumours appears closely correlated with the alkylating potential within this class of chlorination by-products (Daniel et al., 1986). This suggests that the carcinogenic activity of the HANs may be related to mutagenic effects, despite the fact that cytotoxicity limits the capability of test systems to detect such activity. Cytotoxicity actually appears to inhibit the tumour-initiating activity responses rather than to amplify them, as has been seen with other DBPs. This suggests that the HANs retain some specificity for inducing cytotoxic responses in initiated cells.

Another concern in this class is the ability of certain members to induce developmental delays. At present, interpretation of these results is somewhat clouded by the issues of interactions in the toxicity of the test compound with its vehicles, as discussed in the recent publication of Christ et al. (1996). No satisfactory explanation has been offered for these results. Such effects may be the result of fairly subtle changes in the pharmacokinetics and metabolism of the compound, or, as Christ et al. (1996) suggest, TCAN may have acted synergistically with a subthreshold effect of tricaprylin on developmental processes. This is suggested by a minimal, but consistent, response in treatment groups that received tricaprylin only relative to a group of naive controls.

The potential importance of the HANs as cyanogens has not been extensively explored. As noted above, Pereira et al. (1984) indicated that significant portions of the dose of the HANs are eliminated as thiocyanate in the urine. Thus, cyanide release could be contributing significantly to the effects of these chemicals at high doses.

4.5   Halogenated hydroxyfuranone derivatives

The halogenated hydroxyfuranones were first identified in the bleaching of pulp (Holmbom et al., 1984). The first member of this class, MX, was found because of its high mutagenic activity in *Salmonella* tester strains. In the same time frame, mutagenic activity had been associated with the chlorination of drinking-water (Meier, 1988). The high specific mutagenic activity of MX prompted examination of the possibility that it could contribute to the mutagenic activity that had been identified in chlorinated drinking-water. Subsequent experimentation confirmed this hypothesis. Estimates of the contribution of MX to the mutagenic activity in drinking-water ranged from 3% to 57% (Hemming et al., 1986; Meier et al., 1987a; Kronberg & Vartiainen, 1988). The lower estimates should probably be discounted, because the methods for recovering MX and other mutagens from water have varied. Moreover, it is important to recognize that these estimates apply only to MX itself. A variety of related compounds are produced that are also mutagens (Daniel et al., 1991b; DeMarini et al., 1995; Suzuki & Nakanishi, 1995), but which have received very little toxicological study. The contribution of these related compounds has not been estimated.

The present section will focus on the research subsequent to that which identified MX as an important chlorination by-product. This review will confine itself to newer data that provide some perspective on possible mechanisms of action *in vivo*. To avoid unnecessary redundancy, other furanones will be discussed only as they have been investigated to aid in an understanding of responses to MX.

4.5.1   *General toxicological properties and information on dose–response in animals*

The lack of a commercial source of MX has limited research in experimental animals. However, a number of *in vivo* studies and a carcinogenesis study of MX have been published (Bull et al., 1995; Komulainen et al., 1997). Reported epidemiological associations of drinking-water mutagenicity with cancer of the gastrointestinal and urinary tracts (Koivusalo et al., 1994b, 1996, 1997) provided additional impetus for investigating the compound.

Three studies explicitly examined the acute toxicity of MX. The oral LD_{50} for MX in Swiss-Webster mice was determined to be 128 mg/kg of body weight when MX was administered for 2 consecutive days by gavage (Meier et al., 1987b). Doses of 70% of the LD_{50} and less (≤ 90 mg/kg of body weight) had no significant effect on body weight of the mice, nor were they lethal. Most mice died within 24 h of receiving the first dose. Mice that died were found to have enlarged stomachs with moderate haemorrhagic areas in the forestomach. Very limited mortality was observed in weanling CD-1 mice administered a single dose of 144 mg/kg of body weight (Mullins & Proudlock, 1990). In this study, focal epithelial hyperplasia was observed in the stomach, and some vacuolation of the superficial villus epithelium was observed in the duodenum and jejunum. Evidence of increased numbers of mitotic figures was observed in the liver, and the possibility of some cytotoxicity was identified in the urinary bladder. Komulainen et al. (1994) administered MX in distilled water to male Wistar rats. Rats tolerated doses of 100 mg/kg of body weight but displayed severe symptoms, including dyspnoea, laborious breathing, depressed motor activity and cyanosis. At necropsy, gastrointestinal inflammation was observed, and oedema was noted in the lungs and kidneys.

The study of Meier et al. (1996) examined the effects of a 14-day course of MX treatment by gavage at a dose of 64 mg/kg of body weight per day on a number of enzyme activities in the liver of rats. MX treatment reduced hepatic levels of catalase, cytochrome P450 reductase, aminopyrine demethylase and aromatic hydrocarbon hydroxylase. It did not affect fatty acyl CoA oxidase, glutamylcysteine synthetase, GST or glutathione peroxidase. The main result of such effects would be potential modifications of metabolism of various xenobiotics and endogenous biochemicals.

A more extensive study of the effect of MX on enzyme activities in various tissues was conducted by Heiskanen et al. (1995) in Wistar rats. This study employed a constant daily dose of 30 mg/kg of body weight administered by gavage for 18 weeks as the low dose, whereas the higher dose was achieved by initiating treatment at 45 mg/kg of body weight (7 weeks) and raising it to 60 mg/kg of body weight (2 weeks) and to 75 mg/kg of body weight (5 weeks). A dose-related decrease in ethoxyresorufin-*O*-deethylase activity was observed in liver and kidney. MX appears to inhibit this enzyme's activity directly based upon *in vitro* experiments conducted by the authors. However, the high concentrations required (0.9 mmol/litre) are unlikely to be approached systemically from the very low levels found in chlorinated drinking-water. The treatment also increased the activities of two phase 2 enzymes, uridine diphosphate-glucuronosyltransferase and GST, in the kidneys in a dose-dependent manner, but only in female rats. The health consequences of such modifications are uncertain, but could reflect an effect on physiological mechanisms associated with differences in sex. Again, it is important to recognize that these effects were produced at doses that were chronically, as well as acutely, toxic and unlikely to be remotely approached at the low concentrations found in chlorinated drinking-water.

In a subchronic (14–18 weeks) toxicity study, Wistar rats (15 per sex per group) were given MX by gavage, 5 days per week, at doses of 0 or 30 mg/kg of body weight (low dose) for 18 weeks or, in the high-dose group, at doses increasing from 45 to 75 mg/kg of body weight over 14 weeks. The high dose was finally lethal (two males and one female died) and caused hypersalivation, wheezing respiration, emaciation and tangled fur in animals. Increased water consumption, decreased body weights and food consumption, elevated plasma cholesterol and triglycerides, and increased urine excretion were noted in high-dose male rats. Urine specific gravity was decreased and the relative weights of the liver and kidneys were increased in both sexes at both doses in comparison with the controls. At both doses, duodenal hyperplasia occurred in males and females, and slight focal epithelial hyperplasia in the forestomach was observed in males. Splenic atrophy and haemosiderosis were seen in two high-dose females, and epithelial cell atypia was seen in the urinary bladder of one high-dose male and female. The frequency of bone marrow polychromatic erythrocytes with micronuclei was slightly increased only in low-dose male rats (Vaittinen et al., 1995).

4.5.2 Toxicity in humans

There have been no studies of the effects of these compounds in humans.

4.5.3 Carcinogenicity and mutagenicity

4.5.3.1 Studies in bacteria and mammalian cells in vitro

There have been extensive studies of the mutagenic activity of MX and related chemicals. *In vitro* studies have extended knowledge beyond the initial characterization of simple mutagenic responses to (i) demonstrate effects in higher test systems, (ii) extend the data to other genotoxic end-points, (ii) characterize the mutagenic lesions produced in DNA and (iv) develop structural correlates. At higher levels of biological organization, a limited number of studies have been conducted to document that the genotoxic form of MX reaches the systemic circulation and to measure mutagenic effects in particular cell types *in vivo*.

Meier et al. (1987b) demonstrated that MX induced chromosomal aberrations in CHO cells at concentrations as low as 4 µg/ml *in vitro*. However, these authors were unable to demonstrate an increased frequency of micronuclei in the bone marrow of Swiss-Webster mice following two consecutive daily doses administered by gavage at 70% of the LD_{50} (90 mg/kg of body weight × 2). Treatment with 30–300 µmol of MX per litre (1 h) induced DNA damage in a concentration-dependent manner in suspensions of rat hepatocytes. DNA damage was induced in V79 Chinese hamster cells and in isolated rat testicular cells at the same concentrations as in hepatocytes. V79 cells exposed to 2–5 µmol of MX per litre (2 h) showed an increased frequency of SCE, whereas no significant effect on hypoxanthine-guanine phosphoribosyltransferase mutation induction was observed (Brunborg et al., 1991).

Watanabe et al. (1994) found that the mutagenic activity of MX was effectively inhibited by sulfhydryl compounds such as cysteine, cysteamine, GSH, dithiothreitol and 2-mercaptoethanol. Pre-incubation of 0.5 µg of MX with 15 µg of cysteine in a phosphate buffer at 37 °C for 15 min prior to exposure of bacterial cells depleted the mutagenic activity of MX. Together with the result showing a change in the UV spectra, the authors suggested that sulfhydryl compounds inactivate MX by direct chemical interaction before MX induces DNA damage. On the other hand, a variety of antioxidants other than the sulfhydryl compounds showed no inhibitory effects. Investigation using structural analogues of cysteine revealed that the thiol moiety was indispensable for antimutagenic activity, and the amino moiety appeared to enhance the MX-inactivating reaction of the sulfhydryl group.

Incubation of both rat and mouse hepatocytes with MX *in vitro* resulted in a dose-dependent increase in UDS at subcytotoxic concentrations (1–10 µmol of MX per litre; 20-h incubation). Depletion of GSH stores by pretreatment of rat hepatocytes with buthionine sulfoximine did not result in a significant increase in UDS produced by MX. In contrast, MX did not induce UDS in mouse hepatocytes *ex vivo* either 3 or 16 h following administration of a single oral dose of 100 mg of MX per kg of body weight. Despite the ability of MX to produce repairable DNA damage, restricted access of MX to the liver may prevent a measurable UDS response *in vivo* (Nunn et al., 1997).

Jansson et al. (1995) examined MX and a related compound, 3,4-(dichloro)-5-hydroxy-2(5H)-furanone (MA, also known as mucochloric acid), in the CHO hypoxanthine phosphoribosyl transferase (*hprt*) locus assay system where 6-thioguanine resistance (TG^r) is the parameter measured. Both MX and MA induced TG^r mutants. Indirect evidence was provided to suggest that the difference in sensitivity in the bacterial systems was related to differential ability to repair bulky adducts hypothesized to be induced by MX versus smaller adducts suggested to occur as a result of MA treatment. These results are interesting, considering the fact that Daniel et al. (1991b) found that MX and MA were of approximately equivalent potencies in inducing nuclear anomalies in gastrointestinal cells of the B6C3F$_1$ mouse.

Harrington-Brock et al. (1995) recently examined MX in the L5178/TK$^{+/C}$3.7.2C mouse lymphoma system. A mutant frequency of 1027 per 10^6 surviving cells was found. There was, however, a predominance of small-colony mutants. Small colonies more commonly arise from clastogenic effects than from point mutations. In parallel experiments, MX was found to have clastogenic effects (chromatid breaks and rearrangements). Point mutations and clastogenic effects were both observed at a medium concentration of 0.75 µg/ml.

MX and MA also induced micronuclei when applied to inflorescences of pollen mother cells of *Tradescantia* (Helma et al., 1995). MX was approximately 5 times as potent as MA in this assay system.

DeMarini et al. (1995) compared the mutation spectra induced by MX and extracts of water treated with chlorine, chloramine, ozone or ozone followed by chlorine or chloramine in *Salmonella typhimurium* strains TA98 and TA100. The mutation spectra induced in the *hisG46* codon displayed a predominance of the GAC mutation with MX, but there were also significant increases in the CTC and to a lesser extent ACC mutations. These latter mutations are not typical of MX. Since MX has never been identified as a by-product of ozonation, it is somewhat surprising that extracts of ozonated water produced a similar spectrum, even though these extracts are much less potent than those obtained from chlorinated or chloraminated water (i.e., they produced net increases in mutant colonies that are only about twice the spontaneous rate). The mutation spectra induced in the TA98 *hisD3052* allele more clearly differentiated between ozone and chlorinated or chloraminated water. In this case, virtually all of the frameshift mutations induced by raw and ozonated water extracts involved hotspot mutations, whereas only 30–50% of those induced by MX or extracts from water that had been treated with chlorine or chloramine involved the hotspot. Thus, the TA98 mutations are consistent with the hypothesis that the chemicals responsible for mutagenic effects of ozonated water are distinct from those induced by chlorination by-products.

Hyttinen et al. (1996) found that MX and MA induce different mutation spectra in the DNA of *Salmonella typhimurium hisG46* codons (target codon sequence is CCC). The predominant mutation was GAC followed by ACC in MX-treated colonies, whereas CTC dominated the spectra produced by MA. MX primarily induced G:C → T:A transversions, whereas MA produced G:C → A:T transitions in the second base of the codon. The G:C → T:A transversion in *Salmonella* was also observed in the *hprt* gene of CHO cells (Hyttinen et al., 1996). Knasmuller et al. (1996) found the same difference in the mutation spectra of MX and MA in *S. typhimurium* mutants. These latter authors further found that 3-chloro-4-(chloromethyl)-5-hydroxy-2(5H)-furanone (CMCF) produced the same transversion as MX, while chloromalonaldehyde produced the same transition found with MA.

Some complex structure–activity relationships appear to occur with these two types of halofuranones. Kronberg et al. (1993) found that MA forms ethenocarbaldehyde derivatives with adenosine and cytidine, with chloroacetaldehyde being an intermediate. As pointed out by Knasmuller et al. (1996), ethenocytosine adducts formed by vinyl chloride cause G:C → A:T transitions as reported for MA. The mutations induced by MX are similar to those produced by carcinogens that form bulky adducts, such as benzo[*a*]pyrene and 4-aminobiphenyl. Bulky adducts block replication leading to base substitutions according to the "adenine rule" (Strauss, 1991). As a consequence, there may be some significant differences in the health impact (e.g., tumour site or character if they are found to be carcinogenic) of the mutagenic activities of these two chlorohydroxyfuranone derivatives.

Ishiguro et al. (1988) examined structure–activity relationships for MX and related compounds. Their studies identified the chlorine substitution on C_3 as being very important to the mutagenic activity of MX. Association of similar losses in mutagenic activity by removing the analogous chlorine from an open-ring structure compound, 3-(dichloromethyl)-4,4-dichloro-2-chlorobutenoic acid, strongly supported this hypothesis.

LaLonde and co-workers (LaLonde et al., 1991a,b, 1992; LaLonde & Xie, 1992, 1993) conducted a series of experimental and computational studies to relate the electronic structure of MX and related compounds with mutagenic activity within the class. Substitutions for the hydroxyl group led to reduction of mutagenic activity by a factor of 100. Removal of the C_3 or C_6 chlorines from the structure reduced mutagenic activity by a factor of 10. Removal of the second chlorine at C_3 caused a very large further reduction of mutagenic activity (by a factor of 1000) (LaLonde et al., 1991b). The mutagenicity appears to depend on the electron density at C_2, C_3 or C_4 based upon ^{13}C chemical shifts observed by nuclear magnetic resonance. Expansion of these studies supported the hypothesis that the mutagenic properties of the class paralleled the electrophilic character of chemicals within the class and the ability to stabilize a radical anion following acceptance of a single electron.

Another difference in the chemistry of MA and MX, which might have biological implications, is that GSH readily displaces the chlorine on C_4 of MA, greatly reducing its electrophilicity. On the other hand,

GSH or *N*-acetylcysteine reacts with MX to produce mixtures that are intractable to analysis, with the release of hydrogen sulfide (LaLonde & Xie, 1993).

4.5.3.2   Studies in experimental animals

In vivo studies are of two types: those that use bacterial systems to document absorption of MX (or mutagenic metabolite), and those in which effects on the test animal are directly measured.

Fekadu et al. (1994) injected mixtures of repair-competent and repair-deficient *Escherichia coli* K-12 cells intravenously into mice as test cells, and the animals were subsequently treated with 200 mg of test chemical per kg of body weight. Two hours later, the mice were sacrificed and cells recovered from various organs. MX, CMCF and MA were the test chemicals. The differential survival of the DNA repair-deficient strain versus a repair-competent variant is used to detect mutagenic activity. All three compounds significantly reduced recovery of the repair-deficient strain in the stomach, lung, intestine, liver, kidney and spleen. In a further experiment, the effects of lower doses of MX (4.3, 13 and 40 mg/kg of body weight) were investigated. Significantly depressed recovery was seen with MX doses as low as 4.3 mg/kg of body weight. MA did not modify recovery of the repair-deficient strain at doses less than or equal to 40 mg/kg of body weight. These data suggest that significant amounts of MX or a mutagenic metabolite reach the systematic circulation and at least reach the extra-cellular water. They do not clearly demonstrate effects in the target tissue of the experimental animal.

Meier et al. (1996) found that only 0.3% of the original dose was excreted in a genotoxically active form in the urine of rats administered MX at a dose of 64 mg/kg of body weight for 14 days by gavage. No evidence of micronuclei induction was detected in peripheral blood erythrocytes in mice treated with a similar protocol. Whereas muta-genic activity was observed in urine at doses of 64 mg/kg of body weight, no significant mutagenic activity was observed at doses of 32 mg/kg of body weight and below.

Brunborg et al. (1990, 1991) studied DNA damage induced by MX and other compounds in organs of rats using the alkaline elution assay (to detect strand breaks). While clear evidence of strand breaks was obtained with dibromochloropropane and 2-amino-3,4-dimethyl-imidazo[4,5-*f*]quinoline, no significant effects were observed with MX after an intraperitoneal dose of 18 mg/kg of body weight or at oral doses of up to 125 mg/kg of body weight. The organs examined included the small and large intestine, stomach, liver, kidney, lung, bone marrow, urinary bladder and testis.

Nishikawa et al. (1994) investigated cell proliferation and lipid peroxidation in the glandular stomach mucosa in Wistar rats given 0, 6.25, 12.5, 25 or 50 mg of MX per litre in their drinking-water for 5 weeks. Statistically significant cell proliferation increased in a dose-dependent manner up to 25 mg/litre. The MX treatment was also associated with increased lipid peroxidation levels in the gastric mucosa as well as in the urine, with loose dose dependence, although not at 50 mg/litre. Histopathologically, gastric erosion was noted in rats receiving 25 mg of MX per litre or more. These results suggest that MX may exert a gastric tumour-promoting action in rats, even at low doses that do not give rise to toxic effects, because of the clear dose–response relationship evident at low levels.

The peripheral lymphocytes of male and female Han:Wistar rats exposed to MX at 30 or 45–75 mg/kg of body weight per day by gavage, 5 days a week for 14–18 weeks, showed significant dose-related increases in SCEs at both levels of exposure in both sexes (Jansson et al., 1993).

The peripheral lymphocytes of male Han:Wistar rats exposed to MX (25–150 mg/kg of body weight) by gavage on 3 consecutive days showed a significant dose-related increase in chromosomal damage measured as micronuclei, in addition to SCEs. Moreover, MX produced a significant dose-related increase in SCEs in the kidney cells of the exposed rats. However, the magnitude of the genotoxic responses observed was relatively weak (Maki-Paakkanen & Jansson, 1995).

Daniel et al. (1991b) found that MX and MA induced nuclear anomalies in the epithelial cells of the gastrointestinal tract of B6C3F$_1$ mice. Doses of 0.37 mmol/kg of body weight (approximately 80 mg/kg of body weight) produced a modest increase in nuclear anomalies in the duodenum. There was no effect at 0.28 mmol/kg of body weight. Mullins & Proudlock (1990) and Proudlock & Crouch (1990) also found insignificant increases in nuclear anomalies in the non-glandular stomach, urinary bladder, jejunum and ileum. These latter authors noted that at the top dose at which nuclear anomalies were observed (144 mg/kg of body weight), there was significant irritation, inflammation and evidence of apoptotic cells in the gastrointestinal tract. These changes render the significance of the observed nuclear anomalies uncertain.

MX was administered to Wistar rats (50 per sex per group) in drinking-water for 104 weeks at 0, 0.4, 1.3 or 5.0 mg/kg of body weight per day for males and 0, 0.6, 1.9 or 6.6 mg/kg of body weight per day for females. Dose-dependent increases in the incidence of some tumours were observed in rats, while the same MX doses had no obvious toxic effects on animals. Increases in tumours of the lung, mammary gland, haematopoietic system, liver, pancreas, adrenal gland and thyroid were observed, but few showed a clear dose–response (Table 21) (Komulainen et al., 1997).

4.5.4   Comparative pharmacokinetics and metabolism

There are very few data on the metabolism and pharmacokinetics of MX or related compounds. Ringhand et al. (1989) examined the distribution of radioactivity derived from 3-^{14}C-MX in male F344 rats. Approximately 35% of the radiolabel was eliminated in the urine and 47% in the faeces, with about 6% remaining in the body after 48 h. Neither the parent compound nor any specific metabolites were identified in any body compartment or fluid.

Horth et al. (1991) studied the disposition of 3-^{14}C-MX in male CD-1 mice. [14]C was rapidly absorbed, reaching peak values in blood within 15 min of its administration. There was some evidence for binding to protein and retention of label within tissues, but no attempt was made to identify the chemical form in which the ^{14}C was bound, so it was not clear whether MX was binding by virtue of its electrophilic character or whether this represented metabolic incorporation of metabolites of MX. Approximately 57% of the radioactivity was eliminated in the urine and 28% in the faeces. Less than 1% of the initial dose was retained in the carcass 120 h after administration, but most of this was associated with the stomach. It was stated that the urinary metabolites were polar, but no specific identifications were made.

Table 21. Summary of primary tumours observed in selected tissues in male rats after exposure to 3-chloro-4-(dichloromethyl)-5-hydroxy-2(5H)-furanone (MX) in drinking-water for 104 weeks[a]

Tissue	Control	MX (mg/kg of body weight per day)			P[b]
		0.4	1.3	5.0	
Integumentary system					
Skin, subcutaneous tissue[c]	50	50	50	50	
Basal cell tumour[d]	1 (2%)		1 (2%)	3 (6%)	0.0314
Mammary glands[c]	50	50	50	49	
Adenocarcinoma[d]			1 (2%)		0.3162
Fibroadenoma[d]		1 (2%)	3 (6%)	1 (2%)	0.2996
Fibroma[d]		1 (2%)			0.4749
Respiratory system					
Lungs[c]	50	50	50	50	
Alveolar & bronchiolar carcinomas[d]	1 (2%)				
Alveolar & bronchiolar adenomas[d]	2 (4%)	1 (2%)	1 (2%)	7 (14%)	0.0015
Haematopoietic system					
Multiple tissues[c]	50	50	50	50	

Table 21 (Contd).

Lymphoma & leukaemia[d]		3 (6%)	4 (8%)	3 (6%)	0.1527
Digestive system					
Liver[c]	50	50	50	50	
Carcinoma[d]			2 (4%)	1 (2%)	0.1605
Hepatocholangiocarcinoma[d]		1 (2%)	1 (2%)		0.4897
Cholangioma[d]			1 (2%)	4 (8%)	0.0009
Adenoma[d]		1 (2%)	2 (4%)	4 (8%)	0.0142
Pancreas[c]	50	50	50	50	
Langerhans' cell carcinoma[d]	4 (8%)	3 (6%)	5 (10%)	4 (8%)	0.3769
Langerhans' cell adenoma[d]	5 (10%)	8 (16%)	8 (16%)	12 (24%)	0.0116
Acinar cell adenoma[d]	2 (4%)	3 (6%)	2 (4%)	4 (8%)	0.1243
Endocrine system					
Adrenal glands[c]	50	50	50	50	
Pheochromocytoma, malignant[d]			1 (2%)		0.3213
Pheochromocytoma, benign[d]	5 (10%)	2 (4%)	9 (18%)	3 (6%)	0.4830

Table 21 (Contd).

Tissue	Control	MX (mg/kg of body weight per day)			P^b
		0.4	1.3	5.0	
Cortical carcinoma[d]	2 (4%)	1 (2%)		14 (28%)	0.9447
Cortical adenoma[d]	5 (10%)	2 (4%)	7 (14%)	14 (28%)	0.0001
Thyroid glands[c]	49	50	50	50	
Follicular carcinoma[d]		1 (2%)	9 (18%)	27 (55%)	0.0000
Follicular adenoma[d]	2 (4%)	20 (40%)	34 (68%)	21 (43%)	0.0045
C-cell carcinoma[d]			2 (4%)		0.4478
C-cell adenoma[d]	11 (22%)	7 (14%)	10 (20%)	11 (22%)	0.2459

[a] From Komulainen et al. (1997).
[b] P value from the one-sided trend test. A statistically positive trend at $P \leq 0.05$ or lower.
[c] Values (reading across) = number of animals analysed.
[d] Values (reading across) = number of animals with one or more indicated tumours (frequency of animals with tumour as percentage of examined animals).

Komulainen et al. (1992) evaluated the pharmacokinetics of MX after a single oral or intravenous administration in Han:Wistar rats using ^{14}C-labelled compound. Approximately 20–35% of the dose was absorbed into circulation from the gastrointestinal tract. The mean elimination half-life of the radioactivity in blood was 3.8 h. Traces of radioactivity remained in the blood for several days. The tissues lining the gastrointestinal and urinary tracts, kidney, stomach, small intestine and urinary bladder contained the highest radioactivity. The activity declined most slowly in the kidneys. Urine was the main excretion route, with 77% of the total radioactivity appearing in urine in 12 h and 90% in 24 h. No radioactivity was exhaled in air. After an intravenous administration of ^{14}C-MX, the mean elimination half-life was much longer, 22.9 h, and the total elimination half-life was 42.1 h. Results indicate that MX is absorbed from the gastrointestinal tract to a considerable degree and is excreted in urine very rapidly. A fraction of MX or its metabolites is retained in blood for a longer period of time.

No data are available in the scientific literature on the metabolism of MX or related compounds in humans.

In conclusion, there are data to suggest that MX or a mutagenically active metabolite reaches the systemic circulation in experimental animals. Mutagenic activity has been detected in various organs and tissues using doses as low as 4.3 mg/kg of body weight (Fekadu et al., 1994). If these data are to have application to estimation of the hazards that MX presents to humans consuming chlorinated drinking-water, it is essential to understand whether MX or a metabolite reaches critical targets in the human body. An essential component of the information required would be an understanding of the metabolism and pharmacokinetics of MX and those of critical metabolites. The available data are too limited to provide much more than very general guidance in this area.

4.6 Chlorite

4.6.1 General toxicological properties and information on dose–response in animals

Concerns over chlorite in drinking-water first arose as chlorine dioxide began to play a role in the primary disinfection of drinking-water. Chlorite is the principal by-product of oxidative reactions of chlorine dioxide, but acidification of chlorite solutions is one method for generating chlorine dioxide for purposes of water disinfection (Aieta & Berg, 1986).

Unless otherwise noted, references to chlorite will generally be to the sodium salt. This is the form most frequently studied. The term chlorite will be used if the authors expressed their doses in terms of chlorite; if dose levels were expressed as sodium chlorite, they will be identified as such. There is no reason to suspect that other salts of chlorite would exert inherently different toxicological effects, so this convention should not lead to confusion. A preparation of sodium chlorite with lactic acid is specifically excluded from consideration here because the actual composition of the product has not been specified (Scatina et al., 1984). Consequently, it is not clear that the data on this product have any relevance to chlorite or vice versa.

Early investigations of chlorite's toxic properties focused almost entirely on it potential ability to produce methaemoglobin and haemolysis. Heffernan et al. (1979a) examined the ability of sodium chlorite to induce methaemoglobinaemia in cats and Sprague-Dawley rats. When administered to cats as an oral bolus, as little as 20 mg of sodium chlorite per kg of body weight resulted in formation of significant amounts of methaemoglobin. Intraperitoneal doses of 20 mg/kg of body weight in rats also induced methaemoglobin formation. However, when administered in drinking-water, no significant elevation in methaemoglobin was observed in cats (up to 1000 mg/litre as sodium chlorite) or rats (up to 500 mg/litre). Thus, chlorite must enter into the systemic circulation at a rapid rate, i.e., as a bolus dose, to induce methaemoglobin formation.

Short-term toxic effects of chlorite were more systematically assessed in rats using gavage doses ranging from 25 to 200 mg/kg of body weight (Harrington et al., 1995a). Minor effects were observed at 25 and 50 mg/kg of body weight. At 100 mg/kg of body weight and above, signs of haemolytic anaemia became apparent, with decreases in red blood cell count, haemoglobin concentration and haematocrit. These data support the idea that bolus doses were necessary to determine substantial effects on oxidative stress.

Treatment of both cats and rats with sodium chlorite in drinking-water for extended periods (up to 90 days) resulted in decreases in red blood cell counts, haemoglobin concentrations and packed cell volume. These effects were observed with 500 mg of sodium chlorite per litre in cats (equivalent to 7 mg/kg of body weight per day) and with as little as 100 mg/litre in rats (equivalent to 10 mg/kg of body weight per day) (Heffernan et al., 1979a). The changes in these blood parameters appeared to generally decrease in severity as the treatment was extended from 30 to 90 days, suggesting that adaptation to the treatment was occurring. In rats, however, red blood cell glutathione concentrations remained significantly depressed and 2,3-diphosphoglycerate levels elevated through 90 days of treatment with concentrations of sodium chlorite as low as 50 mg/litre (5 mg/kg of body weight per day). In the cat, increased turnover of erythrocytes was detectable at concentrations of 100 mg/litre, with no significant effect being observed at 10 mg/litre. This latter concentration resulted in a daily dose of 0.6 mg/kg of body weight per day. Red blood cells drawn from rats treated with 100 mg/litre had significantly less ability to detoxify hydrogen peroxide that was generated by the addition of chlorite *in vitro*. These data show that while the anaemia caused by haemolysis was largely compensated for in subchronic treatment of healthy rats, there was still evidence of oxidative stress being exerted by the chlorite treatment. Depletion of this reserve capacity could be of importance in individuals who are in a more compromised state (e.g., glucose-6-phosphate dehydrogenase deficiency) or who might be exposed to other haemolytic agents. The lowest concentration at which GSH was depleted significantly from control levels in rats was 50 mg/litre, and no effect was observed at 10 mg/litre (equivalent to 1 mg/kg of body weight per day).

The results of Heffernan et al. (1979a) have been generally confirmed by subsequent studies in a variety of species. Abdel-Rahman et al. (1980) and Couri & Abdel-Rahman (1980) obtained very similar effects in rats treated for up to 11 months. Moore & Calabrese (1980, 1982) produced similar results in mice, and Bercz et al. (1982) demonstrated reduced red blood cell counts and decreased haemoglobin levels at similar doses in African green monkeys. These studies tended to identify altered forms of erythrocytes that are commonly associated with oxidative damage at treatment doses below those that produced actual anaemia (most consistently at a concentration of 100 mg/litre, with hints of such effects at lower doses).

A more recent study employed doses of sodium chlorite administered by gavage to male and female Crl: CD (SD) BR rats (15 per sex per group) (Harrington et al., 1995a). Doses of 0, 10, 25 or 80 mg of sodium chlorite per kg of body weight per day were administered daily by gavage for 13 weeks (equivalent to 0, 7.4, 18.6 or 59.7 mg of chlorite per kg of body weight per day). This study is important because it included many of the standard parameters of subchronic toxicological studies, whereas previous studies had focused almost entirely on blood parameters. A gavage dose of 80 mg/kg of body weight per day produced death in a number of animals. It also resulted in morphological changes in erythrocytes and significant decreases in haemoglobin concentrations. Red blood cell counts were reduced slightly, but not significantly, at doses of 10 mg/kg of body weight per day in male rats, with further decreases being observed at 80 mg/kg of body weight per day. Red blood cell counts were significantly depressed in female rats at doses of 25 mg/kg of body weight per day and above. As would be expected where haemolysis is occurring, splenic weights were increased. Adrenal weights were increased in females at 25 and 80 mg/kg of body weight per day, whereas statistically significant changes were observed only at 80 mg/kg of body weight per day in males. Histopathological examination of necropsied tissues revealed squamous cell epithelial hyperplasia, hyperkeratosis, ulceration, chronic inflammation and oedema in the stomach of 7 out of 15 males and 8 out of 15 females given 80 mg/kg of body weight per day doses. This effect was observed in only 2 out of 15 animals at the 25 mg/kg of body weight per day dose and was not observed at all at 10 mg/kg of body weight per day. Microscopic evaluations were made in 40 additional tissues, and no treatment-related abnormalities were found.

The Harrington et al. (1995a) study confirms the essential findings of previous studies and, in retrospect, justifies their focus on the blood cells as the critical target for chlorite toxicity. It also confirmed negative results of other studies that failed to identify significant effects in investigations of particular target organs (Moore et al., 1984; Connor et al., 1985).

4.6.2 Reproductive and developmental toxicity

Sodium chlorite did not exert any spermatotoxic effects in short-duration (1–5 days) tests (Linder et al., 1992).

Moore et al. (1980b) reported that sodium chlorite administered at a concentration of 100 mg/litre throughout gestation and through 28 days of lactation reduced the conception rate and the number of pups alive at weaning in A/J mice. A significantly reduced pup weight at weaning was interpreted as indicating that chlorite retarded growth rate.

Groups of 4–13 Sprague-Dawley rats were treated on gestation days 8–15 with sodium chlorite at concentrations of 0, 100, 500 or 2000 mg/litre in drinking-water, by injection of 10, 20 or 50 mg/kg of body weight per day intraperitoneally or by gavaging with 200 mg/kg of body weight per day. Calculated daily doses of sodium chlorite administered to pregnant rats in drinking-water were 0, 34, 163 or 212 mg. Rats body weights were approximately 0.3 kg, giving estimated doses of 0, 110, 540 or 710 mg/kg of body weight per day. Sodium chlorite at 20 or 50 mg/kg of body weight per day intraperitoneally or at 200 mg/kg of body weight per day by gavage caused vaginal and urethral bleeding. Doses of 10, 20 and 50 mg/kg of body weight per day intraperitoneally caused 0%, 50% and 100% mortality of dams, respectively. No deaths were caused by sodium chlorite in the drinking-water, but the body weight and food consumption of the dams were decreased at 500 and 2000 mg/litre. Blood smears from the dams injected intraperitoneally with all doses or drinking water containing 2000 mg of sodium chlorite per litre showed irregular, bizarre and ruptured erythrocytes. Injection of 10 or 20 mg/kg of body weight per day or drinking a solution containing 2000 mg/litre resulted in a decrease in litter size and an increase in stillbirths and resorption sites. Drinking 100 or 500 mg of sodium chlorite per litre did not produce any significant embryotoxicity. With all treatments, no significant gross soft tissue or skeletal malformations were observed. Postnatal growth of the pups was not affected by any treatment of the dams during the gestation period (Couri et al., 1982a,b).

The effects of chlorite at 1 or 10 mg/litre in drinking-water for 2.5 months prior to mating and throughout gestation were studied in Sprague-Dawley rats (Suh et al., 1983). This study indicated an increase in the incidence of anomalies in fetuses at both concentrations in two separate experiments; however, because the treatment groups were small (6–9 pregnant females per group), the effects were not considered statistically significant. Moreover, there were no consistent differences in either skeletal or soft tissue anomalies.

Male and female Long-Evans rats were given 0, 1, 10 or 100 mg of sodium chlorite per litre of drinking-water. Males were exposed for 56 days before mating and during 10 days of mating; females were treated for 14 days prior to mating, throughout the 10-day breeding period and gestation and through to day 21 of lactation. Males were evaluated for sperm parameters and reproductive tract histopathology following the breeding period. Dams and pups were necropsied at weaning. There was no effect on fertility, litter size or survival of neonates or on the weight of the testis, epididymis or cauda epididymis when males treated as described above were mated with these females. Decreases in the concentrations of triiodothyronine and thyroxine in blood were observed on postnatal days 21 and 40 in male and female pups exposed to 100 mg/litre. There were no effects at lower doses. Additionally, groups of males were exposed to 0, 10, 100 or 500 mg of sodium chlorite per litre for 72–76 days to confirm subtle observed changes in sperm count, morphology and movement. A significant increase in the percentage of abnormal sperm morphology and a decrease in the progressive sperm motility were observed for adult males at 100 and 500 mg/litre (Carlton et al., 1987).

Mobley et al. (1990) exposed groups of female Sprague-Dawley rats (12 per group) for 9 weeks to drinking-water containing 0, 20 or 40 mg of sodium chlorite per litre (0, 3 or 6 mg of chlorite per kg of body weight per day) beginning 10 days prior to breeding with untreated males and until the pups were sacrificed at 35–42 days post-conception. Animals exposed to a dose of 6 mg/kg of body weight per day exhibited a consistent and significant depression in exploratory behaviour on post-conception days 36–39. Exploratory activity was comparable between treated and control groups after post-conception day 39.

In a two-generation study conducted by CMA (1997) and described in TERA (1998), Sprague-Dawley rats (30 per sex per dose) received drinking-water containing 0, 35, 70 or 300 mg of sodium chlorite per litre for 10 weeks and were then paired for mating. Males were exposed through mating, then sacrificed. Exposure for the females continued through mating, pregnancy, lactation and until necropsy following weaning of their litters. Twenty-five males and females from each of the first 25 litters to be weaned in a treatment group were chosen to produce the F_1 generation. The F_1 pups were continued on the same treatment regimen as their parents. At approximately

14 weeks of age, they were mated to produce the F_{2a} generation. Because of a reduced number of litters in the 70 mg/litre F_1–F_{2a} generation, the F_1 animals were remated following weaning of the F_{2a} generation to produce the F_{2b} generation. Doses for the F_0 animals were 0, 3.0, 5.6 or 20.0 mg of chlorite per kg of body weight per day for males and 0, 3.8, 7.5 or 28.6 mg of chlorite per kg of body weight per day for females. For the F_1 animals, doses were 0, 2.9, 5.9 or 22.7 mg of chlorite per kg of body weight per day for males and 0, 3.8, 7.9 or 28.6 mg of chlorite per kg of body weight per day for females. There were reductions in water consumption, food consumption and body weight gain in both sexes in all generations at various times throughout the experiment, primarily in the 70 and 300 mg/litre groups; these were attributed to a lack of palatability of the water. At 300 mg/litre, reduced pup survival, reduced body weight at birth and throughout lactation in F_1 and F_2, lower thymus and spleen weights in both generations, lowered incidence of pups exhibiting a normal righting reflex, delays in sexual development in males and females in F_1 and F_2, and lower red blood cell parameters in F_1 were noted. Significant reductions in absolute and relative liver weights in F_0 females and F_1 males and females, reduced absolute brain weights in F_1 and F_2, and a decrease in the maximum response to an auditory startle stimulus on postnatal day 24 but not at postnatal day 60 were noted in the 300 and 70 mg/litre groups. Minor changes in red blood cell parameters in the F_1 generation were seen at 35 and 70 mg/litre, but these appear to be within normal ranges based on historical data. The NOAEL in this study was 35 mg/litre (2.9 mg/kg of body weight per day), based on lower auditory startle amplitude, decreased absolute brain weight in the F_1 and F_2 generations, and altered liver weights in two generations.

Harrington et al. (1995b) examined the developmental toxicity of chlorite in New Zealand white rabbits. The rabbits (16 per group) were treated with 0, 200, 600 or 1200 mg of sodium chlorite per litre in their drinking-water (equal to 0, 10, 26 or 40 mg of chlorite per kg of body weight per day) from day 7 to day 19 of pregnancy. The animals were necropsied on day 28. There were no dose-related increases in defects identified. Minor skeletal anomalies were observed as the concentration of chlorite in water was increased and food consumption was depressed.

4.6.3   Toxicity in humans

The effects of chlorite have received some attention in toxicological and epidemiological investigations in human subjects. All of these studies were conducted at doses within an order of magnitude of concentrations of chlorite that might be expected in water supplies disinfected with chlorine dioxide. None pushed the limit of tolerance such that clear effects were observed. As a consequence, they are not informative for establishing a margin of safety.

An experimental epidemiological study was conducted in the USA in a small city that had been using chlorine dioxide for some time in the summer months (April to October) to avoid taste and odour problems associated with the use of chlorine (Michael et al., 1981). Chlorine dioxide was generated from sodium chlorite that was mixed with chlorine gas and metered into the water. During the active use of chlorine dioxide, the chlorite concentrations in the water averaged 5.2 mg/litre (range about 3–7 mg/litre). Subjects were monitored for 11 parameters: haematocrit, haemoglobin, red cell count, white cell count, mean corpuscular volume, methaemoglobin, BUN, serum creatinine, total bilirubin, reticulocyte count and osmotic fragility of red blood cells. No effects could be associated with the switch of treatment from chlorine to chlorine dioxide disinfection. A total of 197 people were monitored in the exposed population, and there were 112 non-exposed individuals. Each person served as his/her own control.

Chlorine dioxide, free chlorine, chloramine and chlorate concentrations were also measured and were found to be 0.3–1.1, 0.5–0.9, 0.9–1.8 and 0.3–1.8 mg/litre, respectively. The sampling for clinical measurements was done 1 week before chlorine dioxide disinfection began and 10 weeks into the cycle. Water samples taken during weeks 10–13 had chlorite levels that were systematically somewhat below those observed in the prior 9 weeks of sampling, and the same general trend was observable in other measures of chlorine dioxide and chlorate. This was not observed with chlorine or chloramines, suggesting that some change in water treatment had occurred. The authors provided no explanation for this change in water quality, but, since clinical samples were taken in week 10, this change in water quality could have resulted in lower exposure to chlorite and chlorate.

The second set of evaluations of chlorite in humans involved direct administration of sodium chlorite in a rising-dose tolerance study and a follow-up study in which volunteers were treated for 12 weeks, which were reported on in several publications. Lubbers et al. (1981, 1982) provided an overview of the studies. The detailed results of the rising-dose tolerance study were reported in Lubbers & Bianchine (1984), and those of the repeated-dose study in Lubbers et al. (1982, 1984a). A fourth paper (Lubbers et al., 1984b) reported results for three male volunteers that had glucose-6-phosphate dehydrogenase deficiency.

The rising-dose tolerance study (Lubbers & Bianchine, 1984) involved administration of progressively increasing single doses of chlorite (0.01, 0.1, 0.5, 1.0, 1.8 or 2.4 mg/litre) in two 500-ml portions to a group of 10 healthy adult male volunteers. Doses were administered on days 1, 4, 7, 10, 13 and 16. In the interval between doses, clinical evaluations of the subjects were performed and a battery of clinical chemistry tests was performed on blood and urine samples. These latter tests were primarily directed at potential haematological effects of chlorite, but serum thyroxine and uptake of triiodothyronine were also determined. In addition, blood pressure, ECGs and other physiological parameters were monitored. No treatment-related effects were observed.

In the repeated-dose study (Lubbers et al., 1984a), 10 male volunteers were administered 5 mg of chlorite per litre in a 500-ml portion for 12 weeks (0.036 mg/kg of body weight per day). Physical examinations and blood and urine analyses were conducted throughout the duration of treatment and for 8 weeks following the last dose of the solutions. None of the parameters investigated was found to fall outside the normal range; although there were some consistent changes in values with time, none of these appeared to be related to chlorite treatment.

Three individuals with glucose-6-phosphate dehydrogenase deficiency were identified in the course of the study. This genetic disorder makes individuals more sensitive to oxidative damage, which is frequently manifested as increased methaemoglobin production and haemolysis when the individuals are exposed to oxidative chemicals in sufficient doses. All three individuals were treated with chlorite in the same concentrations and in the same manner as described for the study of normal individuals (Lubbers et al., 1984b). No clinically significant changes were found in these individuals.

A study (Ames & Stratton, 1987) was conducted of renal dialysis patients in California (USA) after a water district introduced chlorine dioxide as a drinking-water disinfectant but failed to inform the clinic for 12 months. Water treatment at the clinic consisted of ion exchange, GAC, 5-µm filtration and reverse osmosis. Chlorite levels measured after this treatment were 0.02–0.08 mg/litre, but there were periods during which no chlorine dioxide was added, and exposures to the patients may have been lower. Measures for 28 serum and haematological parameters were available for 17 renal dialysis patients for a period of 3 months before and 1 month after exposure. Methaemoglobin measures were not available. Only one measure was statistically associated with the use of water disinfected by chlorine dioxide: serum uric acid declined by 10% after exposure to disinfected water, a change that was not considered clinically important. The study found no evidence of anaemia or other adverse effects of chlorine dioxide-disinfected water for these renal dialysis patients, but the interpretation of these results is severely limited because of the small sample size and apparently very low exposures.

Collectively, these studies suggest that humans are probably not sensitive to the concentrations of chlorite that are likely to be found in water disinfected with chlorine dioxide. Some safety factor is present in these data, because it is unlikely that concentrations of chlorite would exceed 1 mg/litre with new methods of application. However, these studies provide little information relative to the actual margin of safety that exists between those concentrations seen or administered and concentrations that would lead to clear adverse effects. Consequently, these studies do not imply that the concentrations of chlorite in drinking-water should be without limits.

4.6.4 Carcinogenicity and mutagenicity

Sodium chlorite was reported to produce a concentration-dependent increase in revertants in *Salmonella typhimurium* strain TA100 in both the presence and absence of rat liver S9 fraction (Ishidate et al., 1984). A linear dose–response curve was observed, and the net number of revertants produced at 0.3 mg per plate was 88. The S9 mix used for metabolic activation was from the liver of F344 rats pretreated for 5 days with polychlorinated biphenyls at 500 mg/kg of body weight.

Meier et al. (1985b) evaluated chlorite in the mouse micronucleus assay, the mouse bone marrow cytogenetics assay and the mouse sperm head abnormality assay. The doses administered were 0.2, 0.5 or 1 mg per mouse or approximately 40 mg/kg of body weight at the highest dose. No statistically significant results were found in any of the tests. In a later reference, it was indicated that chlorite also induced chromosomal aberrations (Kurokawa et al., 1986b), but the data were not provided. Hayashi et al. (1988, 1989) found an increase in micronuclei in the bone marrow of mice given 0, 7.5, 15, 30 or 60 mg/kg of body weight by intraperitoneal injection at doses of 15 and 30 mg/kg of body weight. In a repeat study in which mice were given 0 or 15 mg/kg of body weight on 4 successive days, no increase in micronuclei was observed. In a study using the oral route with doses of 0, 37.5, 75, 150 or 300 mg/kg of body weight, a significant increase in micronuclei was observed only at 150 mg/kg of body weight.

In a carcinogenicity study, sodium chlorite was administered to F344 rats (50 per sex per dose) at concentrations of 0, 300 or 600 mg/litre of drinking-water (equivalent to 0, 18 or 32 and 0, 28 or 41 mg of chlorite per kg of body weight per day in males and females, respectively) and to B6C3F$_1$ mice (50 per sex per dose) at concentrations of 250 or 500 mg/litre (equivalent to 0, 36 or 71 mg/kg of body weight per day) for 85 weeks (Kurokawa et al., 1986b). The rats became infected with a Sendai virus in all groups, which resulted in the termination of the study after only 85 weeks. There was a statistically significant increase in the incidence of hyperplastic nodules in male mice treated with 250 mg/litre, but not in females. The incidence of these lesions did not increase when the dose of chlorite was increased to 500 mg/litre. Hepatocellular carcinomas were too few for their observation to add anything substantive to the evaluation. There were no other treatment-related changes in the incidence of other tumours in either male or female mice.

Groups of 50 male and female B6C3F$_1$ mice were given 0, 250 or 500 mg of sodium chlorite per litre in the drinking-water for 80 weeks (0, 36 or 71 mg of chlorite per kg of body weight per day). A small, but statistically significant ($P < 0.05$), increase in the incidence of lung adenomas was observed at 500 mg/litre. The authors noted that this was not accompanied by the appearance of lung adeno-carcinomas and that the incidence was within the range of historical controls; thus, it was not possible to conclude from these data that chlorite induced lung tumours (Yokose et al., 1987).

In an associated experiment, Kurokawa et al. (1984) assessed the ability of sodium chlorite to promote skin tumours in a group of 20 female Sencar mice. These mice were initiated with a single topical application of 20 nmol (5.1 µg) of dimethylbenzanthracene in acetone followed by 0.2-ml applications of sodium chlorite at 20 mg/ml in acetone twice weekly for 51 weeks. A group of 15 female mice given a single application of dimethylbenzanthracene followed by applica-tions of acetone were used as controls. This treatment resulted in 5 of 25 mice having squamous cell carcinomas at 52 weeks. No tumours were found in the corresponding initiated control mice. Both TPA and benzoyl peroxide produced increased tumour incidence in dimethyl-benzanthracene-initiated mice. These data indicate the potential for a weak tumour-promoting activity for sodium chlorite. However, no dose–response information has been forthcoming in the literature.

4.6.5 *Comparative pharmacokinetics and metabolism*

Some limited data on the absorption, distribution and excretion of chlorite have been developed in rats using ^{36}Cl-labelled chlorite. The label was absorbed with a half-life of about 3.5 min and eliminated with a terminal half-life of 35.2 h (Abdel-Rahman et al., 1982b, 1984b). In 72 h, approximately 35% of the label was recovered in the urine and another 5% in the faeces. In the urine, 32% of the admin-istered dose was determined to be chloride, whereas 6% was found to be chlorite, utilizing a fractionation procedure developed in a prior study (Abdel-Rahman et al., 1980). While these studies did not deter-mine the form of the radiolabel found in blood, plasma and tissues, it was clear that there were significant differences in the behaviour of the label derived from chlorite and chlorate. However, the efforts in this area have been seriously hampered by the lack of an analytical method to discriminate between chlorine dioxide, chlorite, chlorate and chlor-ide *in vivo*.

4.6.6   *Mode of action*

The adverse effects of chlorite appear to be mediated through its activity as an oxidant. However, this question has received very limited attention, except for the involvement of oxidation in its haematological effects. Heffernan et al. (1979b) demonstrated that chlorite was consumed during the oxidation of haemoglobin to methaemoglobin *in vitro*. It was also observed that, unlike methaemoglobin induction by nitrite, the action of chlorite also depleted the red blood cells of GSH, and that this could be partially counteracted by including glucose in the incubation medium. The oxidative action of chlorite could be associated with the production of hydrogen peroxide as measured by the formation of complex I with catalase. This production of hydrogen peroxide was associated with oxidative damage by demonstrating that it could also be attenuated by the inclusion of glucose in the medium. In a dose–response comparison, it could be demonstrated that the loss of GSH and the loss of catalase activity paralleled one another and occurred at concentrations an order of magnitude lower than those required for methaemoglobin formation. This is consistent with the behaviour of other oxidants that produce haemolytic anaemia. These observations also appear to explain why destruction of the red blood cell (measured as decreased haematocrit, decreased haemoglobin concentrations and increased red blood cell turnover) is a much more sensitive and important measure of chlorite toxicity than methaemoglobin formation.

4.7   Chlorate

4.7.1   *General toxicological properties and information on dose–response in animals*

Toxicological data on chlorate in the open scientific literature are limited to two short-term studies in dogs (Sheahan et al., 1971; Heywood et al., 1972) and a series of studies that focused primarily on its ability to induce oxidative damage in the blood of rats and chickens (Abdel-Rahman et al., 1980; Couri & Abdel-Rahman, 1980) and African green monkeys (Bercz et al., 1982). Two short-term studies, one in dogs and one in rats, carried out by Bio/Dynamics Inc. in 1987, were reviewed by WHO (1996). In the dog study, a NOAEL of 360 mg/kg of body weight was identified based on no significant effects on any measured parameter. In the rat study, a NOAEL of

100 mg/kg of body weight was identified based on haematological effects at the highest dose (1000 mg/kg of body weight). There is also a single subchronic study of toxicity conducted in rats in which histopathological examination of tissues was performed (McCauley et al., 1995). This limited data set has hindered attempts to establish a guideline value for chlorate in drinking-water (WHO, 1993).

The studies in dogs documented the fact that high acute doses of 1 or 2 g/kg of body weight induce methaemoglobinaemia (Sheahan et al., 1971; Heywood et al., 1972). In addition, Heywood et al. (1972) administered lower doses (200–300 mg/kg of body weight) for 5 days and observed no clinical signs at doses lower than 300 mg/kg of body weight per day. Those doses that produced some evidence of met-haemoglobinaemia were also found to have produced some discoloration of the kidneys and haematogenous cases in renal tubules at necropsy.

No consistent effects were observed when chlorate was administered to rats at concentrations of 10 or 100 mg/litre (equivalent to 1 or 10 mg/kg of body weight per day) for 12 months (Couri & Abdel-Rahman, 1980). These authors documented some loss of the normal sensitivity of erythrocytes to osmotic shock at these doses, however.

Bercz et al. (1982) administered drinking-water containing sodium chlorate to African green monkeys for a total of 8 weeks in a rising-dose experiment. Drinking-water concentrations were 25, 50, 100, 200 or 400 mg/litre, equivalent to 4, 7.5, 15, 30 or 58.4 mg/kg of body weight per day. Chlorate was found to be without significant effect on a number of serum parameters related to oxidative damage and thyroid hormone levels at concentrations of up to 400 mg/litre.

In the subchronic study (McCauley et al., 1995), concentrations of chlorate of 3, 12 or 48 mmol/litre in drinking-water were provided to both male and female Sprague-Dawley rats for 90 days. These concentrations correspond to 250, 1000 and 4000 mg of chlorate per litre, equal to 30, 100 or 510 mg/kg of body weight per day in males and 42, 164 or 800 mg/kg of body weight per day in females, based on measured water consumption of each group. Body weight gain was sharply curtailed in both sexes at the highest concentration. These effects were generally paralleled by smaller organ weights (except for brain and testes). Some decreases in haemoglobin, haematocrit and red blood cell counts were observed at this same dose. Pituitary lesions (vacuolization in the cytoplasm of the pars distalis) and thyroid gland colloid depletion were observed in both the mid- and high-dose groups of both sexes. The NOAEL in this study was 30 mg/kg of body weight per day.

4.7.2 Reproductive and developmental toxicity

Suh et al. (1983) examined the effects on fetal development of chlorate at 0, 1 or 10 mg/litre administered to rats for 2.5 months prior to mating and throughout gestation. This was a very limited study, involving only six female rats per treatment group. Therefore, the apparent increase of anomalous fetuses from 30.7% in the control group to 52% and 55.2% in the groups receiving 1 and 10 mg/litre, respectively, was not statistically significant. The abnormalities were limited to relatively mild skeletal defects (missing sternebra and rudimentary ribs).

A teratogenicity study carried out by Bio/Dynamics Inc. in 1987 was reviewed by WHO (1996). In this study, rats given 0, 10, 100 or 1000 mg of chlorate per kg of body weight per day on days 6–15 of gestation showed no effects on maternal or fetal health.

4.7.3 Toxicity in humans

There have been sporadic reports of poisoning with sodium or potassium salts of chlorate (Temperman & Maes, 1966; Mengele et al., 1969; Yoshida et al., 1977; Bloxham et al., 1979; Helliwell & Nunn, 1979; Steffen & Seitz, 1981). Most of these cases involved ingestion of preparations of sodium chlorate used for pesticidal purposes. The symptomatology observed is consistent with that observed in the acute studies in dogs identified above. There was generally evidence of oxidative damage to erythrocytes, methaemoglobin formation and the renal complications of haemolytic anaemia. The lethal dose to humans has been estimated to be in the range 20–30 g.

A study in 10 male human volunteers was conducted by administering solutions of 0.01–2.4 mg of chlorate per litre in two 500-ml portions (highest dose 0.034 mg/kg of body weight per day) in a 6-day rising-dose tolerance design (Lubbers & Bianchine, 1984). No adverse effects were noted. This test of acute studies was followed by an experiment (Lubbers et al., 1981) that provided 500 ml of water containing 5 mg of chlorate per litre per day to 10 subjects for 12 weeks (average dose 0.036 mg/kg of body weight per day). Volunteers in both studies were monitored using a battery of clinical and physiological parameters and routine physical examinations throughout the course of the study and for 8 weeks following termination of treatments. Again, no adverse effects were observed.

4.7.4 Carcinogenicity and mutagenicity

There are no published studies of the carcinogenic potential of chlorate administered alone. Sodium and potassium chlorate were evaluated as promoters of renal tumours in *N*-ethyl-*N*-hydroxyethyl-nitrosamine (EHEN)-initiated F344 rats. Sodium chlorate and potassium chlorate were administered in the drinking-water for 28 weeks. There was an increased incidence of renal cell tumours (7/15 rats) in the EHEN-initiated group treated with sodium chlorate, but no effect was observed with potassium chlorate (1/5) relative to control rats (2/15). The small numbers of animals used in this study make the treatment groups indistinguishable from one another statistically (Kurokawa et al., 1985b).

Chlorate has long been known to select nitrate reductase-deficient mutants of *Aspergillus nidulans* (Cove, 1976). However, Prieto & Fernandez (1993) demonstrated that there is also a mutagenic effect of chlorate in *Chlamydomonas reinhardtii* and *Rhodobacter capsulatus*. Chlorate failed to induce mutations in the BA-13 strain of *Salmonella typhimurium*. The positive mutagenic effects were separated from simple selection of nitrate reductase mutants by incubating cells in nitrogen-free media. Lack of nitrogen prevents cell division during the treatment period. In the case of *C. reinhardtii*, significant increases in mutants were observed at concentration of 4–5 mmol/litre and above.

Meier et al. (1985b) examined chlorate in assays for micronuclei and chromosomal aberrations in bone marrow and sperm head anomalies, but all findings were negative.

4.7.5 Mode of action

Some research has been directed towards establishing the mechanisms by which chlorate oxidatively damages erythrocytes and their contents. There is a characteristic delay in the production of met-haemoglobin by chlorate when erythrocytes are incubated in the presence of chlorate (Singelmann et al., 1984). It has been suggested that this delay was due to the conversion of chlorate to chlorite (Heubner & Jung, 1941; Koransky, 1952), but there is no direct evidence to support this view. A competing hypothesis suggested that chlorate formed a complex with methaemoglobin, which autocatalytically increased methaemoglobin formation. This suggestion is supported by experiments demonstrating that the formation of methaemoglobin accelerates the further formation of methaemoglobin in the presence of chlorate (Huebner & Jung, 1941; Jung, 1947, 1965). It is further supported by the observation that compounds that compete for binding of chlorate to methaemoglobin (e.g., azide or cyanide) block the effect.

The properties of the erythrocyte membrane are also modified by chlorate. Increased resistance to haemolysis is the most readily observed effect (Singelmann et al., 1984). These effects appear to be related to the formation of high molecular weight complexes of erythrocytic proteins (Singelmann et al., 1984). These changes could not be reversed by disulfide reduction. The formation of these complexes was associated with the loss of activity of several enzymes, the most sensitive being glucose-6-phosphate dehydrogenase (Singelmann et al., 1984; Steffen & Wetzel, 1993). The inactivation of this enzyme accounts for the insensitivity of chlorate-induced methaemoglobin-aemia to treatment with methylene blue. Reduction of nicotinamide adenine dinucleotide phosphate (NADP) by the pentose pathway is necessary for methylene blue to be effective. The cross-linking of protein is not limited to cytosolic proteins and methaemoglobin, because cross-linking of membrane proteins has also been demonstrated (Steffen & Wetzel, 1993). The cross-linking requires the presence of haemoglobin. Similar changes are induced by hypochlorite, but in this case haemoglobin is not necessary.

The oxidative damage to the erythrocyte appears to be the basis of chlorate's renal toxicity. This hypothesis is supported primarily by the observation that species less sensitive to methaemoglobin formation are also resistant to the nephrotoxic effects of chlorate (Steffen & Wetzel, 1993). The observation is consistent with the finding of haematogenous casts in kidney tubules of dogs treated with doses of chlorate that induce methaemoglobin and their absence in dogs treated with slightly lower doses that did not produce methaemoglobinaemia (Heywood et al., 1972).

4.8 Bromate

4.8.1 *General toxicological properties and information on dose–response in animals*

The acute toxic effects of bromate (administered as either the potassium or sodium salt) have been studied in F344 rats, B6C3F$_1$ mice and Syrian golden hamsters (Kurokawa et al., 1990). The mean LD$_{50}$ values in these species ranged from 280 to 495 mg/kg of body weight, with slightly but consistently lower values found in males than in females of each species. Mice appear to be somewhat more sensitive than the other two species, but the lethal doses are remarkably similar across species. Toxic signs and symptoms at lethal doses included suppressed locomotor activity, ataxia, tachypnoea, hypothermia, diarrhoea, lacrimation and piloerection. Hyperaemia of the stomach and congestion of lungs were observed at autopsy. Damage to renal tubules was seen microscopically, including necrosis in the proximal tubular epithelium. Regenerative changes were observed from 48 h to 2 weeks after treatment. These effects were less marked in mice and hamsters. No glomerular lesions were observed in any species.

Treatment of rats for 10 weeks with potassium bromate concentrations of 250, 500, 1000, 2000 or 4000 mg/litre of drinking-water established a maximally tolerated concentration of less than 1000 mg/litre. As treatments were extended to 13 weeks, elevated levels of glutamate–oxalate transaminase (GOT), glutamate–pyruvate transaminase (GPT), LDH, AP and BUN were observed in blood samples (Onodera et al., 1986; Kurokawa et al., 1990).

Eosinophilic droplets were observed in the cytoplasm of the proximal renal tubule cells in male F344 rats receiving 600 mg of potassium bromate per litre for 12 weeks (Onodera et al., 1986; Kurokawa et al., 1990). These droplets were determined to be eosinophilic bodies rather than hyaline droplets. Lipofuscin pigments were also observed in the proximal tubular epithelium.

Dogs, rats and monkeys were fed bread or flour treated with up to 200 mg of potassium bromate per kg of body weight for up to

17 months (FAO/WHO, 1989). These studies revealed no adverse effects, but, as pointed out by Kurokawa et al. (1990), substantial portions of bromate are presumed to be converted to bromide during the dough-making process. It is also important to note that the numbers of animals included in these studies were quite limited. Subsequent studies conducted for longer periods of time indicated an increase periarteritis in male rats and pathology to the adrenal glands in female rats (Fisher et al., 1979).

Lifetime studies in female rats administered potassium bromate in drinking-water found significant increases in GPT, albumin/globulin ratios, serum potassium ion and cholinesterase activity at concentrations of 500 mg/litre. Slight increases in BUN were also observed at this dose (Kurokawa et al., 1990).

4.8.2 Toxicity in humans

Human poisonings have been associated with the ingestion of sodium bromate and potassium bromate. Many of these poisonings result from accidental or deliberate ingestion of preparations used as neutralizers in permanent wave kits (Warshaw et al., 1985; Lue et al., 1988). Clinical signs of bromate poisoning include anaemia and haemolysis, renal failure and hearing loss. Loss of hearing appears to be more common in adults than in children (Lichtenberg et al., 1989). The hearing loss and renal failure can have a prolonged course in some, but not all, people poisoned by bromate (Kuwahara et al., 1984). Poisoning with bromate is frequently fatal when doses exceed 6 g (Kurokawa et al., 1990).

4.8.3 Carcinogenicity and mutagenicity

IARC evaluated potassium bromate in 1986 and concluded that there is sufficient evidence for its carcinogenicity in experimental animals, whereas no data were available on its carcinogenicity to humans. On this basis, potassium bromate was assigned to Group 2B: the agent is possibly carcinogenic to humans (IARC, 1986, 1987).

In 1992, the Joint FAO/WHO Expert Committee on Food Additives (JECFA) evaluated potassium bromate and concluded that it was genotoxic and carcinogenic. On this basis, JECFA concluded that the use of potassium bromate as a flour treatment agent was not appropriate (FAO/WHO, 1993).

Potassium bromate was found to be weakly mutagenic in *Salmonella typhimurium* strain TA100 when incubated with rat S9 fraction for metabolic activation (Kawachi et al., 1980; Ishidate et al., 1984). Negative results were found in strains TA98, TA1535, TA1537 and TA1538 (Kurokawa et al., 1990). Potassium bromate was also inactive in *Escherichia coli* Wptry⁻ and *E. coli* WP2try⁻his⁻ (Ishidate et al., 1984). Bromate was later found to be active in *S. typhimurium* strains TA102 and TA104, which were developed to detect compounds that generate oxygen radicals (Kurokawa et al., 1990).

Potassium bromate also induced chromosomal aberrations in a Chinese hamster fibroblasts cell line. The concentrations required were, however, very high (>30 mmol/litre) (Ishidate et al., 1984). Such high doses may induce changes by indirect mechanisms.

Bromate appears capable of inducing micronuclei *in vivo*. Significant increases in the frequency of micronuclei were observed in polychromatic erythrocytes when potassium bromate was administered by either the oral or intraperitoneal route (Hayashi et al., 1988; Nakajima et al., 1989). Positive results were obtained at doses of 24 mg/kg of body weight when administered intraperitoneally. Oral doses of less than 100 mg/kg of body weight were negative. Ms/Ae and CD-1 mice were found to be equally sensitive to these effects.

Several reports of bromate-induced cancer in experimental animals are available. The clearest evidence comes from studies in F344 rats (Kurokawa et al., 1983, 1986a, 1987a; DeAngelo et al., 1998). The dose–response curves for the principal target organs, the kidney and peritoneum, are provided in Figure 7. Tumours found in the kidney were of tubular origin, with significantly increased numbers of both adenomas and adenocarcinomas being observed in both males and females (Kurokawa et al., 1983). The peritoneal tumours were mesotheliomas, but treatment-related increases were observed only in male rats. In the Kurokawa et al. (1983) study, concentrations of potassium bromate of 0, 250 or 500 mg/litre correspond to doses of 0, 9.6 or 21.3 mg of bromate per kg of body weight per day in males and 0, 9.6 or 19.6 mg/kg of body weight per day in females (as cited in IARC, 1986 and WHO, 1996). The Kurokawa et al. (1986a) study represented, in part, a repeat of the earlier study, except that more doses were included and only male rats were studied. Concentrations in this study were 0, 15, 30, 60, 125, 250 or 500 mg of potassium bromate per litre, corresponding to 0, 0.7, 1.3, 2.5, 5.6, 12 or 33 mg of bromate per kg of body weight per day (as cited in WHO, 1996). The study provided verification of the ability of potassium bromate to induce both renal cell tumours and mesothelioma. An increased incidence of renal tumours was observed at 125 mg of potassium bromate per litre of drinking-water. Results with mesothelioma were not observed at a dose of 250 mg/litre, but this is partially attributable to the smaller number of animals per treatment group in this experiment. However, the incidences of mesothelioma were very similar at 500 mg/litre in the two studies. Significant increases in the occurrence of dysplastic foci of the kidney (considered to be preneoplastic lesions) were found in groups at doses higher than 30 mg/litre.

The time course of renal tumour development was examined in a third study (dose–response provided in panel C of Figure 7) by Kurokawa et al. (1987a). These experiments were designed to include sacrifices of animals at 13, 26, 39 or 52 weeks as well as the 104-week period examined in prior studies. Additional groups were included, however, that involved treatment for the above periods, but the animals were maintained on bromate-free water until 104 weeks before they were sacrificed. The concentration of potassium bromate was 500 mg/litre during active treatment periods (average dose 32.3 mg of bromate per kg of body weight per day). If animals were held for 104 weeks, 13 weeks of treatment was sufficient to produce the same tumour incidence as was produced by longer treatment periods. Moreover, the same incidence of renal cell tumours was observed in animals that had been treated for 52 weeks and sacrificed at 52 weeks. These data indicate that the tumour yield is not dependent upon the total dose administered, but rather that sufficient time simply had to be provided for the tumours to become evident.

The carcinogenicity of bromate has also been studied in three hybrid strains of mice (B6C3F_1, BDF_1 and CDF_1). Treatments of female mice were conducted at concentrations of 0, 500 or 1000 mg/litre for 78 weeks (average dose 0, 43.5 or 91.6 mg of bromate per kg of body weight per day). No treatment-related increases in tumour incidence were observed (Kurokawa et al., 1986b). Groups of 27 male mice of the same strains were provided 750 mg of potassium bromate

A Renal cell tumours

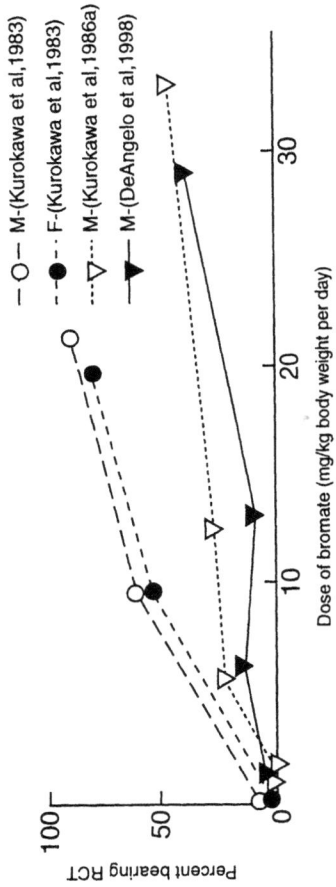

—○— M-(Kurokawa et al,1983)
—●— F-(Kurokawa et al,1983)
····▽···· M-(Kurokawa et al,1986a)
—▼— M-(DeAngelo et al,1998)

Percent bearing RCT

Dose of bromate (mg/kg body weight per day)

B Mesothelioma

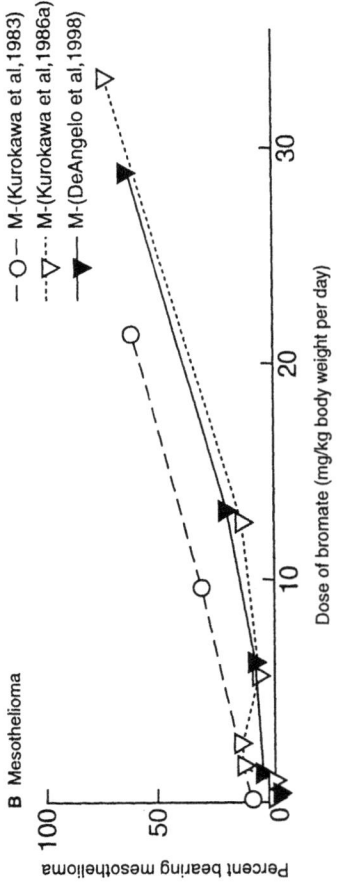

—○— M-(Kurokawa et al,1983)
····▽···· M-(Kurokawa et al,1986a)
—▼— M-(DeAngelo et al,1998)

Percent bearing mesothelioma

Dose of bromate (mg/kg body weight per day)

270

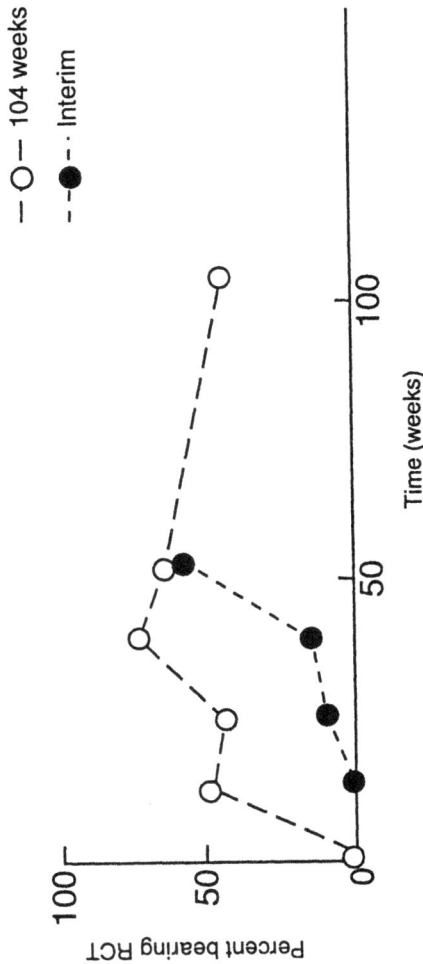

c Renal cell tumours; effect of treatment period

— O — 104 weeks
- - ● - · Interim

Percent bearing RCT

Time (weeks)

WHO 99408

Fig. 7. Bromate carcinogenesis in F344 rats. Data were obtained from four studies: Kurokowa et al. (1983, 1986a, 1987a) and DeAngelo et al. (1998). The effective number of animals per treatment group was 46–53 in the first study, 19–24 in the second, 14–20 in the third and 30–49 in the fourth. Panel A displays the dose–response data for renal cell tumour induction (adenoma plus adenocarcinoma) at terminal sacrifice (up to 104 weeks of treatment). Panel B depicts the induction of mesothelioma in male rats under the same conditions (females did not develop mesothelioma). Panel C depicts the tumour development seen with varying durations of treatment with 500 mg of potassium bromate per litre of drinking-water (29.6–35.5 mg of bromate per kg of body weight per day). Open symbols represent animals that were treated for the indicated period, then placed on distilled water for the remainder of the experiment. All animals were sacrificed at 104 weeks. Solid symbols represent the incidence of tumours when animals were sacrificed at the indicated intervals. Abbreviations used: RCT = renal cell tumours; M = males; F = females.

271

per litre (approximately 60–90 mg/kg of body weight per day, as cited in FAO/WHO, 1993) for 88 weeks. A control group of 15 males per strain was used. Increased numbers of renal cell tumours were not observed in any of the strains. There was, however, an increased frequency of adenomas (14/27 mice) relative to control mice (1/15) of the CDF$_1$ hybrid (Kurokawa et al., 1990).

In a separate study, male Syrian golden hamsters were treated with potassium bromate at concentrations of 0, 125, 250, 500 or 2000 mg/litre of drinking-water for 89 weeks (Takamura et al., 1985). No renal cell tumours were observed in control (0/20) or 125 mg/litre (0/19) groups. At the higher concentrations, the incidences were 1/17 at 250, 4/20 at 500 and 2/19 at 2000 mg/litre.

DeAngelo et al. (1998) administered potassium bromate to male F344 rats and male B6C3F$_1$ mice (78 per group) in drinking-water at concentrations of 0, 20, 100, 200 or 400 mg/litre or 0, 80, 400 or 800 mg/litre, respectively, for 100 weeks. Time-weighted mean daily doses were calculated by the authors from mean daily water consumption and the measured concentrations of potassium bromate. For rats, six animals per group were included for interim sacrifices, which occurred at 12, 26, 52 and 77 weeks. Statistically significant, dose-dependent increases in tumour incidence were observed in the kidney (adenomas and carcinomas combined and carcinomas alone), thyroid (adenomas and carcinomas combined and carcinomas alone) and tunical vaginalis testis (mesotheliomas). Historical control incidences for these tumour sites in male F344 rats are as follows: renal cell tumours, 0.6%; thyroid follicular cell adenomas and carcinomas, 2.1%; and mesotheliomas, 1.5%. The dose–response information for the renal cell tumours and mesotheliomas is provided in Figure 7 to facilitate comparisons with the Kurokawa studies. The combined thyroid cell tumour incidences were 0/36 (0%), 4/39 (10%), 1/43 (2%), 4/35 (11%) and 14/30 (47%) in the 0, 0.1, 6.1, 12.9 and 28.7 mg of bromate per kg of body weight per day dose groups, respectively. Thyroid tumours were not reported in the Kurokawa studies discussed above.

As seen in Figure 7, there is remarkable correspondence in the dose–response relationships for renal cell tumour induction by bromate observed in the DeAngelo et al. (1998) and the Kurokawa et al. (1986a) studies. There was no indication of a positive trend in the dose–response curve at the lowest doses. The DeAngelo et al. (1998)

study produced a positive trend in mesothelioma induction at the lower dose, but this response was not significant until the dose was raised to 6.1 mg/kg of body weight per day, with a strong positive trend in tumour incidence with additional doses. This is different from the Kurokawa studies, in that a significant background incidence of meso-theliomas was observed in one study (Kurokawa et al., 1983), whereas there was no indication of spontaneous lesions in a second study (Kurokawa et al., 1986a). When the studies are combined, a clear positive response is observed at concentrations of 200 mg/litre or more in drinking-water (≥ 12.9 mg/kg of body weight per day).

Tumour responses in male B6C3F$_1$ mice were confined to kidney tumours, but the incidence was not clearly dose-dependent. The tumour incidence at terminal sacrifice was 0/40 (0%), 5/38 (13%), 3/41 (7%) and 1/44 (2%) in mice treated with the equivalent of 0, 6.9, 33 or 60 mg/kg of body weight per day (DeAngelo et al., 1998).

A series of additional studies have evaluated the ability of bromate to act as a tumour promoter in a variety of animal models. Bromate was found to be inactive when applied to the skin of dimethylbenz-anthracene-initiated female Sencar mice in 0.2 ml of acetone at 40 mg of potassium bromate per ml twice per week for 51 weeks (Kurokawa et al., 1984). Potassium bromate was administered for 24 weeks at concentrations of 15, 30, 60, 125, 250 or 500 mg/litre to male F344 rats initiated by EHEN given in the drinking-water for the first 2 weeks at a concentration of 500 mg/litre (Kurokawa et al., 1985b). A dose-related increase in renal cell tumours was observed in rats treated with more than 30 mg of potassium bromate per litre. These changes were apparently not analysed for dose-relatedness, but individual groups were compared using the Student t-test and considered statistically insignificant ($P = 0.05$). There were, however, statistically significant (again compared using the Student t-test) increases in the mean number of dysplastic foci at doses of 30 mg/litre and above ($P < 0.01$) and in the mean number of renal cell tumours observed per cm^2 at 500 mg/li-tre. These data provide evidence that at least some of the carcinogenic activity of bromate can be attributed to its activity as a promoter.

4.8.4   *Comparative pharmacokinetics and metabolism*

The absorption and distribution of bromate and bromide were studied following administration of a single dose of 50 mg of bromate per kg of body weight (Kurokawa et al., 1990). Concentrations of bromate of approximately 4 μg/ml were seen in plasma 15 min after administration. This concentration was quickly reduced to approximately 1 μg/ml within another 15 min and was not detectable in plasma at 2 h. Concentrations of bromate in urine peaked at approximately 1 h after administration. No bromate was detected in urine until doses reached 5 mg/kg of body weight. About 3–6% of the higher doses were recovered in the urine.

These observations are generally consistent with the observed elimination of bromate in human urine following poisonings (Lichtenberg et al., 1989). However, the data available in humans are quite limited and generally involved much higher doses than would be encountered in drinking-water.

4.8.5   Mode of action

Attempts have been made to link the toxic effects of bromate with its oxidant properties. The administration of potassium bromate induces TBARS as a measure of lipid peroxidation (Kurokawa et al., 1987b). Single doses of 77 mg/kg of body weight and higher significantly increased TBARS in the kidney of F344 rats. Mice displayed smaller and less consistent responses, with statistically significant responses being seen in male CDF_1 mice, but not $B6C3F_1$ or BDF_1 mice. Lipid peroxidation was not observed in male Syrian golden hamsters. Treatment of rats with antioxidants (GSH or cysteine) decreased the lethality of potassium bromate. Clinical indicators of kidney damage (non-protein nitrogen, BUN and creatinine) were consistently reduced by GSH or cysteine and increased by co-administration of diethylmaleate, a depletor of GSH. These treatments modified the histopathological changes in renal tubules that were consistent with the clinical findings.

In vitro studies have shown that hydroxyl radical is produced in renal homogenates or kidney cells treated with potassium bromate (Sai et al., 1992a,b). Incubation of hepatocytes or liver homogenates with bromate did not produce evidence of oxygen radicals.

Several studies have demonstrated the formation of 8-OH-dG in the DNA of the kidneys of rats treated with bromate (Kasai et al., 1987;

Sai et al., 1991; Cho et al., 1993). Such modifications in DNA can be produced by oxygen radicals. The formation of 8-OH-dG was not observed in liver DNA of the same animals, paralleling the target organ specificity of the compound. Increases in 8-OH-dG were blocked by parallel treatment with GSH, cysteine or vitamin C (Sai et al., 1992c). Superoxide dismutase and vitamin E were ineffective in modifying DNA damage produced by potassium bromate.

GSH and cysteine administered 30 min before or after bromate significantly inhibited the induction of micronuclei in rat peripheral blood reticulocytes (Sai et al., 1992c). Treatment of superoxide dismutase had no effect on the induction of micronucleated reticulocytes. This suggests that the mechanisms involved in micronuclei formation parallel those involved in production of lipid peroxidation and DNA damage via the production of oxygen radicals.

Chipman et al. (1998) studied the production of DNA oxidation with bromate *in vitro* and with intraperitoneal doses of potassium bromate. Studies with isolated calf thymus DNA demonstrated a GSH-dependent oxidation of guanosine bases. *In vivo* studies indicated that this mechanism was apparently not active. High doses of potassium bromate (100 mg/kg of body weight) administered intraperitoneally induced a statistically significant increase in 8-OH-dG adducts in total cellular DNA. A trend towards an increase was observed at 20 mg/kg of body weight per day.

Studies demonstrating that clastogenic effects of bromate can be suppressed by antioxidant treatments provide evidence that effects in the bone marrow can be attributed to generation of oxygen radicals and the Fenton chemistry that subsequently occurs. The acute doses required to produce evidence of damage to DNA mediated by oxygen radicals generated by bromate have been considerably higher than the daily oral doses required to induce a significant tumour response in the rat kidney (6.1 mg/kg of body weight per day). Consequently, more precise dose metrics and better dose–response information will be necessary to demonstrate the relationship of these effects of bromate with tumour induction. The possibility that increased rates of cell replication could contribute to the renal cancer induced by bromate was investigated by Umemura et al. (1993). Both sodium and potassium salts were utilized and were found to induce significant increases in the cumulative replication fraction of cells in the proximal convoluted tubules of male F344 rats. The effect was significantly smaller in proximal straight or distal tubules. However, female rats did not display elevated rates of replication (Umemura et al., 1993). Thus, these effects in male rats appear to be associated with the formation of bodies that are stained with Mallory-Heidenham stain, used to detect hyaline droplets. These bodies were not seen in female rats. The absence of these responses in female rats, despite a very similar incidence of renal tumours in lifetime exposures (Figure 7), renders an argument of α-2u globulin in the target tissue immaterial. While such pathology could contribute to the tumorigenic response in the male, it is clearly unnecessary for the response in females.

4.9 Other DBPs

Many other DBPs can be found in drinking-water, as indicated in chapter 2. Most of these are present at very low concentrations. Several were considered by WHO (1993, 1996, 1998) in the *Guidelines for drinking-water quality*. Those considered in the Guidelines but not in this document include formaldehyde, chlorophenols, chloropicrin and cyanogen chloride. There are no new data that materially change those evaluations.

5. EPIDEMIOLOGICAL STUDIES

This chapter reviews observational and experimental epidemiological studies that have been conducted to determine associations between disinfected drinking-water and adverse health outcomes. Disinfection practices vary throughout the world. Applied and residual concentrations have varied over the years and from country to country.

Epidemiological study designs, sources of systematic and random error (bias), and guidelines for assessing the causality of associations are discussed in section 5.1. Epidemiological studies of exposures to disinfected drinking-water and to specific DBPs are evaluated in sections 5.2 and 5.3, respectively.

Observational epidemiological studies have been conducted to determine possible associations between adverse health-related outcomes and drinking-water disinfected with chlorine and chloramine. Chlorinated drinking-water was studied most often, and studies primarily compared health risks associated with chlorinated drinking-water from surface water sources with those associated with unchlorinated drinking-water from groundwater sources. Also studied were specific DBPs, including chloroform and other THMs. Only one study considered DBPs other than THMs. Two studies considered risks that may be associated with chloraminated water and chlorine dioxide. The mutagenic activity of drinking-water, which may represent exposure to the non-volatile, acid/neutral fraction of chlorinated organic material in water, was also considered. Health effects studied included cancer, cardiovascular disease and adverse reproductive and developmental outcomes. Most of the studies focused on bladder cancer risks. Also studied were risks of colon, rectal and other cancers.

5.1 Epidemiological study designs and causality of epidemiological associations

Both observational and experimental epidemiological studies have been conducted to assess the health risks associated with drinking-water disinfection (Table 22).

Table 22. Types of epidemiological studies[a]

I.	Experimental		
	A.	Clinical	
	B.	Population	
II.	Observational		
	A.	Descriptive	
		1.	Disease surveillance and surveys
		2.	Ecological
	B.	Analytical	
		1.	Longitudinal
			a. Cohort (follow-up)
			b. Case–control (case–comparison)
		2.	Cross-sectional

[a] Adapted from Monson (1990).

5.1.1 Experimental studies

Results of experimental epidemiological studies, which include clinical trials, are reported in chapter 4 as appropriate under toxicity in humans. These studies consider the effect of varying some characteristic or exposure that is under the investigator's control, much like in a toxicological study. Comparable individuals are randomly assigned to a treatment or intervention group and observed for a specific health-related outcome. Ethical concerns must be fully addressed. Several clinical trials have evaluated changes in lipid, thyroid and haematological parameters that may be affected by consumption of disinfected drinking-water.

5.1.2 Observational studies

Two basic kinds of observational epidemiological studies have been conducted to determine risks associated with disinfection of drinking-water: ecological and analytical. These two study approaches differ primarily in the supportive evidence they can provide about a possible causal association. Unlike the analytical study, an ecological study does not link individual outcome events to individual exposure or confounding characteristics, and it does not link individual exposure and confounding characteristics to one another. In an ecological study, information about exposure and disease is available only for groups of people, and critical information can be lost in the process of aggregating these data (Piantadosi, 1994). Results from ecological studies are difficult to interpret, and serious errors can result when it is assumed that inferences from an ecological analysis pertain either to the individuals within the group or to individuals across the groups (Connor & Gillings, 1974; Piantadosi et al., 1988). Theoretical and empirical analyses have offered no consistent guidelines for the interpretation of ecological associations (Greenland & Robins, 1994a,b; Piantadosi, 1994). Investigators (Greenland & Robins, 1994a,b; Piantadosi, 1994; Poole, 1994; Susser, 1994a,b) have examined the limitations of ecological studies and determined when and under what assumptions this type of study may be appropriate.

Analytical studies can provide the necessary information to help evaluate the causality of an association and estimate the magnitude of risk. For each person included in the study, information is obtained about their disease status, their exposure to various contaminants and confounding characteristics. Analytical studies are either longitudinal or cross-sectional. In a longitudinal study, the time sequence can be inferred between exposure and disease; in other words, exposure precedes disease. In a cross-sectional study, exposure and disease information relate to the same time period; in these studies, it may not always be correct to presume that exposure preceded disease. The cross-sectional study design was used to investigate possible risks of cardiovascular disease and reproductive and developmental risks.

Longitudinal studies are of two opposite approaches: the cohort study and the case–control study. The cohort study begins with the identification of individuals having an exposure of interest and a non-exposed population for comparison; disease consequences or other health-related outcomes are then determined for each group. In a case–control study, the investigator identifies individuals having a disease or health outcome of interest and a control or comparison group of individuals without the disease of interest; exposures and risk factors are evaluated in these persons. In a case–control study, a variety of exposures can be studied, whereas in a cohort study, a variety of diseases can be studied.

The cohort or follow-up study can be either retrospective or prospective, and sometimes a combination retrospective–prospective approach is used. Two or more groups of people are assembled for study strictly according to their exposure status. Incidence or mortality rates for the disease of interest are compared between exposed and unexposed groups. Multiple disease end-points can be evaluated, but a disadvantage is that large numbers of people must be studied, especially for environmental exposures. Because of the lengthy latent period for cardiovascular disease and cancer, a long follow-up period is required for a prospective cohort, and this is usually not feasible. The retrospective cohort study design was used to evaluate the possible association of chlorinated drinking-water with cancer and cardiovascular disease risks.

In a case–control study, persons with the disease of interest (the cases) and persons without this disease (the controls or comparison group) are sampled from either the general population or a special population (e.g., hospitals or a select group) within a specified geographic area. Exposures among the cases are compared with exposures among non-diseased persons. Multiple exposures can be evaluated, and a relatively small number of study participants is needed to obtain reasonably precise estimates of risk associated with environmental exposures. Retrospective exposures must be considered, and, because of the lengthy latency period for cancer and cardio-vascular disease, exposures to water sources and contaminants must be assessed over the previous 20–30 years, or perhaps even a person's lifetime. It may be difficult to assess these exposures accurately. Two types of case–control studies have been conducted to investigate associations between disinfected drinking-water and cancer:

- Decedent cases and controls without interviewing next-of-kin or survivors for information about residential histories, risk factors and possible confounding characteristics.

- Decedent and incident cases and controls using interviews or other methods to obtain information about possible confounding characteristics and document long-term mobility and changes in residences to allow documentation of lifetime exposure to disin-fected water. In several studies, a person's intake of tapwater and historical exposures to chlorinated water, chloroform or other THMs were assessed.

5.1.3   *Random and systematic error*

Biases that occur during the design and conduct of a study can lead to a false or spurious association or a measure of risk that departs systematically from the true value. All reported epidemiological associations require evaluation of random and systematic error so that results can be interpreted properly. Systematic error (bias) affects the validity of a study's observed association; random error affects the precision of the estimated magnitude of the risk. Random error is governed by chance and is influenced by the size of the study. The likelihood that a positive association is due to random error can be assessed by calculating the level of statistical significance ("*P*" value) or confidence interval (CI). A small *P* value or a CI that does not include unity (1.0) suggests that chance may be an unlikely explanation for an observed association, but the association may, nevertheless, be spurious because of systematic error. Statistical significance does not imply causality or biological significance, nor does it mean that random error or chance can ever be completely ruled out as a possible explanation for the observed association. Many epidemiologists believe that strict reliance on statistical significance testing is not appropriate (US EPA, 1994a).

Potential sources of systematic error include observation, selection, misclassification and confounding biases. When information on exposure and disease is collected by methods that are not comparable for each participant (e.g., selective recall), an incorrect association will be due to observation bias. When the criteria used to enrol individuals in the study are not comparable, the observed association between exposure and disease will be due to selection bias. A wrong diagnosis of disease or assessment of exposure can result in misclassification bias. This type of bias may be randomly distributed (non-differential misclassification bias), which almost always biases study results towards the direction of not observing an effect (or observing a smaller change in risk than may actually be present), or it may be non-random (differential misclassification bias), which can result in either higher or lower estimates of risk, depending on how the misclassification is distributed. Lynch et al. (1989) examined the effects of misclassification of exposure using empirical data from an interview-based case–control study of bladder cancer in Iowa (USA). Bladder cancer risk estimates were found to be higher when more information was known about the study participants' residential history and their possible exposure to chlorinated water sources. This suggests that misclassification bias in epidemiological studies of chlorinated water may be primarily non-differential, underestimating the risk; however, in study areas where residential mobility is different from that in Iowa, the magnitude of risk may be overestimated rather than underestimated.

Confounding bias may convey the appearance of an association; that is, a confounding characteristic rather than the putative cause or exposure may be responsible for all or much of the observed association. Although negative confounding bias may occur, concern is usually with positive effects of confounding bias — is confounding bias responsible for the observed association? Confounding bias is potentially present in all epidemiological studies and should always be evaluated as a possible explanation for an association. Information on known or suspected confounding characteristics is collected to evaluate and control confounding during the analysis. In the design of case–control studies, matching is a technique that is used to prevent confounding bias. For example, if smoking is thought to be a possible confounding characteristic, an equal number or proportion of smoking cases and controls can be selected for study in order to avoid confounding bias by this exposure. Techniques are also available to assess and control confounding during the data analysis. In an experimental epidemiological study, randomization is possible; that is, each individual in the study has an equal or random chance of being assigned to an exposed or unexposed group. Because of this random assignment of exposure, all characteristics, confounding or not, tend to be distributed equally between the selected study groups of different exposure.

Procedures in the study's design and conduct are used to prevent or reduce possible bias. If bias has been identified in a study, the direction of the bias can often be determined, but its effect on the magnitude of the association may not. For example, information may be available to determine whether the bias was responsible for an increased or decreased likelihood of observing an association, but its magnitude usually cannot be estimated.

Two basic measures of an association between exposure and disease in analytical studies are the rate ratio or relative risk (RR) and exposure odds ratio (OR). A mortality odds ratio (MOR) is reported when mortality is studied. An RR or OR of 1.0 indicates no association; any other ratio signifies either a positive or negative association. For example, an RR or OR of 1.8 indicates an 80% increased risk among the exposed. Decreased risk and protective effects are indicated by an RR or OR that is less than 1.0. The size of the relative risk and odds ratio is also used to help assess if an observed association may be spurious (Table 23). Based on Monson's (1990) experience, an RR or OR of 0.9–1.2 indicates essentially no association. Associations in this range are generally considered too weak to be detected by epidemiological methods. It is difficult to interpret a weak association, i.e., an RR or OR of 1.2–1.5. One or more confounding characteristics can easily lead to a weak association between exposure and disease, and it is usually not possible to identify, measure or control weak confounding bias. On the other hand, a large relative risk is unlikely to be completely explained by some uncontrolled or unidentified confounding characteristic. When the study has a reasonably large number of participants and the relative risk or odds ratio is large, random variability and confounding bias are much less likely to be responsible for an observed association.

Table 23. Guide to the strength of an epidemiological association[a]

Relative risk	Strength of association
1.0	None
>1.0–<1.5	Weak
1.5–3.0	Moderate
3.1–10.0	Strong
>10.0	Infinite

[a] Adapted from Monson (1990).

Another measure of effect is the standardized mortality ratio (SMR). An SMR of 100 indicates no association; an SMR of 150 indicates a 50% increased risk.

5.1.4   *Causality of an epidemiological association*

Epidemiological associations may be causal; however, before causality can be assessed, each study must be evaluated to determine whether its design is appropriate, the study size is adequate and systematic bias has not influenced the observed association. In addition, the association should be consistent with prior hypotheses and previous study results, and its magnitude should be moderately large. Causality requires sufficient evidence from several well designed and well conducted epidemiological studies in various geographic areas. Supporting toxicological and pharmacological data are also important. Guidelines are available to help epidemiologists assess the possible causality of associations observed in well designed and well conducted studies. Epidemiological data should be interpreted with caution and in the context of other available scientific information. Epidemiologists apply the following guidelines to assess evidence about causality (Hill, 1965; Rothman, 1986):

*   *Biological plausibility.* When the association is supported by evidence from clinical research or toxicology about biological behaviour or mechanisms, an inference of causality is strengthened.

*   *Temporal association.* Exposure must precede the disease, and in most epidemiological studies this can be inferred. When exposure and disease are measured simultaneously, it is possible that exposure has been modified by the presence of disease.

*   *Study precision and validity.* Individual studies that provide evidence of an association are well designed with an adequate number of study participants (good precision) and well conducted with valid results (i.e., the association is not likely due to systematic bias).

*   *Strength of association.* The larger the relative risk or odds ratio, the less likely the association is to be spurious or due to unidentified confounding. However, a causal association cannot be ruled out simply because a weak association is observed.

- *Consistency.* Repeated observation of an association under different study conditions supports an inference of causality, but the absence of consistency does not rule out causality.

- *Specificity.* A putative cause or exposure leads to a specific effect. The presence of specificity argues for causality, but its absence does not rule it out.

- *Dose–response relationship.* A causal interpretation is more plausible when an epidemiological gradient is found (e.g., higher risk is associated with larger exposures).

- *Reversibility or preventability.* An observed association leads to some preventive action, and removal of the possible cause leads to a reduction of disease or risk of disease.

5.2 Epidemiological associations between disinfectant use and adverse health outcomes

Studies of water disinfected with chlorine and chloramine are reviewed in this section. Chlorinated drinking-water was studied most often. Studies primarily compared health risks associated with ingestion of chlorinated drinking-water from surface water sources with those associated with ingestion of unchlorinated drinking-water from groundwater sources, but risks were also compared among populations using chloraminated and chlorinated surface water supplies. Studies that considered exposures to specific DBPs are reviewed in section 5.3. Studies that considered exposures to both disinfected drinking-water and specific by-products are described in either section 5.2 or 5.3.

One study assessed the effects on haematological and serum chemical parameters that may be associated with the use of chlorine dioxide. Because of their relevance to other experimental studies, results are reported in section 4.6.3.

5.2.1 *Epidemiological studies of cancer and disinfected drinking-water*

Since 1974, numerous epidemiological studies have attempted to assess the association between cancer and the long-term consumption of disinfected drinking-water. Studies were conducted in various geographic locations with different types of water sources, chemical quality and levels and types of DBPs. Ecological, cohort and case–control studies of incident and decedent cases were conducted. The quality of information about water disinfection exposures and potential confounding characteristics differs dramatically between these studies. In many of the case–control studies, interviews or other methods were used to obtain information about various risk factors, confounding characteristics and residential histories, to determine long-term exposures to disinfected drinking-water supplies; in several studies, individual tapwater consumption was estimated. However, in several other case–control studies, limited information about exposure and confounding factors was obtained only from the death certificates.

In most studies, disease incidence or mortality was compared between populations supplied with chlorinated surface water and those supplied with unchlorinated groundwater. The chemical quality of drinking-water for a number of chemical constituents, including DBPs, differs between surface water and groundwater and also among the various surface waters in the different geographic locations studied. Surface water sources may also be contaminated with non-volatile synthetic organic compounds from industrial, agricultural and residential runoff. Groundwater may be contaminated with volatile synthetic organic compounds and inorganic constituents, such as arsenic and nitrate. It is not feasible to consider epidemiological studies of cancer in populations consuming unchlorinated drinking-water from surface water sources because so few people consume such drinking-water, but exposures to water contaminants in addition to DBPs must be considered. Since the quality of water sources may also affect the concentration and type of DBPs, even when the same disinfectant is used, it is important to assess specific by-products in water systems included in epidemiological studies.

5.2.1.1   *Cancer associations in ecological studies*

Early epidemiological studies analysed group or aggregate data available on drinking-water exposures and cancer. Usually the variables selected for analysis were readily available in published census, vital statistics or public records. Cancer mortality rates, usually obtained for census tracts, counties or other geographic regions, were compared for areas with different water sources and disinfection practices. Differing source waters and their disinfection were usually used as surrogates for drinking-water exposures of the populations. For example, the drinking-water for the area was categorized as being primarily from a surface water or from a groundwater source and as chlorinated or not chlorinated. In some instances, exposure variables included estimates of the proportion of the area's population that received drinking-water from chlorinated surface water or unchlorinated groundwater. In several ecological analyses, the investigators studied the association between cancer mortality and an estimate of population exposures to levels of chlorination by-products based on the measure of THMs or chloroform levels from a limited number of water samples from monitoring studies (see section 5.3.1.1).

The first ecological studies reported higher mortality from several cancers in Louisiana (USA) parishes where the majority of the population used the lower Mississippi River as a source of drinking-water. Lower mortality was reported in parishes where the majority of the population used groundwater sources (Harris, 1974; Page et al., 1976). Additional ecological studies for different geographic areas of the USA, including Louisiana, Ohio, Missouri, Kentucky, New York, Massachusetts and Iowa, reported increased cancer mortality or incidence in areas using chlorinated surface water (Craun, 1991). A wide range of cancer sites was found to be statistically associated with the use of chlorinated surface water. These cancer sites included gall bladder, oesophagus, kidney, breast, liver, pancreas, prostate, stomach, bladder, colon and rectum. These studies have been extensively reviewed (NAS, 1980, 1986; Crump & Guess, 1982; Shy, 1985; Craun, 1991; Murphy & Craun, 1990). The NAS (1980) noted the limitations of these studies and recommended that analytical studies be conducted to further assess the possible association of chlorinated drinking-water and cancer. It was recommended that studies focus on cancers of the bladder, stomach, colon and rectum because they had been most often associated with chlorinated water in ecological studies.

As noted in section 5.1.2, ecological analyses have theoretical deficiencies, and the interpretation of results from these studies is difficult. Associations reported from ecological analyses cannot be evaluated for causality, nor do they provide an estimate of the magnitude of risk. Yet these studies continue to be conducted. An ecological study in Norway reported weak associations between chlorinated drinking-water supplies and cancer of the colon and rectum in men and women (Flaten, 1992). No associations between chlorinated surface water supplies and bladder or stomach cancer were found in Valencia province, Spain (Suarez-Varela et al., 1994). A study in New Jersey found no association between DBPs and either bladder or rectal cancer (Savin & Cohn, 1996). A study in Taiwan, China, reported associations between the use of chlorinated drinking-water and cancer of the rectum, lung, bladder and kidney (Yang et al., 1998). THMs were not found to be associated with breast cancer risk in an ecological study in North Carolina (Marcus et al., 1998).

5.2.1.2 Cancer associations in analytical studies

More case–control studies have been conducted than cohort studies. Case–control studies have included the traditional interview-based study and those where information was obtained only from death certificates or other readily available sources.

1) Cohort studies

Wilkins & Comstock (1981) found no statistically significant associations between the incidence of cancer mortality in Washington County, Maryland, USA, and residence in an area supplied with chlorinated surface water. Information was available for individuals in a well-defined homogeneous cohort that allowed disease rates to be computed by presumed degree of exposure to chlorination by-products. The cohort was established from a private census during the summer of 1963 and followed for 12 years. The source of drinking-water at home was ascertained, and personal and socioeconomic data were collected for each county resident, including age, education, smoking history and number of years lived at the 1963 address.

Potential cases of cancer were obtained from death certificate records, the county's cancer registry and medical records of the county hospital and a regional medical centre. Census data were used to compute age–gender–site-specific cancer mortality incidence rates for 27 causes of death, including 16 cancer sites, cardiovascular disease, vehicular accidents, all causes of death and pneumonia. Three exposure categories were examined: a high-exposure group of residents served by chlorinated surface water, a low-exposure group served by unchlorinated deep wells and a third group served by a combination of chlorinated surface water and groundwater. The average chloroform level from an extensive analysis of chlorinated surface water samples was 107 µg/litre. The third group, which represented an intermediate exposure, was not used in detailed analyses. Confounding bias was controlled and incidence rates were adjusted by multiple regression analysis for age, marital status, education, smoking history, frequency of church attendance, adequacy of housing and number of persons per room. Selected cancer mortality rates for males and females are reported in Table 24. Small increased risks of bladder and liver cancer were reported; these risk estimates are not statistically stable. Although the study was of high quality and well conducted, the associations reported are subject to random error (i.e., all relative risks had a confidence interval that included 1.0 and thus were not statistically significant). Even though over 31 000 people were included in the cohort, estimates of specific cancer risks were based on relatively few deaths.

History of length of residence was used to estimate a person's duration of exposure to chlorinated and unchlorinated water. For bladder and liver cancer in females and bladder cancer in males, the association was stronger for persons who had lived in their 1963 domicile for 12 or more years than for those who had lived in it 3 years or less. Among men who had at least 24 years' exposure to chlorinated surface water, the bladder cancer risk was high (RR = 6.5; 95% CI = 1.0–>100) but very imprecise and statistically unstable (the CI is high). Additional follow-up of the cohort for several more years can possibly provide more meaningful associations. Freedman et al. (1997) and Ijsselmuiden et al. (1992) conducted case–control studies in Washington County, Maryland (USA) to evaluate risks of cancer of the bladder and pancreas. The results of these two studies are given below.

Zierler et al. (1986) examined mortality patterns of Massachusetts (USA) residents at least 45 years of age who died between 1969 and 1983 and whose last residence was in a community where drinking-water was disinfected with either chlorine or chloramine. A standardized mortality study found little differences in the patterns of 51 645 deaths due to cancer in 43 Massachusetts communities with water supplies disinfected with either chlorine or chloramine as

Table 24. Cohort study: Selected cancer mortality, water source and disinfection, Washington County, Maryland (USA)[a]

Cause of death	Chlorinated surface water		Unchlorinated groundwater		Risk	
	Deaths	Incidence rate[b]	Deaths	Incidence rate[b]	RR	95% CI
Females						
Liver cancer	31	19.9	2	11.0	1.8	0.6–6.8
Kidney cancer	11	7.2	2	7.1	1.0	0.3–6.0
Bladder cancer	27	16.6	2	10.4	1.6	0.5–6.3
Males						
Liver cancer	9	6.4	2	9.0	0.7	0.2–3.5
Kidney cancer	15	10.6	3	13.6	0.8	0.3–2.7
Bladder cancer	46	34.6	5	19.2	1.8	0.8–4.8

[a] From Wilkins & Comstock (1981).
[b] Adjusted incidence rate per 100 000 person–years.

compared with all cancer deaths reported in Massachusetts. The mortality rate of residents from these selected communities with chlorinated drinking-water was slightly higher than expected for stomach cancer (SMR = 109; 95% CI = 104–114) and lung cancer (SMR = 105; 95% CI = 103–107). Mortality rates in selected communities served by chloraminated drinking-water was slightly less than expected for bladder cancer (SMR = 93; 95% CI = 88–98) but greater than expected for lung cancer (SMR = 104; 95% CI = 102–106). Because residence at death was used to assign the exposure status of persons to either chlorinated or chloraminated drinking-water, there is a serious potential for exposure misclassification bias. In addition, errors in death certificate classification of the cause of death may also affect the interpretation of these findings.

Bean et al. (1982) conducted a cohort study of municipalities in Iowa (USA) that were classified into groups based on the source of their drinking-water — surface water or groundwater of various depths. Municipalities included were those with a 1970 population of more than 999 and a public water supply that used exclusively either surface water or groundwater sources that had remained stable for at least 14 years. All of the surface water sources were chlorinated; groundwater was less frequently chlorinated, especially as the depth of the well increased. In the regression analysis, each group was considered a single population, and age-adjusted, sex-specific cancer incidence rates were determined for the years 1969–1978. Indicators of socioeconomic status were obtained for the municipalities to determine if they could explain any observed differences in cancer incidence, and detailed information about residential mobility, water usage and smoking, collected from a sample of non-cancer controls in a large bladder cancer case–control study, was used to assess exposure misclassification and confounding. Municipalities supplied by chlorinated surface water had higher lung and rectal cancer incidence rates than those using groundwater sources for all population groups (<10 000; 10 000–50 000; >50 000); no differences were found for colon and bladder cancer incidence between surface water and groundwater sources. Using information reported by Bean et al. (1982), Poole (1997) estimated a single relative risk for lung cancer (RR = 1.1; 95% CI = 1.1–1.2) and rectal cancer (RR = 1.2; 95% CI = 1.1–1.3).

Selected results from a prospective cohort study of 41 836 post-menopausal women in Iowa are reported in Table 25. The study compared risks among users of groundwater and surface water sources; an assessment of exposure to chloroform and other THMs was also included (Doyle et al., 1997). In 1989, the participants were asked about their source of drinking-water and the length of time this source had been used. Information on potential confounding characteristics was obtained from the baseline questionnaire. Analyses were limited to those who reported drinking municipal or private well-water for more than the past 10 years (*n* = 28 237). Historical water treatment and water quality data were used to ascertain exposure to THMs (see section 5.3.1.2). No increased risks were found for women who used private wells. In comparison with women who used 100% municipal groundwater sources, women who used 100% municipal surface water sources were at a statistically increased risk of all cancers combined (RR = 1.3; 95% CI = 1.1–1.6), colon cancer and breast cancer. No increased risk was observed for bladder cancer or cancer of the rectum and anus; however, only two and six cases of cancer were observed in the cohort. No increased risks were found for cancer of the kidney and six other sites. Reported relative risks were adjusted for age, education, smoking status, physical activity, fruit and vegetable intake, total energy intake, body mass index and waist to hip ratio. Limitations of this study include the relatively short period (8 years) of follow-up of the cohort and possible misclassification of exposure because the source of drinking-water was assessed at only one point in time.

2)   Decedent case–control studies without interviews or residential histories

Six case–control studies where no information was obtained from next-of-kin interviews (Alavanja et al., 1978; Struba, 1979; Brenniman et al., 1980; Gottlieb et al., 1981, 1982; Young et al., 1981; Zierler et al., 1986) considered only information that was routinely recorded on death certificates or readily available from vital statistics, such as occupation, race, age and gender. Deceased cases of cancer of interest were identified, and controls were non-cancer deaths from the same geographic area. In four of these studies, controls were matched for certain characteristics, including age, race, gender and year of death, to prevent possible confounding bias by these characteristics. In

Table 25. Cohort study: Selected incidence of cancer in post-menopausal women and water source in Iowa (USA)[a]

Cancer	100% municipal groundwater		Mixed municipal surface water and groundwater			100% municipal surface water		
	Cases	RR[b]	Cases	RR[b]	95% CI	Cases	RR[b]	95% CI
Bladder	23	1.0	16	2.4	1.3–4.6	2	0.7	0.2–2.9
Colon	106	1.0	47	1.5	1.1–2.2	23	1.7	1.1–2.7
Rectal	53	1.0	20	1.3	0.8–2.2	6	0.9	0.4–2.1
Breast	381	1.0	106	0.9	0.8–1.2	65	1.3	1.03–1.8
Kidney	21	1.0	5	0.8	0.3–2.2	3	1.1	0.3–3.8
Lung	95	1.0	30	1.1	0.7–1.1	17	1.4	0.9–2.4
Melanoma	29	1.0	12	1.4	1.7–2.8	4	1.1	0.4–3.2
All cancers	631	1.0	223	1.2	1.04–1.4	112	1.3	1.1–1.6

[a] From Doyle et al. (1997).
[b] Reported relative risks were adjusted for age, education, smoking status, physical activity, fruit and vegetable intake, total energy intake, body mass index and waist to hip ratio.

studies where matching was not employed, these characteristics were controlled in the analysis. Other possible confounders considered included occupation listed on the death certificate and a measure of urbanization of the person's residence. Information about important potential confounders, such as diet and smoking, was not available and could not be assessed. In one study, smoking was indirectly controlled by assessing lung cancer risks among those exposed to chlorinated water.

A single address (address at death or usual address) or combination of addresses (address at birth and death) was used to determine place of residence for assessing exposure to disinfected water. This place of residence was linked to public records of water source and treatment practices to classify the type of water source and drinking-water disinfection. Exposures considered were surface water or groundwater sources and chlorinated or unchlorinated water sources at the residence (Shy, 1985); in one study, chlorinated and chloraminated water were evaluated (Zierler et al., 1986). In three studies, a statistically significant increased risk of bladder cancer was found to be associated with chlorinated surface water; an increased risk of colon cancer was found in three studies, and an increased risk of rectal cancer was found in four studies (Shy, 1985; Zierler et al., 1986).

Alavanja et al. (1978) studied 3446 deaths due to total urinary tract and total gastrointestinal cancers in seven New York (USA) counties during 1968–1970. The comparison group was non-cancer deaths from the same period matched on age, race, gender, county of birth and county of residence; occupation and the urban nature of the county were considered as potential confounders. Statistically significant increased risks of colon (OR = 2.0) and bladder (OR = 2.0) cancer mortality were found to be higher in men but not women who resided in communities with chlorinated surface water. Other statistically significant increased risks in men who resided in communities with chlorinated surface water were for liver and kidney (OR = 2.8), oesophagus (OR = 2.4) and pancreas (OR = 2.2) cancer mortality; stomach cancer risks were increased for both men (OR = 2.4) and women (OR = 2.2). A study by Struba (1979) of bladder, colon and rectal cancer deaths (700–1500 cases per site) and a comparison group of deaths matched on age, race, gender and region of residence in North Carolina (USA) during 1975–1978 also found statistically significant increased risks for bladder (OR = 1.5), rectal (OR = 1.5) and colon (OR = 1.3) cancer mortality associated with chlorinated water. In studies of similar design, Brenniman et al. (1980), Young et al. (1981) and Gottlieb et al. (1981, 1982) did not find significant increased risks of bladder or colon cancer mortality associated with chlorinated water.

Gottlieb et al. (1981, 1982) found increased risks for rectal (OR = 1.7) and breast (OR = 1.6) cancer mortality associated with chlorinated water in Louisiana (USA). In Illinois (USA), Brenniman et al. (1980) found an increased risk of rectal cancer mortality, but only for females (OR = 1.4). Young et al. (1981) reported an association between colon cancer mortality in Wisconsin (USA) and the average daily chlorine dosage of drinking-water over a 20-year period. The study included 8029 cancer deaths and 8029 non-cancer deaths in white women matched on county of residence, age and year of death. Urbanization, marital status and occupation were considered as potential confounders. Logistic regression analysis was used to evaluate risks for a number of site-specific cancer deaths associated with drinking-water classified by investigators as high, medium and low chlorine-dosed water. Only cancer of the colon was found to be statistically associated with the use of chlorine, but the risk did not increase with higher chlorine dosages. Young et al. (1981) found no association between chlorinated drinking-water and mortality from cancer of the bladder, liver, kidney, oesophagus, stomach, pancreas, lung, brain or breast.

Zierler et al. (1986) evaluated exposures to surface water supplies disinfected with either chlorine or chloramine among 51 645 persons aged 45 years and older who died from cancer and 214 988 controls who died from cardiovascular, cerebrovascular or pulmonary disease or from lymphatic cancer in 43 Massachusetts (USA) communities. Using lymphatic cancer deaths as the comparison group, bladder cancer mortality was found to be moderately increased (OR = 1.7; 95% CI = 1.3–2.2) among residents who died in communities with chlorinated drinking-water as compared with those who died in communities with chloraminated water. This analysis controlled for the potential effects of differences in population density, poverty, age at death and year of death between the communities treated with different disinfectants. Because smoking is a known risk factor for bladder cancer, a special comparison group of lung cancer deaths was enrolled to evaluate this potential cause of confounding bias. Results suggested that smoking did not explain all of the excess mortality from bladder cancer; thus, chlorinated drinking-water may present some risk. However, because residence at death is a poor measure of long-term exposure to disinfected water, an interview-based case–control study was designed to further evaluate the possible association between chlorinated water and bladder cancer (see below).

Although not subject to all of the design limitations of ecological studies, these decedent case–control studies are, nevertheless, still limited in their ability to provide information about the causal nature of the associations observed. Interpretation of results reported by these studies is limited because of likely systematic bias due to misclassification and uncontrolled confounding. Use of decedent instead of incident cancer cases means that differential survival among cases may also influence the observed association. Selection bias is also likely in the control group. Insufficient information was available in these studies to adequately assess historical, long-term exposures to chlorinated water, and use of a single residential address can result in exposure misclassification bias, which may lead to risk being underestimated or overestimated. While the magnitude of risk may be underestimated, as was the case in Iowa (Lynch et al., 1989), risk may also be overestimated as a result of possible different residential mobility patterns. Thus, these studies can provide very limited information about causality and the magnitude of cancer risks of chlorinated water. The findings from these studies should be interpreted with caution because of study design limitations.

3)   Case–control studies with interviews or residential histories

Two additional decedent case–control studies included more complete information about residential histories for a better assessment of exposure to disinfected water. Lawrence et al. (1984) studied the relationship of THMs and colo-rectal cancer among a cohort of white female teachers in New York State (USA) who died of either colo-rectal cancer or non-cancer causes. A case–control study (Zierler et al., 1990) of individuals who had died of primary bladder cancer and other causes was conducted in selected Massachusetts (USA) communities that obtained drinking-water from surface water sources disinfected by either chlorine or chloramine. Eleven case–control studies assessed risks of cancer incidence and included interviews with study participants or a surrogate to obtain information about complete residential histories, long-term drinking-water exposures to chlorinated or chloraminated water and potential confounding characteristics (Cantor et al., 1985, 1987, 1990, 1995, 1997, 1998; Cragle et al., 1985; Young et al., 1987, 1990; Lynch et al., 1990; Ijsselmuiden et al., 1992; McGeehin et al., 1993; Vena et al., 1993; King & Marrett, 1996; Freedman et al., 1997; Hildesheim et al., 1998). In seven of these studies (Cantor et al., 1987, 1990, 1995, 1997, 1998; McGeehin et al., 1993; Vena et al., 1993; King & Marrett, 1996; Hildesheim et al., 1998), information about tapwater consumption was also obtained. In six studies (Young et al., 1987, 1990; McGeehin et al., 1993; Cantor et al., 1995, 1997, 1998; Hildesheim et al., 1998; King & Marrett, 1996), THM exposure was evaluated (see also section 5.3.1.2).

Bladder cancer risk

Chlorinated water studies. Cantor et al. (1985) reported results from a national study of water chlorination and bladder cancer in the USA, the largest case–control study of water chlorination risks reported to date. The study included 2982 people between the ages of 21 and 84 diagnosed with bladder cancer in 1978 and residing in five states and five metropolitan areas of the USA and 5782 population-based comparison subjects, randomly selected and frequency matched on gender, age and study area. The primary purpose of the study was to evaluate the possible association of bladder cancer and artificial sweeteners; however, because of its case–control design, it was possible to include an assessment of drinking-water exposures. Participants were interviewed for information about past residences, smoking, occupation, artificial sweetener use, coffee and tea consumption and use of hair dyes. A lifetime residence history categorized individuals according to water sources and chlorination status on a year-by-year basis. Information was obtained on use of bottled water and fluid consumption. Logistic regression analysis was used to control for potential confounding bias. Overall, no association was found between bladder cancer risk and duration of exposure to chlorinated water. In all study areas combined, no increased risk was found among participants who lived in areas with chlorinated water supplies for <20, 20–39, 40–59 and 60 or more years (Table 26A). However, an increased bladder cancer risk was found among persons who never smoked, were never employed in a high-risk occupation and resided

Table 26. Bladder cancer risks and duration of exposure to chlorinated surface water in five interview-based incident case–control studies

Years of exposure to chlorinated surface water	Odds ratio	95% CI	Comments	Reference
A. Ten areas of the USA			Whites only; adjusted for age, gender, smoking, usual employment as a farmer, study area	Cantor et al. (1985)
0	1.0			
1–19	1.1	0.8–1.4		
20–39	1.0	0.8–1.3		
40–59	1.0	0.8–1.3		
≥60	1.1	0.8–1.5		
B. Ontario, Canada			Adjusted for age, gender, smoking, education, calorie intake	King & Marrett (1996)
0–9	1.0			
10–19	1.0	0.7–1.5		
20–34	1.2	0.9–1.5		
≥35	1.4	1.1–1.8		
C. Colorado			Whites only; adjusted for gender, smoking, coffee consumption, tapwater intake, family history of bladder cancer, medical history of bladder infection or kidney stone	McGeehin et al. (1993)
0	1.0			
1–10	0.7	0.4–1.3		
11–20	1.4	0.8–2.5		
21–30	1.5	0.8–2.9		
>30	1.8	1.1–2.9		
D. Iowa			Adjusted for age, gender, smoking, education, high-risk employment, study area	Cantor et al. (1998)
0	1.0			
<19	1.0	0.8–1.2		
20–39	1.1	0.8–1.4		
40–59	1.2	0.8–1.7		
≥60	1.5	0.9–2.6		
E. Washington County, Maryland			Adjusted for age, gender, smoking, urbanicity	Freedman et al. (1997)
0	1.0			
1–10	1.0	0.6–1.5		
11–20	1.0	0.6–1.6		
21–30	1.1	0.6–1.8		
31–40	1.1	0.6–2.2		
>40	1.4	0.7–2.9		

in areas served by chlorinated surface sources (Table 27A). There was little evidence of an exposure–response relationship among persons who had never smoked. Only in the low-risk group of non-smokers who had resided 60 or more years in an area served by chlorinated water was the increased bladder cancer risk statistically significant (RR = 2.3; 95% CI = 1.3–4.2). Although the study included a large number of cases and controls, this subgroup analysis included relatively few study participants (Table 27A). Only 46 cases and 77 controls were included in the analysis, which found a doubling of risk among non-smokers who had resided 60 or more years in an area served by chlorinated water.

Lynch et al. (1990) conducted a separate analysis of the Iowa (USA) portion of the national bladder cancer study. Included were 294 primary, histologically confirmed cases of bladder cancer in whites and 686 comparison subjects, all of whom had spent more than 50% of their lifetimes on primary water sources with known chlorination exposure. Study participants exposed to chlorinated water sources for more than 40 years were found to have twice the risk of bladder cancer (OR = 2.0; 95% CI = 1.3–3.1) compared with participants exposed to unchlorinated groundwater sources. Unadjusted risks were higher (OR = 9.9; 95% CI = 2.6–38.0) when the analysis was restricted to study participants who used, for more than 40 years, water sources that had been chlorinated prior to filtration, a water treatment practice known to result in higher THM levels. However, for both of these chlorination practices, no statistically significant risks were found to be associated with the use of chlorinated water for 40 or fewer years. The risk of bladder cancer was also increased for cigarette smokers with longer duration of exposure to chlorinated drinking-water. Unadjusted risks were 4 times as great in heavy smokers (OR = 9.9; 95% CI = 2.6–38.0) as in non-smokers (OR = 2.7; 95% CI = 1.2–5.8) who were exposed to chlorinated water for more than 30 years. A greater risk of bladder cancer was also seen in heavy smokers (OR = 4.0; 95% CI = 2.0–8.4) who were exposed to chlorinated water for 30 or fewer years.

King & Marrett (1996) conducted a population-based case–control study in Ontario (Canada). Cases were residents between 25 and 74 years of age with a histologically confirmed diagnosis of primary cancer or carcinoma *in situ* of the bladder, diagnosed between

Table 27. Bladder cancer risks for smokers and non-smokers exposed to chlorinated water

Years at a residence served by chlorinated water	Cases	Controls	Odds ratio (95% CI)	Cases	Controls	Odds ratio (95% CI)	Reference/comments
A. Males and females, 10 areas of the USA	**Never smoked**			**Current smoker**			Cantor et al. (1985)
0	61	268	1.0	87	109	1.0	Whites, adjusted for study area, gender, age, usual employment as a farmer, smoking
1–19	29	110	1.3 (0.7–2.2)	63	71	0.9 (0.6–1.5)	
20–39	73	236	1.5 (0.9–2.4)	136	186	0.7 (0.4–1.1)	
40–59	108	348	1.4 (0.9–2.3)	166	211	0.7 (0.5–1.2)	
≥60	46	77	2.3 (1.3–4.2)	27	37	0.6 (0.3–1.2)	
B. Males and females, Colorado	**Non-smokers**			**Smokers**			McGeehin et al. (1993)
0	19	45	1	85	57	1	Whites only; adjusted for gender, smoking, coffee consumption, tapwater intake, family history of bladder cancer, medical history of bladder infection or kidney stone
1–11	7	21	0.8 (0.2–2.4)	36	33	0.8 (0.4–1.4)	
12–34	11	34	0.9 (0.3–2.3)	70	34	1.4 (0.8–2.4)	
>34	21	25	2.9 (1.2–7.4)	77	25	2.1 (1.1–3.8)	

Table 27 (Contd).

C. Males and females, Washington County, Maryland

	Never smoked			Smoker (past/present)			(Freedman et al., 1997)
0	32	331	1.0	47	391	1.3 (0.8–2.2)	Adjusted for age, gender, and urbanicity
1–10	21	232	0.8 (0.4–1.6)	70	469	1.4 (0.8–2.5)	
11–20	15	147	0.9 (0.5–1.9)	41	285	1.4 (0.8–2.5)	
21–30	6	89	0.6 (0.2–1.5)	32	177	1.7 (0.9–3.2)	
31–40	3	53	0.5 (0.1–1.5)	13	54	2.2 (1.0–4.7)	
>40	5	51	0.9 (0.3–2.3)	8	27	2.8 (1.0–6.9)	

D. Males, Iowa

	Never smoked			Current smoker			Cantor et al. (1998)
0	112	332	1.0	188	156	3.5 (2.5–4.7)	Adjusted for age, study period, education, high-risk population
1–19	27	75	1.0 (0.6–1.6)	73	62	3.5 (2.3–5.3)	
20–39	6	22	0.8 (0.3–2.0)	37	20	5.7 (3.1–10.4)	
>40	5	26	0.7 (0.3–1.9)	29	16	5.8 (3.0–11.3)	

1 September 1992 and 1 May 1994. Of 1694 eligible cases, 250 patients were not included in the study because an appropriate physician could not be identified or the patients were recently deceased or too ill to be contacted. Of the remaining 1444 patients, consent was received to contact 1262 (87%). The remaining 13% of cases did not participate because the physician refused to participate, did not provide consent or did not respond. Controls were an age–sex frequency matched sample of the general population from households randomly selected from a computerized database of residential telephone listings in the same area. Since the control subjects were also used to study cancers of the colon and rectum with respect to the same exposures (results not yet published), they were selected to have the expected age–sex distribution of these three cancer sites combined. In over 90% of the 2768 households with an eligible resident, the person selected for the study agreed to participate. The overall response rate considering actual participation was 73% for cases and 72% for controls.

Relevant exposure and confounding variables were collected using a mailed questionnaire in combination with a computer-assisted telephone interview. Interviewers were blinded as to the case or control status of the subject. Questions were included on demographics (e.g., gender, date of birth and education), other potentially important confounding variables (e.g., smoking history and usual diet prior to diagnosis) and information pertaining to the primary exposures of interest (e.g., residence and water source history and usual water consumption prior to diagnosis). Persons reported their drinking-water source and other household water sources at each residence as municipal, household well, bottled water or other. Volume of tapwater was calculated from the reported daily frequency of consuming beverages containing water during the 2-year period before the interview and usual source of water (tap or bottled) used to make hot and cold beverages. The water supply for each participant was characterized by source (surface water vs. groundwater) and chlorination status (chlorinated vs. unchlorinated).

The analysis considered the 696 cases (75%) and 1545 controls (73%) for whom water source characteristics were available for at least 30 of the 40 years ending 2 years before the person's interview. To reduce possible misclassification of exposure, only persons with 30 or more years of known water history were included in a separate analysis. Logistic regression was used to estimate bladder cancer risks. Potentially important confounders considered were age, gender, smoking, education, consumption of alcoholic beverages, coffee consumption, total fluid consumption and dietary intake of energy (total calories), protein, fat, cholesterol, fibre and vitamin A.

The study found a pattern of increasing bladder cancer risk with increasing number of years exposed to chlorinated surface water, but a statistically significant association was found only for lengthy exposures (Table 26B). For persons exposed to a chlorinated surface water source for 35 years or more, the bladder cancer relative risk was increased by 40% in comparison with those exposed for less than 10 years. An analysis restricted to those who had relatively homogenous water exposures found that exposure to chlorinated surface water for 30 or more years was associated with a weak increased risk (OR = 1.4; 95% CI = 1.1–1.8) compared with exposure to a groundwater source. King & Marrett (1996) found higher relative risk estimates for non-smokers associated with many years of exposure to chlorinated drinking-water from surface water sources, but the difference in risk compared with smokers was not statistically significant, nor was the pattern of higher risks in non-smokers observed consistently.

McGeehin et al. (1993) conducted a case–control study to assess the relationship between chlorinated or chloraminated drinking-water and bladder cancer in Colorado. Study participants were identified from a population-based cancer registry; 327 histologically confirmed incident bladder cancer cases and 261 randomly selected controls with other cancers, except colo-rectal and lung, were interviewed by a single blinded interviewer about demographic data, drinking-water source, fluid consumption and personal habits. Persons with colo-rectal and lung cancers were excluded from the control group because of a possible association with chlorinated surface water reported in earlier studies. Of the originally identified cases, 38% could not be interviewed because permission was denied by the physician, cases were dead or persons refused to participate. For controls, 47% were not interviewed for these reasons. Because of the large number of excluded study participants, selection bias is a concern. Bias could be present if the excluded persons were different from participating persons in ways that are related to the exposure and outcome.

Information was collected from individuals on tapwater consumption and from local water utilities regarding water source and method of disinfection in order to construct individual lifetime profiles of exposure to disinfected drinking-water. Although 91% of person-years of community exposure to specific water sources could be determined, only 81% of disinfection methods, 60% of THM levels and 55% of residual chlorine levels could be determined for use in assessing exposures.

Logistic regression analysis, adjusting for coffee consumption, smoking, tapwater intake, family history of bladder cancer, sex and medical history of bladder infection or kidney stone, found no statistically significant increased risk of bladder cancer for persons exposed to chlorinated drinking-water for 1–10, 11–20 or 21–30 years compared with those with no exposure to chlorinated drinking-water (Table 26C). The increased relative risk (OR = 1.8; 95% CI = 1.1–2.9) of bladder cancer for persons exposed to chlorinated drinking-water for more than 30 years was statistically significant. A trend of increasing risk with increasing duration of exposure was reported (trend $P < 0.01$), but no association was found between THM levels and bladder cancer (also see section 5.3.1.2). The authors reported that these results support the hypothesis that prolonged (i.e., more than 30 years) exposure to chlorinated drinking-water from surface water sources is associated with an increased risk of bladder cancer. However, incomplete characterization of the exposure profiles for water sources and disinfection, potential bias from non-participation and potential confounding bias from undetermined confounders tend to limit this interpretation. An increased risk of bladder cancer was seen among both smokers and non-smokers with more than 34 years of exposure to chlorinated water (Table 27B).

Freedman et al. (1997) conducted a population-based case–control study in Washington County, Maryland (USA) to evaluate the association between the incidence of bladder cancer and use of chlorinated surface water (Table 26E). The study included 294 bladder cancer cases in white residents enumerated in a 1975 county census and reported to the county cancer registry between 1975 and 1992;

2326 white controls, frequency matched by age and gender, were randomly selected from the census. Duration of exposure to chlorinated surface water was based on length of residence in the census household before 1975, and relative risks were calculated using logistic regression methods adjusting for age, gender, tobacco use and urbanicity. Nearly all municipal sources in 1975 were supplied by surface waters that had been chlorinated for more than 30 years. Bladder cancer risk was found to be weakly associated with municipal water and duration of exposure to municipal water (for exposure to municipal water for more than 40 years, OR = 1.4; 95% CI = 0.7–2.9). The association was limited, however, to those who smoked cigarettes (Table 27C), primarily male smokers. Male smokers who had resided more than 40 years in an area with municipal water supplies had a 3-fold greater risk than male smokers who had not resided in an area with municipal water supplies or had resided in such an area for 20 years or less (OR = 3.2; 95% CI = 1.1–8.6). No increased relative risk was found for female smokers; in fact, relative risks for exposure to municipal water for 1–30 years were less than those for no exposure to municipal water (OR ranged from 0.4 to 0.6; 95% CI ranged from 0.1 to 2.9). A limitation of this study is that duration of exposure was based solely on place of residence in 1975. Also, there was no information on prior or subsequent domiciles, but the authors felt that because the population was relatively stable, residential mobility was not a major concern. No water consumption data were available, nor were data on DBPs available. As previously reported, however, chloroform analyses in 1975 found an average chloroform concentration of 107 µg/litre in chlorinated surface waters used by the cohort (Wilkins & Comstock, 1981).

Cantor et al. (1998) and Hildesheim et al. (1998) conducted a population-based case–control study in Iowa (USA) in 1986–1989 to evaluate cancer risks that may be associated with chlorinated water; results have been reported for bladder, colon and rectal cancer. Information about residential history, drinking-water source, beverage intake and other factors was combined with historical data from water utilities and measured THM levels to create indices of past exposure to chlorinated by-products. The bladder cancer study was composed of 1123 incident cases who were residents of Iowa, aged 40–85 years and diagnosed with histologically confirmed bladder cancer in 1986–1989 and 1983 randomly selected controls from driver's licence records and US Health Care Financing Administration listings for whom data relating to at least 70% of their lifetime drinking-water source were available. Of 1716 eligible bladder cancer cases, 85% participated. Adjusted odds ratios were determined using unconditional logistic regression analysis. Where appropriate, risks were adjusted for gender, age, cigarette smoking, years of education and employment in an occupation with elevated bladder cancer risk, including in the analysis persons with at least 70% of lifetime years with available information on drinking-water source. No increased risk was observed for men and women combined (Table 26D). Risk increased among men, with duration of chlorinated surface water exposure, duration of chlorinated groundwater exposure and duration of exposure to any chlorinated water source. For women, risks did not increase, and a protective effect for duration of exposure to chlorinated surface water was suggested, with OR values of less than unity; OR values ranged from 0.7 to 0.9, and 95% CIs ranged from 0.2 to 2.4. The increased relative risks in men were restricted to current smokers (Table 27D) and past smokers. No increased risk was found for men who had never smoked. Among non-smoking men and women, regardless of their previous smoking habit, there was no association between duration of exposure to chlorinated water and bladder cancer risk. Little or no association of risk was found for either total daily tapwater intake or intake of all beverages for men or women (Table 28A).

Chloraminated water studies. In Massachusetts (USA), a number of towns have used surface water disinfected only with chlorine or chloramine since 1938, providing an opportunity to compare cancer risks between these two disinfectants. In a previous study, Zierler et al. (1986) found bladder cancer mortality to be weakly associated with residence at death in Massachusetts communities using chlorine for water disinfection; however, because of the concern that residence at time of death is a poor measure of historical exposure to a water disinfectant and likely resulted in misclassification bias, an analytical study (Zierler et al., 1988, 1990) was also conducted. Eligible for the study were all persons who were over 44 years of age at death and who died during 1978–1984 from bladder cancer, lung cancer, lymphoma, cardiovascular disease, cerebrovascular disease or chronic obstructive pulmonary disease while residing in 43 selected communities. Included were 614 persons who died of primary bladder cancer and 1074 individuals who died of other causes. Possible confounding bias

Table 28. Bladder cancer risks associated with daily tapwater consumption

Tapwater consumption (litres/day)	Odds ratio	95% CI	Comments	Reference
A. Males and females, Iowa			Beverages from tapwater; adjusted for gender, age, study period, education, high-risk occupation, smoking	Cantor et al. (1998)
<1.58	1.0			
1.58–<2.13	1.2	0.9–1.5		
2.13–2.85	1.3	1.0–1.6		
>2.85	1.2	0.9–1.5		
B. Males and females, 10 areas of the USA			Adjusted for age, gender, smoking, high-risk occupation, population size, usual residence	Cantor et al. (1985, 1987, 1990)
<0.80	1.0			
0.81–1.12	1.1	0.9–1.3		
1.13–1.44	1.1	1.0–1.3		
1.45–1.95	1.3	1.1–1.5		
>1.95	1.4	1.2–1.7		

by age, gender, smoking, occupation and socioeconomic status was controlled by multiple logistic regression. Detailed information on each person's residential history and possible confounding characteristics was obtained from survivors and census records. Analyses included a person's usual exposure (at least 50% of their residence since 1938 was in a community where surface water was disinfected by only one of the two disinfectants, either chlorine or chloramine) or lifetime exposure to water disinfected with only one of the two disinfectants.

An association was found between bladder cancer mortality and both usual and lifetime exposure to chlorinated drinking-water. The bladder cancer mortality risk was higher for lifetime exposure than for usual exposure; a 60% increased risk of bladder cancer mortality (MOR = 1.6; 95% CI = 1.2–2.1) was found among lifetime residents of communities where only chlorinated surface water was used. The association is statistically significant, and the estimate of risk is precise (i.e., the CI is small). Bias is not likely present, but the magnitude of the association is not large and may be subject to residual confounding by unknown, unmeasured characteristics. The magnitude of the association found by Zierler et al. (1988, 1990), however, may be even larger than a 60% increased risk. Using only lymphatic cancers as the comparison group, the risk of bladder cancer mortality among lifetime consumers of chlorinated water was 3 times the risk for consumers of chloraminated drinking-water (MOR = 2.7; 95% CI = 1.7–4.3). This suggests that one or more causes of death in the comparison group may also be associated with water chlorination.

McGeehin et al. (1993) also found that the risk of bladder cancer decreased with increasing duration of exposure to chloraminated surface water (trend $P < 0.01$). Persons who consumed chloraminated water for 21–40 years had a decreased, but not statistically significant, bladder cancer risk (OR = 0.7; 95% CI = 0.1–1.1). Those who consumed chloraminated water for more than 40 years also had a slightly decreased risk of cancer (OR = 0.6; 95% CI = 0.4–1.0). However, neither of these risks was statistically significant. McGeehin et al. (1993) reported that their results do not imply that chloraminated water conveys a protective effect, because there is no plausible biological explanation for suggesting that choramination inhibits neoplastic transformation of the bladder epithelium. Zierler et al. (1988, 1990) found that lifetime users of chloraminated surface water had a lower bladder cancer mortality risk than lifetime users of chlorinated surface water, and the findings of McGeehin et al. (1993), if real and not due to bias, provide additional evidence to support the conclusion that bladder cancer risks may be lower in persons using chloraminated drinking-water for long periods of time.

Water and fluid consumption studies. Studies have reported both increased (Claude et al., 1986; Jensen et al., 1986) and decreased (Slattery et al., 1988) risk of bladder cancer associated with a high total fluid intake. Vena et al. (1993) conducted a case–control study that investigated the relationship between the incidence of bladder cancer and fluid intake and consumption of drinking-water. The study included 351 white males with histologically confirmed transitional cell carcinoma of the bladder and 855 white male controls with cancer of one of six other sites (oral cavity, oesophagus, stomach, colon, rectum and larynx).

Study subjects were interviewed about diet and their total daily fluid intake of alcoholic beverages, bottled beverages, soda, milk, coffee, tea, all juices and glasses of tapwater. A dose–response relationship was found between daily intake of total liquids and risk of bladder cancer when a number of potential confounding factors were controlled (trend $P < 0.001$). For persons under the age of 65, up to a 6-fold increased risk of bladder cancer was found for those who drank more than 7 cups of fluids compared with those who drank 2–7 cups of total fluids daily (the lowest quartile studied). The OR ranged from 2.6 (95% CI = 1.2–5.7) for those who drank 8–10 cups of total fluids per day to 3.7 (95% CI = 1.7–8.2) for those who drank 11–13 cups and 6.3 (95% CI = 2.8–14.1) for those who drank 14–49 cups of total fluids daily. These ORs are adjusted for age, education, cigarette smoking, coffee, carotene and sodium by logistic regression. Statistically significant but slightly smaller risks were observed for those 65 and older. Total fluid consumption was divided into tapwater and non-tapwater consumption. Tapwater beverages included coffee, tea (hot and iced), 75% reconstituted orange juice, all other juices and glasses of water taken directly from the tap. A dose–response relationship was observed between increased tapwater consumption and bladder cancer (trend $P < 0.001$), but no statistically significant increased risk of bladder cancer, regardless of age, was found for persons consuming either 6–7 or 8–9 cups of tapwater per day compared with persons consuming 0–5 cups. Only in the highest group (10–39 cups of tapwater per day) was the association between tapwater consumption and bladder cancer statistically significant (OR = 2.6, 95% CI = 1.5–4.5, for those under the age of 65; OR = 3.0, 95% CI = 1.8–5.0, for those 65 and older). Increased bladder cancer risk was also found among persons under the age of 65 with the highest quartile of non-tapwater intake.

The results provide additional hypotheses for further study, but limitations of this study preclude definitive conclusions regarding a potential water chlorination–cancer association. Over a third of potential cases were excluded for reasons including death (3%), refusal to be interviewed (24%) and extreme illness (11%). Selection bias would be present if the excluded cases were different from the participating cases in ways that are related to the exposure and outcome. Recall bias may also have been present, as bladder cancer cases were asked to recall usual dietary habits for the year before onset of cancer symptoms, whereas the controls, other cancer patients, were asked to recall dietary habits for the year before their interview for the study. Assessing fluid consumption in the year before onset of symptoms may not reflect historical or lifetime patterns, and increased consumption may occur during the early stages of bladder cancer.

Since increased risks were seen primarily in total fluid consumption, it is also possible that total fluid consumption may be relevant in the pathogenesis of bladder cancer. Total daily fluid intake may be a marker for some unmeasured risk factor, and it is important to determine the biological relevance of increased fluid intake, independent of chlorinated tapwater, in the pathogenesis of bladder cancer (US EPA, 1994a).

Since over 70% of the study population spent more than 90% of their lives using chlorinated surface water from public water supplies in western New York State, it is possible that the observed increased risks for bladder cancer may be associated with a high consumption of chlorinated tapwater. However, limited information was available with which to determine a study participant's duration of exposure to specific municipal water systems, and risks were not compared for populations using chlorinated surface water supplies.

Cantor et al. (1987, 1990) conducted a further analysis of the national bladder cancer study to include beverage consumption information that was available for 5793 men and 1983 women. After correcting for age, smoking and other potential confounding characteristics, it was found that people who drank the most chlorinated tapwater had a bladder cancer relative risk about 40% higher than people who drank the least (Table 28B). When tapwater consumption was analysed separately for men and women, however, the association between water consumption and bladder cancer risk was statistically significant only among males. Bladder cancer risk was also evaluated for the combined effects of tapwater consumption and duration of chlorinated surface water use. No increased risk was associated with a high consumption of chlorinated drinking-water from surface water sources for less than 40 years. Increased bladder cancer risk (OR = 3.2; 95% CI = 1.2–8.7) was seen primarily in populations who had resided 60 or more years in areas served by chlorinated surface water and whose tapwater consumption was above the median of greater than 1.4 litres per day. Among non-smoking men, a risk gradient was apparent for those who consumed more than the population median of tapwater (Table 29), but a higher risk was also seen for non-smoking

Table 29. Bladder cancer risks among non-smokers according to daily tapwater consumption and exposure to chlorinated surface water in 10 areas of the USA[a]

Years at residence with chlorinated water	Odds ratio (95% CI)[b]			
	Tapwater consumption below 1.4 litres		Tapwater consumption above 1.4 litres	
	Males	Females	Males	Females
0	1.0	1.0	1.0	1.0
1–19	1.6 (0.7–4.0)	1.2 (0.4–3.7)	0.8 (0.3–2.5)	1.7 (0.5–5.4)
20–39	1.0 (0.4–2.6)	1.5 (0.5–4.4)	2.1 (0.9–5.2)	1.8 (0.6–5.4)
40–59	0.7 (0.3–1.9)	2.1 (0.8–5.9)	2.5 (0.9–6.6)	1.8 (0.6–5.9)
≥60	1.3 (0.4–4.4)	4.3 (1.3–14.5)	3.7 (1.1–12.0)	3.6 (0.8–15.1)

[a] From Cantor et al. (1987, 1990).
[b] Adjusted for age, gender, smoking, high-risk occupation, population size, usual residence.

311

women who consumed less than the median amount. The increasingly smaller numbers of participants available for these subgroup analyses generally lead to statistically unstable estimates, making it difficult to evaluate trends in these data.

In Colorado (USA) (McGeehin et al., 1993), the risk of bladder cancer (OR = 2.0; 95% CI = 1.1–2.8) was found to be elevated among persons who consumed more than five glasses of tapwater per day, and a dose–response trend was found (P < 0.01). However, tapwater consumption appeared to be an independent risk factor for bladder cancer. There was no evidence of an increased relative risk of bladder cancer when both the volume of water consumed and years of exposure to chlorinated water were considered in the analysis. For example, similar estimates of risk were found for those who consumed more than five glasses of chlorinated water for fewer than 12 years (OR = 2.0; 95% CI = 0.8–4.7) and those who consumed more than five glasses of chlorinated water for 12 years or more (OR = 2.4; 95% CI = 1.0–5.9). Similar to the study in western New York (Vena et al., 1993), tapwater consumption in Colorado was assessed for the year prior to diagnosis for cancer and controls and thus may not reflect historical patterns.

King & Marrett (1996) also evaluated the combined effects of tapwater consumption and duration of exposure to chlorinated water (see also section 5.3.1.2). Overall, the pattern of risk estimates did not provide evidence for the interdependence of water consumption and years of exposure to THMs at levels above 49 µg/litre to increase bladder cancer risks (P for interaction = 0.775). Similar low, but not statistically significant, estimated relative risks are observed for those with less than 19 years' exposure to high THM levels, regardless of the volume of water they consumed. For persons with 20–34 years of exposure to THMs at levels above 49 µg/litre, the estimated relative risk of bladder cancer was also similar for those who consumed less than 1.54 litres per day (OR = 1.7; 95% CI = 1.1–2.7) and those who consumed more than 2.08 litres per day (OR = 1.7; 95% CI = 1.1–2.7). For persons with 35 or more years of exposure to high THM levels, statistically significant risk estimates representing more than a doubling of estimated relative risk are observed for those who consumed between 1.54 and 2.08 litres of tapwater per day (OR = 2.6; 95% CI = 1.3–5.2) or more than 2.08 litres per day (OR = 2.3; 95% CI =

1.1–4.7). Cantor et al. (1998) studied tapwater consumption in Iowa (USA) and found little or no association of risk for either total daily tapwater intake or intake of all beverages for men or women (Table 28A).

Colon cancer risk

Cragle et al. (1985) investigated the relationship between water chlorination and colon cancer using 200 incident cases from seven hospitals and 407 hospital-based comparison subjects without evidence of cancer who had been North Carolina (USA) residents for at least 10 years. Comparison subjects were matched on age, race, gender, vital status and hospital to prevent potential confounding by these characteristics. Additional information on potential confounders, including alcohol consumption, genetic risk (number of first-degree relatives with cancer), diet, geographic region, urbanicity, education and number of pregnancies, was obtained by either mailed questionnaire or telephone interview. Water exposures were verified for each address and categorized as chlorinated or unchlorinated. Logistic regression analysis showed genetic risk, a combination of alcohol consumption and high-fat diet, and an interaction between age and chlorination to be positively associated with colo-rectal cancer. Risks for people who drank chlorinated water at their residences for 16 or more years were consistently higher than risks for those exposed to chlorinated water for less than 16 years, but a statistically significant association between water chlorination and colo-rectal cancer, controlling for possible confounding bias, was found only for those above age 60 (Table 30). For example, 70- to 79-year-old participants who drank chlorinated water for more than 15 years had twice the relative risk of colo-rectal cancer, but for 70- to 79-year old participants who drank chlorinated water for less than 16 years, the risk of colon cancer was only about 50% higher. Confusing the interpretation of the results is an apparent protective effect of chlorinated water for colo-rectal cancer found in age groups under age 50 (Table 30). For example, 40- to 49-year-old persons who drank chlorinated water for less than 16 years had about half the relative risk, and 20- to 29-year-old persons who drank chlorinated water for less than 16 years had about one-quarter the risk. These apparent protective effects may indicate lack of control for an important confounding characteristic.

Table 30. Colon cancer risks associated with exposure to chlorinated water supplies in North Carolina[a]

Age	Odds ratio (95% CI)[b]	
	1–15 years exposure	>15 years exposure
20–29	0.2 (0.1–0.5)	0.5 (0.2–1.0)
30–39	0.4 (0.2–0.7)	0.6 (0.3–1.1)
40–49	0.6 (0.4–0.9)	0.8 (0.5–1.2)
50–59	0.9 (0.8–1.1)	0.9 (0.7–1.3)
60–69	1.2 (0.9–1.5)	1.4 (1.1–1.7)
70–79	1.5 (1.2–1.8)	2.2 (1.7–2.7)
80–89	1.8 (1.3–2.5)	3.4 (2.4–4.6)

[a] From Cragle et al. (1985).
[b] Adjusted for various confounders, including gender, race, diet, alcohol consumption, education, region and medical history of intestinal disorder.

The colon cancer association in Wisconsin (USA) was further pursued in an interview-based study (Young et al., 1987, 1990) of incident cases of colon cancer and population-based comparison subjects where historical exposures to THMs were estimated. When water disinfection within only the most recent 10-year exposure period was considered, colon cancer cases were more likely supplied with chlorinated rather than with unchlorinated water (OR = 1.6; 95% CI = 1.0–2.4) and used municipal groundwater rather than private groundwater (OR = 1.7; 95% CI = 1.1–2.4). Increased risks were not found for use of chlorinated water or municipal groundwater for 20 or 30 years prior to diagnosis of cancer. THMs are not usually found in chlorinated municipal groundwaters in Wisconsin, but contaminants such as tetrachloroethylene, trichloroethylene and 1,1,1-trichloroethane have been found. Lawrence et al. (1984) studied the relationship of THMs and colo-rectal cancer in New York (USA) where THM exposure was higher than in Wisconsin (see section 5.3.1.2 for details about these studies).

Hildesheim et al. (1998) conducted a population-based case–control study in Iowa (USA) in 1986–1989 to evaluate cancer risks that may be associated with chlorinated water; results have been reported for colon and rectal cancer. Information about residential history, drinking-water source, beverage intake and other factors was combined with historical data from water utilities and measured THM levels to create indices of past exposure to chlorinated by-products. The colon cancer study was composed of 560 incident cases who were residents of Iowa during March–December 1987, aged 40–85 years and with histological confirmation and 2434 age and gender frequency matched controls for whom water exposure information was available for at least 70% of their lifetime. Of the 801 eligible colon cancer cases, 685 (86%) participated; of these cases, 560 (82%) had sufficient information about water exposures. Unconditional multiple logistic regression analysis was used to estimate odds ratios for risks associated with chlorinated surface water and groundwater, THM exposure and tapwater consumption, while adjusting for potentially confounding factors. For colon cancer and subsites, no increase in risk was associated with duration of exposure to chlorinated surface water or chlorinated groundwater (Table 31A). A slight decrease in colon cancer risk was found with increased tapwater consumption. Those who drank 2.9 litres or more of tapwater daily had a 25% reduced risk of colon cancer compared with those who drank less than 1.5 litres per day.

Table 31. Colo-rectal cancer risks associated with exposures to chlorinated water supplies in Iowa (USA)[a]

Years of exposure to chlorinated surface water	Odds ratio	95% CI	Comments
A. Colon cancer risks			Adjusted for age, gender
0	1.0		
1–19	1.0	0.8–1.3	
20–39	1.0	0.7–1.5	
40–59	1.2	0.8–1.8	
≥60	0.8	0.4–1.7	
B. Rectal cancer risks			Adjusted for age, gender
0	1.0		
1–19	1.1	0.8–1.4	
20–39	1.6	1.1–2.2	
40–59	1.6	1.0–2.6	
≥60	2.6	1.4–5.0	

[a] From Hildesheim et al. (1998).

Rectal cancer risk

Hildesheim et al. (1998) conducted a population-based case–control study in Iowa (USA) in 1986–1989 to evaluate cancer risks that may be associated with chlorinated water; results have been reported for colon and rectal cancer. Information about residential history, drinking-water source, beverage intake and other factors was combined with historical data from water utilities and measured THM levels to create indices of past exposure to chlorinated by-products. The study was composed of 537 incident rectal cancer cases aged 40–85 years who were residents of Iowa from January 1986 to December 1988 and whose cancer was confirmed histologically and 2434 age and gender frequency matched controls for whom water exposure information was available for at least 70% of their lifetime. Of the 761 eligible rectal cancer cases, 655 (86%) participated; sufficient information about water exposures was available for 537 (82%) of these 655 cases. Unconditional multiple logistic regression analysis was used to estimate odds ratios for risks associated with chlorinated surface water, chlorinated groundwater, THM exposure and tapwater consumption, while adjusting for potentially confounding factors. An increasing rectal cancer risk was associated with both increasing cumulative THM exposure and duration of exposure to chlorinated surface water (Table 31B). However, the amount of tapwater consumed did not confound the risk, as the authors reported that little association (no data provided) was found between water consumption and rectal cancer after adjustment for age and gender. Larger relative risks for rectal cancer were found among persons with low dietary fibre intake and longer-duration exposure to chlorinated surface water source compared with persons with high-fibre diets and no exposure to chlorinated surface water.

Pancreatic cancer risk

A population-based case–control study (Ijsselmuiden et al., 1992) was conducted in Washington County, Maryland (USA), the same area in which an earlier cohort study had been conducted by Wilkins & Comstock (1981). Included in the study were 101 residents who were identified by the county cancer registry with a diagnosis of pancreatic cancer from July 1975 to December 1989 and 206 controls randomly chosen from the county population defined by a specially conducted census in 1975. Drinking-water source obtained from the 1975 census was used to assess exposure. Multivariate analysis found an increased risk of pancreatic cancer (RR = 2.2; 95% CI = 1.2–4.1) associated with chlorinated municipal surface water after adjusting for cigarette smoking; however, the authors recommended caution in the interpretation of this finding because of limitations in the assessment of exposure for study participants. Exposure was assessed at only one point in time, 1975, and this may not accurately reflect long-term exposure to chlorinated water. No increased risk of pancreatic cancer (RR = 0.8; 95% CI = 0.4–1.5) was found by Wilkins & Comstock (1981) in an earlier cohort study in the same county. Ijsselmuiden et al. (1992) did not report the reason for studying pancreatic cancer rather than evaluating further the previous findings of Wilkins & Comstock (1981) of increased, but not statistically significant, risks for bladder, liver or kidney cancer.

Brain cancer risk

In an abstract, Cantor et al. (1996) described the results of a population-based case–control study of 375 incident brain cancer patients, diagnosed in 1984–1987, and 2434 controls in Iowa. After controlling for age, farm occupation and other potential confounding characteristics, brain cancer risk among men, but not women, was associated with increased duration of exposure to chlorinated surface water. The risk was greatest for over 40 years of exposure (OR = 2.4; no CI reported) compared with 20–39 years of exposure (OR = 1.8) and 1–19 years of exposure (OR = 1.3). Historical exposures to chlorination by-products in drinking-water were also estimated from recent measures of THMs, other water quality data and information from study participants, but results of these analyses were not presented.

5.2.1.3 Meta-analysis of cancer studies

Meta-analysis is the application of quantitative techniques to literature reviewing. Two complementary approaches may be taken (US EPA, 1994a). One is an aggregative approach to summarize the compiled research on a given topic. This summary typically provides a measure of overall statistical significance or a consolidated estimate of effect, such as a relative risk. In practice, "when the world's literature on a topic is declared to be statistically significant," results of this type of meta-analysis are usually interpreted as an indication that research should cease and action should begin (US EPA, 1994a).

The other approach to meta-analysis is an analytical or explanatory approach (Greenland, 1994), in which the goal is to see whether differences among the studies can explain differences among their results. A formal analysis of the explanatory type might take the form of a meta-regression (Greenland, 1987), in which the dependent variable is the measure of effect, as estimated by each study, and the independent variables are the potentially explanatory factors that might yield higher or lower estimates of effect. The strength of explanatory meta-analysis is that it produces an enhanced understanding and appreciation of the strengths and weaknesses of the studies that have been conducted on the selected topic (US EPA, 1994a).

In the case of chlorinated drinking-water and cancer, a meta-analysis that used the aggregative approach was published by Morris et al. (1992). The authors conducted significance tests for several cancers and reported two, bladder cancer and rectal cancer, as statistically significant. Emphasized were the summary estimates of effect: pooled RRs of 1.2 (95% CI = 1.1–1.2) for bladder cancer and 1.4 (95% CI = 1.1–1.9) for rectal cancer. In conjunction with crude data on population exposure to chlorinated surface water, an attributable risk was estimated by the authors, suggesting that about 4200 cases (9%) of bladder cancer per year and 6500 cases (18%) of rectal cancer per year may be associated with consumption of chlorinated surface water in the USA. The meta-analysis and its quantitative estimate of risk have caused considerable controversy because there are significant differences in the design of the 10 individual epidemiological studies included (IARC, 1991; Risch et al., 1992; Craun et al., 1993; Murphy, 1993; Bailar, 1995). Reported quality scores for the individual studies were low (43–78 of a possible 100), and their study populations, research methods and results are not homogeneous. Several of the included studies were well designed and attempted to assess historical exposures to chlorinated water and possible confounding characteristics, but most did not adequately assess historical exposures and confounding bias. Only three studies adjusted or matched for smoking (one bladder cancer study, one colon cancer study and a cohort study of bladder, colon and rectal cancer), and only one study considered diet as a potential confounder. In four studies, a single reported address on a death certificate was used to assess the study participants' exposure to chlorinated water.

It is important to ask whether the meta-analysis should have restricted the analysis to those studies that were more homogeneous or those with adequate exposure assessments and control of confounding bias. Bailar (1995) questioned the summary findings for bladder cancer based on his assessment of the weaknesses of the individual studies and concluded that "bias could well explain the whole of the apparently positive findings." A recently completed formal evaluation of the meta-analysis by Poole (1997) concluded that studies should not have been combined into aggregate estimates of relative risk or used as the basis for national attributable risk estimates.

5.2.1.4   Summary of results of cancer studies

Various types of epidemiological studies, primarily in the USA, have attempted to assess the cancer risks associated with chlorinated water systems. Water disinfected with ozone and chlorine dioxide has not been studied for cancer associations, but chloraminated drinking-water was considered in two studies. Many, but not all, ecological studies reported associations between chlorinated water and cancer incidence or mortality and helped develop hypotheses for further study.

Analytical studies reported small relative risks for colon and bladder cancer incidence for populations consuming chlorinated drinking-water for long periods of time. Because of probable bias, interpretation of observed associations is severely limited in case–control studies where information was not obtained from interviews and residence histories. Interview-based case–control epidemiological studies provide a basis for evaluating the potential cancer risk that may be associated with chlorinated drinking-water. Based on Monson's (1980) guide to interpreting the strength of an association, a weak to moderate epidemiological association was found between water chlorination and colon cancer incidence among an elderly population in North Carolina (USA). However, a moderate to strong protective effect was also found among persons 20–49 years of age, confusing the interpretation of these results. The higher risks for those above age

70 in North Carolina suggest that the association may be evident only after a very long duration of exposure to chlorinated surface water. Colon cancer incidence was weakly associated with the use of chlorinated drinking-water for the most recent 10-year period in Wisconsin (USA), but no association was found when 20 or 30 years of exposure were considered. In Iowa (USA), no association was found between colon cancer or any subsites and duration of exposure to chlorinated surface water.

In a national study of 8764 persons in the USA, no overall association was found between chlorinated drinking-water and bladder cancer risk. A moderate association between chlorinated surface water and bladder cancer incidence was observed among an otherwise low-risk population of non-smokers that had received chlorinated surface water for 60 or more years, but this analysis included only 123 persons. In the Iowa portion of this study, moderate to strong associations were found for smokers and non-smokers with at least 30 years of exposure to chlorinated water. Interview case–control studies found a moderate risk of bladder cancer incidence associated with more than 30 years of exposure to chlorinated surface water in Colorado (USA), a weak to moderate risk of bladder cancer incidence associated with more than 35 years of exposure to chlorinated surface water in Ontario (Canada), a weak to moderate risk associated with more than 59 years of exposure to chlorinated surface water in Iowa (USA), and a weak association with more than 40 years of exposure to chlorinated surface water in Washington County, Maryland (USA). Inconsistencies, however, were observed in risks for non-smokers and smokers and in risks for women and men.

In New York State (USA), a dose–response relationship was observed between daily intake of total liquids and risk of bladder cancer and between increased tapwater consumption and risk of bladder cancer. Since increased risks were seen primarily in total fluid consumption, it is possible that total fluid consumption may be relevant in the pathogenesis of bladder cancer. Total daily fluid intake may be a marker for some unmeasured risk factor, and it is important to determine the biological relevance of increased fluid intake, independent of chlorinated tapwater, in the pathogenesis of bladder cancer. Several studies found the risk of bladder cancer to be elevated among persons who consumed more tapwater per day, but increased tapwater consumption appears to be an independent risk factor for bladder cancer. There was no evidence of an increased relative risk of bladder cancer when both the volume of water consumed and duration of exposure to chlorinated water or THMs were considered in the analysis.

In Massachusetts (USA), an increased risk of bladder cancer mortality was observed in a population receiving chlorinated surface water compared with a population receiving chloraminated surface water. These associations are weak to moderate in strength, depending upon the diseases used for comparison, and also considered long exposures, over 40 years' duration. A decreased risk of bladder cancer incidence was also associated with a similar duration of exposure to chloraminated surface water in Colorado (USA), but investigators felt that the results do not imply that chloraminated water conveys a protective effect because there is no plausible biological explanation for suggesting that choramination inhibits neoplastic transformation of the bladder epithelium.

A case–control study reported a large increased risk of rectal cancer among those with long duration of exposure to chlorinated water, but two cohort studies did not find an increased relative risk. A single case–control study reported a moderate to strong risk of pancreatic cancer associated with chlorinated surface water in Washington County, Maryland (USA), but the interpretation of this study is hampered because exposure was assessed at only one point in time, and this may not accurately reflect long-term exposure to chlorinated water. Preliminary results from a study in Iowa (USA) found that a moderate risk of brain cancer among men, but not women, was associated with increased duration of exposure to chlorinated surface water, especially for over 40 years of exposure. Additional details of this study are required to allow these conclusions to be evaluated. A weak increased risk of lung cancer incidence was also seen for users of chlorinated surface water in Iowa.

A controversial meta-analysis study, which statistically combined the results of 10 previously published epidemiological studies, reported a small pooled increased relative risk for bladder and rectal cancer but not for colon cancer. This meta-analysis, however, included a number of low-quality studies with likely bias.

Current evidence from epidemiological studies is insufficient to allow a causal relationship between the use of chlorinated drinking-water and the incidence of bladder cancer to be established. Several studies reported weak to moderate associations of long-duration exposure to chlorinated water and bladder cancer, but risks have differed between smokers and non-smokers in several studies. Inconsistent risks have also been seen when gender and water consumption were considered.

For colon cancer, the epidemiological data appear to be equivocal and inconclusive. For rectal cancer, insufficient data are available with which to evaluate the moderate associations observed in one study. Similarly, single studies of reported associations for pancreatic, lung, brain and breast provide insufficient data.

5.2.2 *Epidemiological studies of cardiovascular disease and disinfected drinking-water*

Several epidemiological studies have evaluated possible risks of cardiovascular disease associated with the chlorination of drinking-water. The cohort study (Wilkins & Comstock, 1981) of 31 000 residents of Washington County, Maryland (USA) found a slightly increased, but not statistically significant, risk (RR = 1.1; 95% CI = 1.0–1.3) of death due to arteriosclerotic heart disease in residents exposed to chlorinated drinking-water from a surface water and springs (average chloroform level was reported as 107 µg/litre) compared with residents of towns where unchlorinated well-water was used. A standardized mortality study (Zierler et al., 1986) found little difference in the patterns of 35 539 and 166 433 deaths (age of death was at least 45 years) due to cerebrovascular and cardiovascular disease, respectively, during 1969–1983 in 43 Massachusetts (USA) communities with water supplies disinfected with either chlorine or chloramine as compared with all deaths reported in Massachusetts due to these causes. The mortality rate in these selected communities with chlorinated drinking-water was slightly higher than expected for cerebrovascular disease (SMR = 108; 95% CI = 106–109) and cardiovascular disease (SMR = 104; 95% CI = 104–105). The mortality rate in selected communities with chloraminated drinking-water was slightly lower than expected for cerebrovascular disease (SMR = 86; 95% CI = 85–88) and about the same as expected for cardiovascular disease

(SMR = 101; 95% CI = 100–101). As noted in section 5.2.1.2, the serious potential for exposure and disease misclassification bias in the Massachusetts study limits the interpretation of these findings.

A cross-sectional study (Zeighami et al., 1990a,b) of 1520 adult residents, aged 40–70 years, in 46 Wisconsin (USA) communities was conducted to determine whether the hardness or chlorination of drinking-water affects serum lipids. The water for the communities contained total hardness of less than or equal to either 80 or 200 mg of calcium carbonate per litre; 858 participants (59% female) resided in 24 communities that provided chlorinated water, and 662 (55% female) resided in 22 communities that did not disinfect water. An age–gender-stratified sampling technique was used to choose a single participant from each eligible household, and a questionnaire was administered to obtain data on occupation, health history, medications, dietary history, water use, water supply and other basic demographic information. Among women who resided in communities with chlorinated, hard drinking-water, mean serum cholesterol levels were found to be higher (249.6 mg/dl, standard error [SE] = 6.4) than for women who resided in unchlorinated, hard-water communities (235.3 mg/dl, SE = 6.4). Among women who resided in communities with chlorinated, soft drinking-water, mean serum cholesterol levels were also found to be higher (248.0 mg/dl, SE = 6.2) than in women residing in unchlorinated, soft-water communities (239.7 mg/dl, SE = 6.3). Mean serum cholesterol levels were also higher for men in chlorinated communities, but the differences in mean cholesterol levels between chlorinated and unchlorinated communities were smaller and not statistically significant. The age-specific and overall risks of elevated serum cholesterol levels (>270 mg/dl) in communities with chlorinated drinking-water were also evaluated for men and women. Statistically significant increased risks of elevated serum cholesterol levels were found among women but not men and primarily in women aged 50–59 (OR = 3.1; 95% CI = 1.5–6.7).

Mean levels of LDL cholesterol in men and women had a similar pattern to total cholesterol. However, mean levels of HDL cholesterol were nearly identical in the chlorinated and unchlorinated communities for each gender, and the implication for increased cardiovascular disease risk in communities with chlorinated water remains unclear. Caution is urged in the interpretation of the results of this study. It is possible that an undetermined confounding characteristic due to life-style differences may be responsible for the observed association in the chlorinated communities.

The relationship between consumption of chlorinated drinking-water in the home and serum lipids was also evaluated in a cohort of 2070 white women, aged 65–93, participating in a study of osteo-porotic fractures in western Pennsylvania (USA) (Riley et al., 1995). Mean serum cholesterol levels (247 mg/dl, SD = 41.3) in 1869 women using chlorinated water sources were similar to levels (246 mg/dl, SD = 41.9) in 201 women using unchlorinated water sources. Women with the largest cumulative exposure to chlorinated water had higher serum cholesterol levels (247 mg/dl, SD = 41.3) than women with unchlorinated water (241 mg/dl, SD = 0.7), but the difference was not statistically significant. There was no evidence that increasing the duration of exposure to chlorinated water influenced LDL or HDL cholesterol, triglycerides or apolipoproteins. In this cohort, women exposed to chlorinated water sources tended to smoke and drink more than women not exposed to chlorinated water sources, suggesting that the reported association in Wisconsin may be due primarily to inade-quate control of lifestyle characteristics differentially distributed across chlorinated exposure groups.

5.2.2.1 Summary of results of cardiovascular studies

A mortality study showed little difference between patterns of death due to cardiovascular and cerebrovascular disease in the general population of Massachusetts (USA) and among residents of communi-ties using either chlorine or chloramine . A cohort study in Washington County, Maryland (USA) found a slightly increased, but not statisti-cally significant, risk of death due to arteriosclerotic heart disease in residents exposed to chlorinated drinking-water. A cross-sectional epidemiological study in Wisconsin (USA) found higher serum choles-terol in those exposed to chlorinated drinking-water than in those not exposed, but the association was confined to women aged 50–59. Mean serum lipids and lipoproteins were found to be similar in elderly white women exposed to chlorinated and unchlorinated drinking-water in western Pennsylvania (USA).

There is inadequate evidence from epidemiological studies that chlorinated or chloraminated drinking-water increases cardiovascular disease risks.

5.2.3 Epidemiological studies of adverse reproductive/developmental outcomes and disinfected drinking-water

After adjustment for potential confounders, Aschengrau et al. (1989) found a statistically significant increase in the frequency of spontaneous abortion in Massachusetts (USA) communities that used surface water sources compared with those that used groundwater sources. No measures of DBPs were available for the communities. When surface water sources are chlorinated, DBPs are typically higher than when groundwater sources are chlorinated, but levels of other water parameters also differ between surface water and groundwater sources. Aschengrau et al. (1993) also conducted a case–control study of late adverse pregnancy outcomes and water quality in Massachusetts community water systems. Among women who delivered infants during August 1977 and March 1980 at Brigham and Women's Hospital, various water quality indices were compared for 1039 congenital anomaly cases, 77 stillbirth cases, 55 neonatal deaths and 1177 controls. Risk of neonatal death or all congenital anomalies was not found to be increased in women exposed to chlorinated surface water supplies compared with chloraminated water supplies. Stillbirth risk was associated with chlorinated water supplies; however, after adjustment for appropriate confounding characteristics, the risk was not statistically significant (OR = 2.6; 95% CI = 0.9–7.5). Water quality measures were available for trace metals, but no water quality measures were available with which to assess risks associated with THMs or other DBPs.

A population-based case–control study of miscarriage, preterm delivery and low birth weight was conducted in three counties in central North Carolina (USA) (Savitz et al., 1995). Preterm deliveries (<37 weeks completed gestation) and low birth weight infants (<2500 g) were identified at hospitals with virtually all births to residents of Orange and Durham counties from September 1988 to August 1989 and Alamance County from September 1988 to April 1991. About 50% of eligible live births were both preterm and low birth weight. All medically treated miscarriages among women in

Alamance County from September 1988 to August 1991 were also identified for study. Full-term, normal-weight births immediately following a preterm or low birth weight delivery were selected as controls. Race and hospital were controlled for in the analysis. Telephone interviews were used to obtain information on a number of potential risk factors, including age, race, education, marital status, income, pregnancy history, tobacco and alcohol use, prenatal care, employment and psychological stress. Questions about drinking-water sources at home, including bottled water, and amount of water consumed around the time of pregnancy were also asked. Only 62–71% participated; the lowest response rate was for miscarriage cases. The analysis, which considered water consumption and THMs, was further restricted to women served by public water sources who reported drinking one or more glasses of water per day, and this limited the analysis to 70% of those participating. Selection bias is of concern in these studies, as is recall bias, where cases are more likely to more accurately recall previous exposures. It was found that water source was not related to miscarriage, preterm delivery or low birth weight. Risk of miscarriage was slightly increased among women who used bottled water compared with those who used private wells, but the risk was not statistically significant (OR = 1.6; 95% CI = 0.6–4.3).

A cross-sectional study (Kanitz et al., 1996) was conducted of 548 births at Galliera Hospital in Genoa and 128 births at Chiavari Hospital in Chiavari (Italy) during 1988–1989 to mothers residing in each city. Women in Genoa were exposed to filtered water disinfected with chlorine dioxide (Brugneto River wells, reservoir and surface water) and/or chlorine (Val Noci reservoir). Women residing in Chiavari used untreated well-water. Assignment to a water source and type of disinfectant was based on the mother's address (undisinfected well-water, chlorine, chlorine dioxide or both). Municipal records were used to determine family income, and hospital records were used to obtain information about mother's age, smoking, alcohol consumption and education level and birth outcomes — low birth weight (≤ 2500 g), preterm delivery (≤ 37 weeks), body length (≤ 49.5 cm), cranial circumference (≤ 35 cm) and neonatal jaundice. Neonatal jaundice was almost twice as likely (OR = 1.7; 95% CL = 1.1–3.1) in infants whose mothers resided in the area where drinking-water from surface water sources was disinfected with chlorine dioxide as in infants whose mothers used undisinfected well-water. No increased risk for neonatal jaundice was found for infants whose mothers lived in an area using chlorinated surface water. Large increased risks of smaller cranial circumference and body length were associated with drinking-water from surface water sources disinfected with chlorine or chlorine dioxide. Infants born to mothers residing in areas where surface water was disinfected with chlorine or chlorine dioxide had smaller cranial circumference (OR = 3.5; 95% CI = 2.1–8.5 for chlorine vs. untreated well-water; OR = 2.2; 95% CI = 1.4–3.9 for chlorine dioxide vs. untreated well water) and smaller body length (OR = 2.0; 95% CI = 1.2–3.3 for chlorine dioxide vs. untreated well-water; OR = 2.3; 95% CI = 1.3–4.2 for chlorine vs. untreated well-water). Risks of low birth weight infants were also increased for mothers residing in areas using water disinfected with chlorine and chlorine dioxide, but these associations were not statistically significant. For preterm delivery, small and not statistically significant increased risks were found among mothers residing in the area using chlorine dioxide. This study suggests possible risks associated with surface water disinfected with chlorine or chlorine dioxide, but the results should be interpreted very cautiously (US EPA, 1997). THM levels were low in both chlorinated water (8–16 µg/litre) and chlorine dioxide-disinfected water (1–3 µg/litre). No information was collected to assess the mothers' water consumption or nutritional habits, and the age distribution of the mothers was not considered. It is important to determine whether municipal or bottled water was consumed by the mothers and how much water was consumed. If mothers routinely consumed untreated municipal well-water but did not consume disinfected municipal surface water, drinking bottled water instead, the observed relative risks would not be associated with the disinfection of surface water. In addition, there are concerns about incomplete ascertainment of births and whether the population may be different in respects other than the studied water system differences. On the other hand, if the observed associations with water source and disinfection are not spurious, a question is raised about what water contaminants may be responsible. Exposures to surface water and groundwater sources are compared in this study, and no information is presented about other possible water quality differences.

Preliminary analyses were available for a cross-sectional study (Nuckols et al., 1995) of births to women in Northglenn, Colorado (USA) who were exposed to chlorinated water from Stanley Lake with high THM levels (32–72 µg/litre) and to women in Westminster who were exposed to chloraminated water from Stanley Lake with low THM levels (<20 µg/litre). Lower, but not statistically significant, relative risks for low infant birth weight and preterm delivery were found in the water district using chlorine. Further analysis in the chlorinated water system found increased, but not statistically significant, relative risks for low birth weight infants and preterm delivery in areas where the THMs were higher. These results must be interpreted with caution because very limited information was provided about the epidemiological methods. Instead, the article focused on water distribution system quality modelling and the use of geographic information systems.

5.2.3.1 Summary of results of reproductive/developmental studies

Results of several exploratory epidemiological studies of adverse reproductive effects/developmental outcomes and chlorinated water should be cautiously interpreted because of limitations of study design and likely bias.

5.3 Epidemiological associations between disinfectant by-products and adverse health outcomes

In this section, studies of specific DBPs are reviewed. In some studies, both water source and disinfectant type were considered in addition to the specific by-products; if this is the case, the details of the study design and any limitations are reported in section 5.2.

5.3.1 Epidemiological studies of cancer and disinfectant by-products

5.3.1.1 Cancer associations in ecological studies

1) Volatile by-products

Cantor et al. (1978) studied the relationship between THM levels and age-standardized cancer mortality for 1968–1971 of white men and women in urban counties in the USA. THM concentrations in drinking-water were estimated at the county level from data obtained in two national surveys of water supplies conducted by the US EPA. The analysis took into account the median number of school years completed by county inhabitants over age 25, the foreign-born and native population of the county, the change in county population from 1950 to 1970, the percentage of each county that is considered urban, the percentage of the county work force engaged in all manufacturing industries, and the geographic region of the USA. Multivariate regression analysis found the variability among these counties for gender-specific and cancer-site-specific mortality rates, and the residual mortality rates were then correlated directly with estimated THM exposure for those 76 counties in which 50% or more of the population was served by the sampled water supplies. Among both men and women, a statistically significant positive correlation was found between non-chloroform THM levels and bladder cancer mortality. No association between THM levels and colon cancer mortality rates was observed after controlling for the ethnicity of the population. Hogan et al. (1979) studied county cancer mortality data for an earlier period and county chloroform levels estimated from the same EPA surveys. Multivariate regression analysis of the county cancer mortality rates included, as independent variables, estimated exposure to chloroform concentrations, 1960 county population, county population density, percentage of county that is urban, percentage of county population that is non-white, percentage of county population that is foreign-born, median number of school years completed by county residents over age 25, median family income of county and percentage of county work force engaged in manufacturing. The results suggested that county cancer mortality rates for the rectum, bladder and possibly large intestine increased with increased levels of chloroform in drinking-water supplies.

McCabe (1975) found that age-adjusted total cancer mortality rates correlated positively with estimated chloroform concentrations in 80 US cities but included no attempt to control for potential confounding bias on a group or aggregate level. Carlo & Mettlin (1980) studied 4255 incident cases of oesophageal, stomach, colon, rectal, bladder and pancreatic cancers reported through the New York State Tumor Registry for Erie County, New York (USA) between 1973 and 1976. Age-adjusted incidence rates were calculated by census tract, and levels of THMs were estimated from a single water survey in July 1978. Statistically significant positive associations were found between consumption of chlorinated drinking-water from surface water sources and oesophageal and pancreatic cancer and between THM levels and pancreatic cancer in white males. The authors placed little credence on these findings, noting that the pancreatic cancer–THMs relationship was found only in one gender–race subgroup, the range of THM concentrations in the study was narrow (the largest variation was only 71 µg/litre) and no data were available with which to estimate historical trends in THM levels.

Tuthill & Moore (1980) studied cancer mortality rates from 1969 to 1976 in Massachusetts (USA) communities supplied by surface water. Chlorination exposure data were assessed by considering past chlorine dosage, recent THM levels and recent chlorine dosage. Stomach and rectal cancer mortality rates were associated with recent THM levels and recent chlorine dosage, but not with past chlorine dosage in the communities. However, when regression models included migration patterns and ethnicity, none of the associations was statistically significant.

Wigle et al. (1986) studied selected contaminants in drinking-water and cancer risks in Canadian cities with populations of at least 10 000. Water quality data from three national surveys of urban drinking-water supplies, demographic data and age-standardized cancer mortality rates for 1973–1979 were analysed by multivariate regression techniques. No statistically significant associations were found between chlorine dosage and risk of death with any disease category. When chlorine dosage was replaced in the model by TOC, a statistically significant association was found between this variable and cancer of the large intestine among males but not females. There were no statistically significant associations when chlorine dosage was replaced by THM, chloroform or non-chloroform THM levels. A recent ecological analysis of cancer cases reported to the New Jersey (USA) cancer registry in 1979–1990 found no association between bladder and rectal cancer incidence and THM or BDCM levels in public drinking-water systems (Savin & Cohn, 1996). Exposure was based on address at the time of cancer diagnosis and the water quality of the public water system from monitoring conducted during the 1980s.

These ecological studies used limited information about current THM levels in drinking-water to estimate exposures for a census tract, county or community, and these exposures may not represent long-term exposures or be relevant for the population whose cancer statistics were studied. Available demographic characteristics were included as group variables to assess or control for confounding bias, but these likely have limited value in controlling for such bias. Because of the ecological design of the study, these results cannot be easily interpreted. Even if the exposure information were accurately assessed, it cannot be determined whether the observed associations were a result of exposure to chloroform, THM levels or other DBPs or were confounded by characteristics that were not assessed (e.g., cigarette smoking) or incorrectly assessed by using available demographic data. Ecological studies where no associations were found suffer from similar limitations.

2) Mutagenicity

Several ecological studies have considered the mutagenic activity of drinking-water, as determined by the *Salmonella*/microsome assay. These mutagenicity tests assess the non-volatile, acid/neutral fraction of chlorinated organic material in a concentrated water sample. A mutagen of particular concern is MX, a potent mutagen, as measured by strain *S. typhimurium* TA100, which may be responsible for up to 57% of the mutagenicity in chlorinated drinking-water (Meier et al., 1986, 1987b).

High levels of mutagenic activity have been observed in Finnish chlorinated drinking-water, and Koivusalo et al. (1994a,b, 1995) investigated the relationship between mutagenic activity in drinking-water and gastrointestinal, urinary tract and other cancers in 56 Finnish municipalities. Included in the analysis were cases of bladder, kidney, stomach, colon, rectum, liver, pancreas and soft tissue cancer, leukaemia (acute, chronic myeloid and chronic lymphatic), Hodgkin's disease and non-Hodgkin's lymphoma obtained from the population-based Finnish Cancer Registry for two periods, 1966–1976 and 1977–1989. The Cancer Registry includes virtually all cancer cases in the country. On an ecological level, information was also obtained for several potential confounding characteristics — social class, urban living, time period, migration and exposures from the chemical industry.

Koivusalo et al. (1994b) discussed the methodology used to estimate the mutagenicity of drinking-water and assess past exposures for the epidemiological studies. Exposure was assessed at the ecological, not the individual, level and was based on the proportion of population served by municipal water and the estimated mutagenicity of the water. Previous drinking-water mutagenic activity was estimated for each community on the basis of an equation derived by Vartiainen et al. (1988), yielding an estimated drinking-water mutagenicity level in net revertants per litre for each community for each of two specific periods, 1955 and 1970. The equation used available historical information on raw water quality (TOC, ammonia, permanganate test for oxidizable organic matter, etc.), pre- and post-chlorine dosages, and water treatment practices obtained by a questionnaire sent to the municipalities. Vartiainen et al. (1988) and Koivusalo et al. (1994b) reported a high correlation between estimated and measured drinking-water mutagenicity after comparing the results of assays of drinking-water mutagenicity in 1985 and 1987 with estimated mutagenicity from their equation.

Observed and expected numbers of cancer cases in each municipality were compared by sex, broad age group and time period, and cancer risk was adjusted for social class as a surrogate for lifestyle and smoking habits. For all 56 municipalities, no statistically significant increases in risks of cancer of the kidney, stomach, colon, rectum, liver, pancreas and soft tissue, leukaemia (acute, chronic myeloid and chronic lymphatic) and non-Hodgkin's lymphoma were found among those exposed to a typically mutagenic drinking-water (3000 net revertants per litre) when adjusted for age, sex, period, main cities and social class. The risks of bladder cancer (RR = 1.2; 95% CI = 1.1–1.3) and Hodgkin's disease (RR = 1.2; 95% CI = 1.0–1.4) were small but statistically significant. When this analysis was restricted to those 34 municipalities with mutagenic drinking-water, risks of non-Hodgkin's lymphoma, Hodgkin's disease and cancer of the liver, pancreas, kidney, stomach and bladder were all found to be slightly increased (RRs ranged from 1.1 to 1.3). As this is an ecological study, the small increased relative risks that were observed preclude definitive conclusions.

5.3.1.2   Cancer associations in analytical studies

1)   Bladder cancer risk

In Colorado (USA), where an increased risk of bladder cancer was found for persons exposed to chlorinated drinking-water for more than 30 years (OR = 1.8; 95% CI = 1.1–2.9), no association was found between THM levels and bladder cancer (McGeehin et al., 1993). The mean 1989 levels for THMs and residual chlorine for each water system were multiplied by the number of years each study participant was exposed to that system and summed to compute lifetime exposure indices for each water quality indicator. Higher risks were found when the cumulative exposure index for THMs was less than 200 or greater than 600 µg/litre-years, but not when it was 201–600 µg/litre-years. No statistically significant trends were found; risks did not increase with increased cumulative THM exposure. In logistic regression models that included water source and disinfection variables and controlled for years of exposure to chlorinated water, THMs assessed by this exposure index were not associated with bladder cancer. Interpretation of these results is limited, however, because only 61% of THM levels and 55% of residual chlorine levels could be determined for use in assessing exposures.

In Ontario (Canada), individual information about water consumption and exposure to chlorinated water was supplemented by water treatment data (e.g., area served, water source and characteristics, and treatment practices for years of operation between 1950 and 1990) collected from a survey of historical treatment practices at water supplies in the study area (King & Marrett, 1996). For each treatment facility, water treatment information was obtained for an average day in August in 5-year intervals, and that observation was used to represent water characteristics for the years surrounding that date. The water supply for each participant was characterized by the estimated annual maximum THM levels for each water facility. Historical THM levels were estimated using a model developed to predict the THM level in treated water from characteristics of the treatment process. The model was developed from water quality measurements recorded by the Ontario Drinking Water Surveillance Program between 1988 and 1992 for 114 water treatment facilities. Predicted THM levels were compared with those observed in 1986–1987, and the correlation between observed and predicted values was 0.76. When observed and predicted THM levels were considered as either above or below 50 µg/litre, the model predicted values with a sensitivity of 84% and a specificity of 76%.

King & Marrett (1996) found an increased bladder cancer risk with increasing duration of exposure to THMs, but the association was statistically significant and of higher magnitude only after 35 or more years of exposure (Table 32). A statistically significant increased bladder cancer risk was also found for the highest quartile of cumulative exposure to THMs (Table 33). The risk of bladder cancer incidence was about 40% higher among persons exposed to greater than 1956 µg of THMs per litre-year in water compared with those exposed to less than 584 µg/litre-year. No association between cumulative exposure to THMs and increased bladder cancer risk was found in Colorado (USA) (McGeehin et al., 1993), but the highest cumulative THM levels in Colorado were much lower than those found in Ontario (Table 34).

Table 32. Bladder cancer risks and estimated maximum annual exposure to trihalomethanes in water in Ontario (Canada)[a]

Years of exposure	Odds ratio (95% CI)[b]		
	THMs >24 µg/litre	THMs >49 µg/litre	THMs >74 µg/litre
0–9	1.0	1.0	1.0
10–19	1.2 (0.9–1.7)	1.1 (0.9–1.4)	1.1 (0.9–1.4)
20–34	1.2 (0.9–1.5)	1.4 (1.1–1.8)	1.3 (0.9–1.8)
>34	1.6 (1.2–2.1)	1.6 (1.1–2.5)	1.7 (1.1–2.7)

[a] From King & Marrett (1996).
[b] Adjusted for age, gender, smoking, education and calorie intake.

A population-based case–control study conducted in 1986–1989 in Iowa (USA) (Cantor et al., 1998) found associations of increased bladder cancer risk with total and average lifetime exposure to THMs (Table 35), but increased relative risks were restricted to men who had ever smoked (see also section 5.2.1.2). These findings were similar to associations found with duration of exposure to chlorinated surface water. Relative risks for women suggested a protective effect for increased lifetime average THM levels; ORs ranged from 0.6 to 0.9,

Table 33. Bladder cancer risks and estimated cumulative exposure to
trihalomethanes in Ontario (Canada)[a]

THMs-years of exposure (µg/litre-year)	Odds ratio (95% CI)[b]
0–583	1.0
584–1505	1.2 (0.9–1.6)
1506–1956	1.1 (0.8–1.4)
1957–6425	1.4 (1.1–1.9)

[a] From King & Marrett (1996).
[b] Adjusted for age, gender, smoking, education and calorie intake.

Table 34. Bladder cancer risks and estimated cumulative exposure to
trihalomethanes in Colorado (USA)[a]

THMs-years of exposure (µg/litre-year)	Odds ratio[b]
0	1.0
<200	1.8
201–600	1.1
>600	1.8

[a] From McGeehin et al. (1993).
[b] 95% CI not available; P for trend = 0.16.

and 95% CIs ranged from 0.3 to 1.3. Past exposure to chlorination by-
products was estimated by combining information about water sources,
historical chlorine use, lifetime residential history, fluid consumption,
THM levels and other water quality data, including volatile organic
compounds, TOC, TOX, pesticides, total dissolved solids and nitrates
(Lynch et al., 1990; Neutra & Ostro, 1992). Data reported thus far
(Cantor et al., 1998) have been restricted to THMs.

2)   Colon cancer risk

A colon cancer association was studied in Wisconsin (USA) in an
interview-based study (Young et al., 1987, 1990) of 347 incident cases
of colon cancer, 611 population-based controls and 639 controls with
cancer of other sites. White males and females between the ages of 35
and 90 were eligible for selection in the study. Lifetime residential and
water source histories and information on water consumption habits,
diet, demographic information, medical and occupational histories,

Table 35. Bladder cancer risks and estimated cumulative exposure to
trihalomethanes in Iowa (USA)[a]

Lifetime THM exposure	Odds ratio (95% CI)[b]
Total lifetime exposure (g)	
<0.04	1.0
0.05–0.12	1.3 (1.0–1.6)
0.13–0.34	1.1 (0.9–1.4)
0.35–1.48	1.1 (0.9–1.4)
1.49–2.41	1.2 (0.8–1.7)
>2.42	1.3 (0.9–2.0)
Lifetime average exposure (µg/litre)	
<0.8	1.0
0.8–2.2	1.2 (1.0–1.5)
2.3–8.0	1.1 (0.8–1.4)
8.1–32.5	1.1 (0.8–1.4)
32.6–46.3	1.3 (0.9–1.8)
>46.3	1.2 (0.8–1.8)

[a] From Cantor et al. (1998).
[b] Adjusted for age, gender, study period, smoking, education and high-risk occupation.

lifestyle and other factors was obtained by a self-administered questionnaire and augmented with information from medical records. Historical exposures to THMs were estimated using a predictive statistical model based on current THM levels and water supply operation records. Multivariate logistic regression analysis was used to estimate the risk of colon cancer adjusted for age, gender and urbanization. Individuals exposed to drinking-water containing more than 40 µg of THMs per litre, the highest exposure category, were found to be at no greater risk of colon cancer than individuals exposed to water with no or trace levels of THMs. Nor did cumulative exposure to THMs present a colon cancer risk (Table 36). Although this analysis suggests that the presence of THMs in Wisconsin drinking-water is not associated with a colon cancer risk, THM levels in Wisconsin are low: 98% of water samples had concentrations less than 100 µg/litre.

Table 36. Colon cancer risks and estimated cumulative exposure to trihalomethanes in Wisconsin (USA)[a]

Lifetime THM exposure (µg/litre-year)	Odds ratio[b]	95% CI
<137	1.0	
137–410	1.1	0.7–1.8
>410	0.7	0.4–1.2

[a] From Young et al. (1987).
[b] Adjusted for age, gender and population of place of residence.

Lawrence et al. (1984) studied the relationship of THMs and colo-rectal cancer in New York State (USA) where THM exposure was higher than in Wisconsin and found no association. Included in the study were 395 white female teachers in New York State who died from colo-rectal cancer and an equal number of teachers who died from non-cancer causes. Cumulative chloroform exposure was estimated by a statistical model that considered water treatment operational records during the 20 years prior to death. The distribution of chloroform exposure was not significantly different between cases and controls, and no effect of cumulative exposure was found in a logistic analysis controlling for average source type, population density, marital status, age and year of death. The risk of cancer was not found to be higher among those using a surface water source containing THMs (OR = 1.1; 90% CI = 0.8–1.4). Mean levels of cumulative THM exposure were similar among cases (635 µg/litre-years) and controls (623 µg/litre-years).

The population-based case–control study conducted from 1986 to 1989 in Iowa (USA) (Hildesheim et al., 1998) found no increased risk of colon cancer or any subsites associated with estimates of exposure to THMs, either total (g) or average lifetime (µg/litre) (Table 37).

A prospective cohort study of 41 836 post-menopausal women in Iowa (USA) (Doyle et al., 1997) included an analysis of women who reported drinking municipal or private well-water for more than the past 10 years ($n = 28$ 237). Historical water treatment and water quality data were used to ascertain exposure to THMs. The primary source of information on THMs was a 1986–1987 water survey. All women who lived in the same community were assigned the same

Table 37. Colon cancer rsks and estimated cumulative exposure to
trihalomethanes in Iowa (USA)[a]

Lifetime THM exposure	Odds ratio (95% CI)[b]
Total lifetime exposure (g)	
<0.04	1.0
0.05–0.12	1.0 (0.7–1.2)
0.13–0.34	0.9 (0.6–1.2)
0.35–1.48	1.2 (0.9–1.6)
1.49–2.41	0.5 (0.3–0.9)
>2.42	1.1 (0.7–1.8)
Lifetime average exposure (µg/litre)	
<0.8	1.0
0.8–2.2	1.0 (0.8–1.3)
2.3–8.0	0.9 (0.7–1.3)
8.1–32.5	1.1 (0.8–1.4)
32.6–46.3	0.9 (0.6–1.5)
>46.3	1.1 (0.7–1.6)

[a] From Hildesheim et al. (1998).
[b] Adjusted for age and gender.

level of exposure to THMs. A dose–response relationship (Table 38) was found with increasing chloroform levels in municipal drinking-water for all cancers combined, colon cancer, lung cancer and melanoma (test for trend $P < 0.05$). The highest exposure covered a wide range of values, and selection of the exposure categories for chloroform is unusual and does not reflect normal high exposures to chloroform. Additional analyses after exclusion of women who reported a history of colo-rectal polyps and adjustment for additional risk or protective factors did not change the dose–response relationship and slightly increased the relative risk estimates. No associations were observed between colon cancer and BDCM, DBCM or bromoform, but levels were low, and many water systems had no detectable levels of these THMs. For example, the geometric mean levels of BDCM and DBCM in surface water were 8.7 and 0.4 µg/litre, respectively. Because water quality data were also available from a 1979 water survey for a national bladder cancer study, analyses were also

Table 38. Risks of cancer incidence associated with chloroform levels in post-menopausal women, Iowa (USA)[a]

| Cancer site | Chloroform concentration (μg/litre) | | | | | | | | | | | |
| | 1–2 | | | 3–13 | | | 14–287 | | |
	Cases	RR[b]	95% CI	Cases	RR[b]	95% CI	Cases	RR[b]	95% CI
Bladder	11	0.9	0.4–2.1	12	1.3	0.6–2.8	7	0.7	0.3–1.7
Colon	41	1.1	0.7–1.7	42	1.4	0.9–2.2	57	1.7	1.1–2.6
Rectal	19	0.8	0.4–1.5	14	0.8	0.4–1.5	22	1.1	0.6–2.0
Breast	151	1.1	0.9–1.3	131	1.2	0.9–1.5	136	1.1	0.9–1.4
Kidney	5	0.6	0.2–1.7	9	1.3	0.5–3.2	7	0.9	0.3–2.4
Lung	35	1.4	0.8–2.3	40	2.0	1.2–3.2	42	1.9	1.1–3.0
Melanoma	15	2.5	1.0–6.5	6	1.3	0.4–3.9	17	3.2	1.3–8.2
All cancers	253	1.1	0.9–1.3	220	1.3	1.05–1.5	268	1.3	1.1–1.5

[a] From Doyle et al. (1997).
[b] Reported relative risks were adjusted for age, education, smoking status, physical activity, fruit and vegetable intake, total energy intake, body mass index and waist to hip ratio.

conducted using these data. Fewer municipalities were sampled for THMs in 1979, and only 16 461 participants were included. In this analysis, colon cancer was found to be associated with increasing exposure to chloroform levels.

3) Rectal cancer risk

The population-based case–control study conducted in Iowa (USA) (Hildesheim et al., 1998) found an increased risk of rectal cancer associated with estimates of exposure to THMs after controlling for age, gender and average population size for men and women. For total lifetime exposure to THMs of greater than 1.48 g, odds ratios were almost double (OR = 1.9; 95% CI = 1.2–3.0) those for total lifetime exposure to THMs of less than 0.05 g. For lifetime average THM concentrations of 32.6–46.3 µg/litre and greater than 46.4 µg/litre, odds ratios (OR = 1.7; 95% CI = 1.1–2.6) were almost 70% greater than those for average exposures of less than 0.8 µg/litre (Table 39). This is the only study to report increased rectal cancer risks associated with THM exposure.

4) Mutagenicity

A cohort study of populations exposed to various levels of mutagenicity in drinking-water and a case–control study of kidney and bladder cancers are currently being conducted in Finland (Tuomisto et al., 1995). No results have yet been reported for the case–control study. The cohort study (Koivusalo et al., 1996, 1997) included 621 431 persons living in the same town in which they were born and having a water connection in 1970. Cancer incidence in the cohort was compared with national cancer incidence stratified by gender, time period and age group. Cases were derived from the population-based Finnish Cancer Registry, and follow-up of the cohort started in 1970. Past exposure to drinking-water mutagenicity and THMs was assessed using historical water quality information. The quantity of mutagenicity was estimated for each 5-year period from 1955 to 1970 using an empirical equation relating mutagenicity and raw water pH, potassium permanganate oxidation and chlorine dose. A good correlation was found between estimated and measured values for the period 1986–1987 when measures of mutagenicity were available. The quantity of mutagenicity is minor in raw waters and predominantly results from

Table 39. Rectal cancer risks and estimated cumulative exposure to trihalomethanes[a]

Lifetime THM exposure	Odds ratio (95% CI)[b]
Total lifetime exposure (g)	
<0.04	1.0
0.05–0.12	1.3 (1.0–1.6)
0.13–0.34	1.3 (0.9–1.8)
0.35–1.48	1.5 (1.1–2.1)
1.49–2.41	1.9 (1.2–3.0)
>2.42	1.6 (1.0–2.6)
Lifetime average exposure (µg/litre)	
<0.8	1.0
0.8–2.2	1.0 (0.8–1.4)
2.3–8.0	1.2 (0.9–1.7)
8.1–32.5	1.2 (0.9–1.7)
32.6–46.3	1.7 (1.1–2.6)
>46.3	1.7 (1.1–2.6)

[a] From Hildesheim et al. (1998).
[b] Adjusted for age and gender.

the chlorination process. The *Salmonella*/microsome assay is used to assess the mutagenicity of the non-volatile, acid/neutral fraction of chlorinated organic material in water. A mutagen of particular concern is MX, a potent mutagen, as measured by strain *S. typhimurium* TA100, which may be responsible for up to 57% of the mutagenicity in chlorinated drinking-water (Meier et al., 1986, 1987). After adjusting for age, time period, urbanization and social status, an average exposure to mutagenicity in chlorinated water of 3000 net revertants per litre was found to be associated with a statistically significant increased risk in women for cancers of the bladder (RR = 1.5; 95% CI = 1.0–2.2), rectum (RR = 1.4; 95% CI = 1.0–1.9), oesophagus (RR = 1.9; 95% CI = 1.0–3.5) and breast (RR = 1.1; 95% CI = 1.0–1.2). Past exposure to THMs, one group of volatile by-products of chlorination, did not result in statistically significant excess risks (Koivusalo et al., 1996). Although this study found a moderate association between cancers of the bladder, rectum and oesophagus in women and high levels of mutagenicity in drinking-water, the results should be interpreted with caution, as this is the only analytical epidemiological study of water mutagenicity. Significantly increased relative risks were found only for women, and the magnitude of the risks suggests that results may be due to residual uncontrolled confounding.

5.3.1.3   Summary of results of cancer studies

Cumulative exposure to THMs was slightly higher in New York (USA) than in Wisconsin (USA), but no increased colon cancer risk associated with THM exposure was observed in either study. Data reported thus far from a study in Iowa (USA) show that colon cancer risk was not associated with estimates of past exposure to THMs, but rectal cancer risk was associated with increasing amounts of lifetime exposure to THMs. Risks were not reported for THM levels found in drinking-water. A cohort study in Iowa found moderately increased risks associated with a wide reported range of chloroform concentrations (14–287 µg/litre).

In Ontario (Canada), the risk of bladder cancer incidence was about 40% higher among persons exposed to greater than 1956 µg of THMs per litre-year in water compared with those exposed to less than 584 µg/litre-year. No association between exposure to THM levels and increased bladder cancer risk was found in Colorado (USA). Data reported thus far from a study in Iowa (USA) show that risk of bladder cancer was not associated with estimates of past exposure to chlorination by-products except among men and smokers, where bladder cancer risk increased with duration of exposure after control for cigarette smoking.

In Finland, an average exposure to mutagenicity in chlorinated water of 3000 net revertants per litre was found to be associated with an increased risk in women for cancers of the bladder, rectum, oesophagus and breast; however, past exposure to THMs did not result in statistically significant excess cancer risks. THM levels in drinking-water were not reported for Finland, and these results were reported only in an abstract.

No increased risk of bladder cancer was associated with THM exposure in Colorado (USA); cumulative exposure to THMs in

Colorado was similar to those in New York (USA) and Wisconsin (USA), where no increased risk was found for colon cancer. In Ontario (Canada), THM exposure was much higher, and a moderate increased risk of bladder cancer was found.

At this time, the evidence for an association between THM exposure in drinking-water and colon cancer must be considered inconclusive. No evidence is available from epidemiological studies to suggest an increased risk of colon cancer, but studies have been conducted in areas where cumulative exposures were generally low. The evidence for an association between chlorinated water or THM exposure in drinking-water and bladder cancer is limited. No association was found in Colorado, but cumulative exposures were low. In Canada, where cumulative THM exposure was much higher, a moderate increased risk of bladder cancer was found.

It is possible that other unmeasured by-products may be associated with bladder cancer risks, as several studies have found an association between chlorinated surface water and bladder cancer but not between THMs and bladder cancer. It is possible that another DBP or a water contaminant other than a DBP is responsible. A plausible alternative explanation for the observed results is that residence in an area served by a chlorinated surface water supply is simply a surrogate for some other unidentified risk factor or characteristic of urban populations that may be associated with an increased risk of cancer. Other potential DBPs may include other volatile organic contaminants, but studies have considered ingestion, not inhalation, exposures, and very few studies have attempted to assess both long-term exposures to chlorinated water and historical water consumption patterns. Accurate long-term exposure assessment is difficult. Exposures to other chlorinated or brominated compounds or HAAs have also not been considered. Additional studies should continue to assess the risk of the non-volatile fraction of organic by-products.

Several studies found an elevated bladder cancer risk among persons who consumed more tapwater per day, but increased tapwater consumption appeared to be an independent risk factor for bladder cancer. The association of water and other fluid consumption and bladder cancer also requires additional study.

Weak associations reported between cumulative THM exposure and bladder cancer risks do not provide adequate evidence that THMs cause bladder cancer. In two studies, no association was found. A moderate association was reported for rectal cancer and cumulative THMs, but only in a single study. There is no evidence for an association between the other cancer sites studied and THM exposure.

5.3.2 Epidemiological studies of cardiovascular disease and disinfectant by-products

A cohort study of 31 000 residents of Washington County, Maryland (USA) found a slightly increased, but not statistically significant, risk (RR = 1.1; 95% CI = 1.0–1.3) of death due to arteriosclerotic heart disease in residents exposed to chlorinated surface water and springs compared with residents of towns where unchlorinated well-water was used. Water sampling during the study found average chloroform levels of 107 µg/litre in the Hagerstown water system, but it is not known if these levels accurately represent long-term exposures. Other observational (Zierler et al., 1988; Zeighami et al., 1990a,b; Riley et al., 1995) epidemiological studies of disinfected water evaluated the possible adverse cardiovascular effects of chlorinated or chloraminated drinking-water, but no by-products were measured.

5.3.2.1 Summary of results of cardiovascular studies

Epidemiological studies have not evaluated associations between specific DBPs and cardiovascular disease, but there is no evidence of an increased risk caused by chlorinated or chloraminated drinking-water.

5.3.3 Epidemiological studies of adverse reproductive/developmental outcomes and disinfectant by-products

In the Savitz et al. (1995) study, dates of pregnancy were used to assign THM levels from the appropriate water supply and for the periods in the pregnancy in which exposures might cause any adverse effect. No associations were reported between THM levels in North Carolina (USA) and estimated dose of THMs with miscarriage, preterm delivery or low birth weight. Savitz et al. (1995) found no increased risk of low infant birth weight or preterm delivery associated with exposure to THM levels of 63–69 µg/litre or a computed dose of

THMs of 170–1171 µg/litre-glasses per day. No increased risk of miscarriage was associated with either (i) THM levels of 60–81.0 or 81.1–168.8 µg/litre or (ii) a computed dose of THMs of 140.0–275.0 or 275.1–1171.0 µg/litre-glasses per day. Although no increased miscarriage risk was found in this categorical analysis, an analysis using a continuous measure for THMs predicted an association (1.7 per 50 µg of THMs per litre increment; 95% CI = 1.1–2.7). This association, however, was not part of an overall dose–response gradient and may be a spurious finding. Another categorical analysis using sextiles of THM exposures showed a much higher miscarriage risk (adjusted OR = 2.8; 95% CI = 1.2–6.1) in the highest sextile but a very low risk or even a possibly protective effect in the next highest sextile (adjusted OR = 0.2; 95% CI = 0.0–0.5).

A population-based case–control study in Iowa (USA) used information from birth certificates from January 1989 to June 1990 and a water supply survey conducted in 1987 to study the association of waterborne chloroform and other DBPs with low birth weight (<2500 g), prematurity (<37 weeks' gestation) and intrauterine growth retardation (Kramer et al., 1992). Cases were not mutually exclusive, but each outcome was analysed separately. Controls were randomly selected from the same birth certificates. The study included 159 low birth weight and 795 normal birth weight infants, 342 premature infants and 1710 controls, and 187 intrauterine growth-retarded infants and 935 controls. Mothers were not interviewed to obtain information about their residential history during pregnancy or possible risk factors, and other exposures were not noted on the certificate, which might potentially confound any observed association or modify its effect. Information on maternal age, parity, adequacy of prenatal care, marital status, education and maternal smoking was available from the birth certificate. Residence of the mother at the time of birth determined which water system was used to assign levels of exposure to THM and TOX measured in a previous municipal water survey. The only statistically significant finding was a moderately increased risk (OR = 1.8; 95% CI = 1.1–2.9) of intrauterine growth retardation associated with chloroform levels of greater than 9 µg/litre in water after controlling for confounding characteristics from the certificate. Prematurity (OR = 1.1; 95% CI = 0.7–1.6) and low birth weight (OR = 1.3; 95% CI = 0.8–2.2) were not found to be associated with chloroform levels. No statistically significant associations were seen with any of these developmental outcomes and BDCM, DBCM, bromoform or organic halides. Interpretation of the results of this study, however, is limited because the study design was more ecological than analytical. The authors considered the results to be preliminary because of possible bias. The ascertainment and classification of exposure to the water contaminants were imprecise and may have resulted in misclassification bias. Municipal measures of by-products assigned to the residences for exposure purposes may have been either higher or lower than actual exposures. Characteristics that were not identified (e.g., alcohol consumption) could be responsible for confounding bias. A cross-sectional epidemiological study (Bove et al., 1992a, 1995) was conducted in four northern New Jersey (USA) counties to explore possible associations between THM levels and 13 developmental and adverse reproductive outcomes: low birth weight (<2500 g), prematurity (<37 weeks), small for gestational age, very low birth weight (<1500 g), stillbirths, surveillance malformations for 33 selected categories, central nervous system defects and subgroups, oral cleft defects and subgroups, and cardiac defects and subgroups. A total of 143 hypotheses were formally evaluated; as the stated objective of the study was to identify promising leads for further research rather than for decision-analytical purposes, each finding was reported as if it were the sole focus of the study without statistical adjustment for multiple comparisons.

Reproductive outcomes over a 4-year period, from January 1985 to December 1988, were obtained from a population-based birth defects registry and vital records, birth certificates and death certificates. A total of 80 938 live births and 594 fetal deaths were studied in 75 towns selected because residents were mostly served by public water systems. All information about reproductive outcomes, potential confounding characteristics and risk factors, such as maternal age, race, education, primipara, previous stillbirth or miscarriage, sex and adequacy of prenatal care, was obtained from vital records. Information on other potential important confounders — maternal occupation, drug use during pregnancy, smoking and alcohol consumption — was not available for analysis. Mothers were not interviewed for information on individual exposures and potentially confounding characteristics.

Information about water quality for the 75 towns was obtained from existing records. Monthly estimates of each water contaminant in a town's water system were used to assign exposure for each gestational month of each live birth and fetal death. A mother's residence at birth was assumed to be her residence throughout her pregnancy. All water systems in the study were chlorinated, but sufficient groundwater sources were available to ensure inclusion of areas with very low levels of THMs. The drinking-water contaminants studied were THMs, trichloroethylene, tetrachloroethylene, dichloroethylenes, 1,1,1-trichloroethane, carbon tetrachloride, 1,2-dichloroethane, benzene and nitrate. Type of water source was also considered. For evaluation of risk with different levels of exposure, THMs were categorized into six different levels of potential exposure: ≤20, >20–40, >40–60, >60–80, >80–100 and >100 μg/litre.

Reported associations with levels of THMs greater than 100 μg/litre included small for gestation age (OR = 1.5; 90% CI = 1.2–1.9) and oral cleft defects (OR = 3.2; 90% CI = 1.2–7.3). Reported associations with levels of THMs above 80 μg/litre included all surveillance defects (OR = 1.6; 90% CI = 1.2–2.0), central nervous system defects (OR = 2.6; 90% CI = 1.5–4.3), neural tube defects (OR = 3.0; 90% CI = 1.3–6.6) and major cardiac defects (OR = 1.8; 90% CI = 1.0–3.3). Moderate to strong associations were found for central nervous system, oral cleft and neural tube defects, but only a small number of cases were studied. The study included 4082 small for gestational age infants, but fewer numbers with birth defects: 56 infants with neural tube defects, 83 with oral cleft defects, 108 with major cardiac defects and 118 with central nervous system defects. The observed increased risk for other reproductive outcomes was smaller, and these weak associations could be due to unidentified confounding bias.

As in the Iowa (USA) study, the ecological study design for assessment of individual exposure and confounding bias limits the interpretation of the results. The investigators noted "the difficulty of interpreting the available water contamination data and the numerous assumptions needed in order to estimate contaminant levels" as a limitation (Bove et al., 1992a). "By itself, this study cannot resolve whether the drinking-water contaminants caused the adverse birth outcomes" (Bove et al., 1995).

Also reported were results of a population-based case–control study in New Jersey (USA) to determine risks of cardiac defects, neural tube defects, oral clefts, very low birth weight and low birth weight associated with exposure to different THM levels (Bove et al., 1992b). A total of 563 mothers of cases and controls were interviewed by telephone some 6–54 months after giving birth. The study included 185 infants with birth defects, 37 of whom had neural tube defects, 97 infants with very low birth weights, 113 infants with low birth weights and 138 infants of normal weight without birth defects. Information was obtained for a potential exposure period 3 months prior to conception through the end of pregnancy and included residences of the mother, sources of drinking-water, tapwater consumption, showering and smoking habits, alcohol consumption, exposures in and around the home, prescription drugs, medical history and previous adverse reproductive outcomes. For neural tube defects, a 4-fold increased risk was found to be associated with THM levels greater than 80 µg/litre (OR = 4.25; 95% CI = 1.0–17.7); however, this estimate is based on only 7 cases and 14 controls. The sample size for the case–control study was small, resulting in low statistical power and a lack of precision in estimating the risk; most importantly, a majority (53.3%) of the mothers of the cases and controls could not be located for interviews, causing possible selection bias. Once contact was established with the mother of the case or control, only 78% agreed to be interviewed. In addition, because of the long period between pregnancy and the interview, inaccurate recall of the mothers may be responsible for incorrect or biased information about both potential exposures and confounding characteristics. An assessment of selection bias by the investigators showed that risk had likely been overestimated for neural tube defects. After correcting for selection bias, the risk associated with THM levels greater than 80 µg/litre was reduced from a 4-fold to a 50% increased risk. The observed risk now represents a weak association where unknown confounding bias might be responsible.

A second population-based case–control study was recently reported in a published abstract (Klotz et al., 1996). Cases were births or fetal deaths after 20 weeks' gestation in 1993 and 1994 with anencephaly, spina bifida or encephalocele reported to the New Jersey Birth Defects Registry or Vital Statistics. Controls were randomly selected by month of birth from birth certificates during the same period as cases. In home interviews, information was obtained on ingestion and non-ingestion exposures, other environmental and occupational exposures, and pregnancy characteristics. Exposures were estimated from water quality monitoring data for the appropriate public water system selected to approximate the critical time for neural closure (fourth week of gestation), similar water quality data from the same source 1 year later, and analysis of residential tapwater collected about 1 year after the critical time. To prevent misclassification of exposure, biological monitoring of urine and exhaled breath from a sample of participants was also conducted. Increased relative risks for neural tube defects were associated with THMs; ORs were generally between 1.5 and 2.1 (Klotz & Pyrch, 1998). The only statistically significant results were observed in infants born with neural tube defects (and no other malformations) and whose mothers' residence in early pregnancy was in an area where the THM levels were greater than 40 µg/litre (OR = 2.1; 95% CI = 1.1–4.0). No association was observed between HAAs, HANs or nitrates in drinking-water and risk of neural tube defects.

A cohort study (Waller et al., 1998; Swan, 1998) of women members of Kaiser Permanente Medical Care Program in California (USA) evaluated associations of THMs and spontaneous abortion, low birth weight, preterm delivery and intrauterine growth retardation. Results of the spontaneous abortion analysis were recently reported. Information about water consumption, water source and THM levels was collected for the participating cohort members. Data for THM levels in tapwater were obtained from each public water supply for a 3-year period when distribution taps were monitored at least quarterly. A woman's exposure to THMs was estimated using the average level of THMs for each water supply of samples collected within the woman's first trimester (77% of the cohort) or within 30 days of the subject's first trimester (4%) or the annual average from the utility's annual water quality report (9%). High first-trimester levels of THMs were based on levels corresponding to the 75th percentile, i.e., ≥ 75 µg of total THMs per litre, ≥ 16 µg of chloroform per litre, ≥ 15 µg of bromoform per litre, ≥ 17 µg of BDCM per litre and ≥ 31 µg of DBCM per litre. Pregnancy outcomes were obtained from hospital records, the California Birth Registry and follow-up interviews. Interviews were also used to obtain information about possible confounding characteristics. The study found that an increased risk of miscarriage was associated with a high consumption of water (five or more glasses of cold tapwater per day) containing high levels of total THMs (≥ 75 µg/litre), especially for waters high in BDCM (≥ 17 µg/litre). In the women with high exposures to total THMs (THM levels ≥ 75 µg/litre and five or more glasses of water consumed per day), the relative risk of a miscarriage was almost twice that of the low-exposure groups (total THM levels below 75 µg/litre and fewer than five glasses of water per day). Of the four THMs, only high exposure to BDCM (≥ 17 µg/litre and five or more glasses of water per day) was associated with a 3-fold increased relative risk of miscarriage. The risk for unemployed women was also found to be greater than that for employed women, suggesting that women with a greater opportunity to consume home tapwater with a high level of THMs may be at greater risk. However, it is not certain that other characteristics of employed women were adequately assessed and controlled for (e.g., a healthy worker effect).

Preliminary analyses were available for a cross-sectional study (Nuckols et al., 1995) of births to women in Northglenn, Colorado (USA) exposed to chlorinated water from Stanley Lake with high THM levels (32–72 µg/litre) and women in Westminster exposed to chloraminated water from Stanley Lake with low THM levels (<20 µg/litre). Gallagher et al. (1997)[1] used a geographic information system and water quality modelling as described by Nuckols et al. (1995) to conduct a retrospective cohort study in the same water districts. Information about developmental outcomes and possible confounding characteristics was obtained from birth certificates, and exposures to THMs were modelled based on hydraulic characteristics of the water system and THM levels obtained from a monitoring program. However, sufficient information was available to estimate THM exposures for mothers in only 28 census blocks, 11 of 26 census blocks from Northglenn and 17 of 60 blocks from Westminster. The exclusion of such a large number of births from the study seriously limits the interpretation of the observed results. Women with high or low THM exposure may have been selectively excluded, but this could not be determined with the information reported. After excluding

---

[1] Gallagher MD, Nuckols JR, Stallones L, & Savitz DA (1997) Exposure to trihalomethanes and adverse pregnancy outcomes in Colorado (Unpublished manuscript).

births to mothers in blocks with no THM data and births less than 400 g, only 25% of births remained for analysis, and the reported epidemiological associations must be considered inconclusive.

5.3.3.1   *Summary of results of reproductive/developmental studies*

No associations were reported in North Carolina (USA) for THM levels and estimated dose of THMs, but associations between chloroform or THM levels in water and adverse reproductive or developmental outcomes were reported in studies conducted in California, Iowa and New Jersey (USA).

A recently completed case–control study (but not yet reported in the peer review literature) in New Jersey (USA) reported increased relative risks for infants born with neural tube defects (and no other malformations) and whose mothers' residence in early pregnancy was in an area where the THM levels were greater than 40 µg/litre (OR = 2.1; 95% CI = 1.1–4.0). Replication of these results in another geographic area is required before causality can be assessed. Previous epidemiological studies in New Jersey reported increased relative risks of neural tube defects associated with the mother's residence in areas with high THMs; however, these studies suffer from methodological limitations, and their results are inconclusive.

The Waller et al. (1998) study is well designed and well conducted; as it is the first study to suggest an adverse reproductive effect associated with a brominated by-product, results should be used to support further research on spontaneous abortion risks and drinking-water contaminants, including THM species, other DBPs and other water contaminants. The authors discussed the weaknesses and strengths of their study. One weakness is that water consumption was not assessed at work, but investigators did consider risks separately for women who worked outside the home, reporting that "results were stronger in women not employed outside the home, for whom our home based exposure assessment should be more precise" (Waller et al., 1998). A major limitation is that DBPs other than THMs and other water contaminants were not studied. A concern is how to interpret the results of the Waller et al. (1998) study in light of the findings of Swan et al. (1998).

Swan et al. (1998) analysed tapwater and bottled water consumption in the same cohort studied by Waller et al. (1998) and reported a dose-related increase in spontaneous abortions among tapwater drinkers in Region I, but not in Region II or III. "Our prior studies suggested that the relation between spontaneous abortion and tapwater was independent of chlorination by-products, since the strongest associations were seen in the two studies conducted in areas served only by unchlorinated groundwater. Additionally, in the two rodent studies we conducted, a trend toward increased rates of fetal resorption was seen in rats drinking unchlorinated groundwater, compared with bottled water. In our current study, as discussed in the study by Waller et al., spontaneous abortion risk was increased by exposure to specific chlorination by-products in all regions. Nevertheless, we believe that the associations with cold tapwater and bottled water presented here, which are specific to Region I, cannot be explained by exposure to chlorination by-products, because the association is seen in the absence of high levels of these chemicals" (Swan et al., 1998). In a letter to the editor, Swan & Waller (1998) suggested that there may be "some constituent in addition to THMs" that is specific to tapwater in Region I but provided a poor explanation of why this may be so. "Bromodichloromethane (or some compound highly correlated with it) was the trihalomethane most strongly associated with SAB [spontaneous abortion]" (Waller et al., 1998). "Swan et al. found a dose-related increase in SABs among tapwater drinkers in Region I, but not in Regions II or III. Exposure to TTHM [total THMs] or bromodichloromethane does not entirely explain this association, since a tapwater effect is still evident among Region I women with low levels of both TTHM and bromodichloromethane. Furthermore, the initial studies in Region I found the strongest effect in areas served only by unchlorinated groundwater. Thus, it is likely that other factors contributed to the tapwater effect described by Swan et al." (Waller et al., 1998). Because of these concerns, judgement about the interpretation of the results of Waller et al. (1998) should be deferred until additional water quality data are analysed for the cohort or another well designed and well conducted epidemiological study finds similar results.

Although the study by Waller et al. (1998) does not provide sufficient evidence for a cause–effect relationship between exposure to THMs and early-term miscarriages, it does provide important new information that should be pursued with additional research. Assessing the causality of an observed epidemiological association requires evidence from more than a single study, and additional information is needed on other water exposures.

Several exploratory epidemiological studies have suggested that certain adverse reproductive effects and developmental outcomes may be associated with chloroform or THMs in drinking-water, but additional studies are required to determine whether these observed associations are spurious or due to possible bias. The latest study from New Jersey (USA) reported a moderate association between neural tube defects and THM levels of more than 40 µg/litre but no associations with HAAs, HANs or nitrates in drinking-water. The Waller et al. (1998) and Klotz & Pyrch (1998) studies require replication in another area before results can be properly interpreted.

5.4 Summary

Epidemiological studies have not identified an increased risk of cardiovascular disease associated with chlorinated or chloraminated drinking-water.

Based on the entire cancer–chlorinated drinking-water epidemiology database, there is better evidence for an association between exposure to chlorinated surface water and bladder cancer than for other types of cancer. However, the latest published study (Cantor et al., 1998) notes several inconsistencies in results among the studies for smokers/non-smokers and males/females, and the evidence is still considered insufficient to allow a judgement as to whether the association is causal and which water contaminants may be important. Evidence for a role of THMs is weak. Poole (1997) also notes that "The basic conclusion of the present report is that the hypothesis of a causal relationship between consumption of chlorination by-products and the risk of any cancer, including bladder cancer and rectal cancer, is still an open question."

The overall findings of Cantor et al. (1998) support the hypothesis of an association between bladder cancer and duration of use of chlorinated surface water or groundwater and estimated THM exposures, but aspects of these results caution against a simple interpretation and raise additional questions about the nature of the association. An increase in bladder cancer risk was found with duration of chlorinated groundwater use, as well as with total duration of chlorinated drinking-water (surface water plus groundwater) use, with relative risks similar to those observed with chlorinated surface water. This finding is unexpected, because the levels of by-products from most chlorinated groundwaters are much lower than those in treated surface water. In addition, risk was found to increase with duration of chlorinated surface water use among ever-smokers, but not never-smokers, and among men, but not women. This raises questions of internal consistency, as well as consistency with other findings. In contrast, Cantor et al. (1998) found associations for both sexes, primarily among never-smokers. Cantor et al. (1985) noted: "In Ontario, King and Marrett noted somewhat higher risk estimates for never-smokers associated with duration of chlorinated surface water. In Colorado, McGeehin et al. reported similar patterns of risk among smokers and never-smokers, and among men and women. Finally, in a case–control study from Washington County, Maryland, Freedman et al. reported results that parallel the current findings, namely that the risk associated with chlorinated surface water was primarily observed among men and among smokers. Reasons for differences among these observations and differences with results from our study are unclear. A possible explanation for the apparent discrepancies in findings for smokers and never-smokers among studies may reside in water quality and water treatment differences in the respective study areas, with resulting variations in the chemical composition of byproduct mixtures. Nevertheless, results should not differ by sex."

The existing epidemiological data are insufficient to allow a conclusion that the observed associations between bladder or any other cancer and chlorinated drinking-water or THMs are causal or provide an accurate estimate of the magnitude of risk.

Any association between exposure to chlorinated surface water, THMs or the mutagenicity of drinking-water and cancer of the colon, rectum, pancreas, brain and other sites cannot be evaluated at this time because of inadequate epidemiological evidence. However, the findings from well conducted studies associating bladder cancer with chlorinated water and THMs cannot be completely dismissed, even though inconsistencies have been noted for risks among men and women and among smokers and non-smokers. Because of the large number of people exposed to chlorinated drinking-water, it is important to resolve this issue using studies designed with sound epidemiological principles. Additional studies to resolve the questions about the associations that have been reported for chlorinated surface water, THMs, fluid and tapwater consumption and bladder cancer and reproductive and developmental effects must focus on the resolution of various problems noted in previous studies, especially consideration of exposures to other DBPs.

The existing epidemiological data are insufficient to allow the importance of the observed associations of chlorinated drinking-water or THMs and adverse pregnancy outcomes to be assessed. Although several studies have suggested that increased risks of neural tube defects and miscarriage may be associated with THMs or selected THM species, additional studies are needed to determine whether the observed associations are spurious.

A recently convened scientific panel (US EPA, 1997) concluded that the results of published epidemiological studies do not provide convincing evidence that DBPs cause adverse pregnancy outcomes. The panel recommended that additional studies be conducted, specifically that the Waller et al. (1998) study be expanded to include additional exposure information about by-products other than THMs and that a similar study be conducted in another geographic area.

6. RISK CHARACTERIZATION

It should be noted that the use of chemical disinfectants in water treatment usually results in the formation of chemical by-products, some of which are potentially hazardous. However, the risks to health from these by-products at the levels at which they occur in drinking-water are extremely small in comparison with the risks associated with inadequate disinfection. Thus, it is important that disinfection not be compromised in attempting to control such by-products.

6.1 Characterization of hazard and dose–response

6.1.1 Toxicological studies

6.1.1.1 Chlorine

A WHO Working Group for the *Guidelines for drinking-water quality* (WHO, 1993) considered chlorine. This Working Group determined a tolerable daily intake (TDI) of 150 µg/kg of body weight for free chlorine. This TDI is derived from a NOAEL of approximately 15 mg/kg of body weight per day in 2-year studies in rats and mice (NTP, 1992), incorporating an uncertainty factor of 100 (10 each for intra- and interspecies variation). There are no new data that indicate that this TDI should be changed.

6.1.1.2 Monochloramine

A WHO Working Group for the *Guidelines for drinking-water quality* considered monochloramine (WHO, 1993). This Working Group determined a TDI of 94 µg/kg of body weight based on a NOAEL of approximately 9.4 mg/kg of body weight per day, the highest dose tested, in a 2-year bioassay in rats (NTP, 1992), incorporating an uncertainty factor of 100 (10 each for intra- and interspecies variation). There are no new data that indicate that this TDI should be changed.

6.1.1.3 Chlorine dioxide

Chlorine dioxide chemistry in drinking-water is complex, but the major breakdown product in drinking-water is chlorite. In establishing a specific TDI for chlorine dioxide, data on both chlorine dioxide and chlorite can be considered, given the rapid hydrolysis to chlorite. Therefore, an oral TDI for chlorine dioxide is 30 µg/kg of body weight, based on the NOAEL of 2.9 mg/kg of body weight per day for neurodevelopmental effects of chlorite in rats (CMA, 1997).

6.1.1.4 Trihalomethanes

Cancer following chronic exposure is the primary hazard of concern for this class of DBPs. Owing to the weight of evidence indicating that chloroform can induce cancer in animals only after chronic exposure to cytotoxic doses, it is clear that exposures to low concentrations of chloroform in drinking-water do not pose carcinogenic risks. The NOAEL for cytolethality and regenerative hyperplasia in mice was 10 mg/kg of body weight per day after administration of chloroform in corn oil for 3 weeks (Larson et al., 1994b). Based on the mode of action evidence for chloroform carcinogenicity, a TDI of 10 µg/kg of body weight was derived using the NOAEL for cytotoxicity in mice and applying an uncertainty factor of 1000 (10 each for inter- and intraspecies variation and 10 for the short duration of the study). This approach is supported by a number of additional studies. This TDI is similar to the TDI derived in the *Guidelines for drinking-water quality* (WHO, 1998), which was based on a 7.5-year study in dogs. In this study, beagle dogs were given chloroform in a toothpaste base in gelatin capsules, 6 days per week for 7.5 years, at 0, 15 or 30 mg/kg of body weight per day. Slight hepatotoxicity was observed at 15 mg/kg of body weight per day (Heywood et al., 1979). Incorporating an uncertainty factor of 1000 (10 each for intra- and interspecies variation and 10 for use of a LOAEL rather than a NOAEL and a subchronic study), a TDI of 13 µg/kg of body weight (corrected for 6 days per week dosing) was derived.

Among the brominated THMs, BDCM is of particular interest because it produces tumours in rats and mice and at several sites (liver, kidney and large intestine) after corn oil gavage (NTP, 1987). The induction of colon tumours in rats by BDCM (and by bromoform) is also interesting because of the epidemiological associations with colorectal cancer (see section 5.3.1). BDCM and the other brominated THMs are also weak mutagens (IARC, 1991, 1999; Pegram et al., 1997). It is generally assumed that mutagenic carcinogens will produce linear dose–response relationships at low dose, as mutagenesis is generally considered to be an irreversible and cumulative effect.

In a 2-year bioassay, BDCM given by corn oil gavage induced tumours (in conjunction with cytotoxicity and increased proliferation) in the kidneys of mice and rats at doses of 50 and 100 mg/kg of body weight per day, respectively (NTP, 1987). The large intestine tumours in rats occurred after exposure to both 50 and 100 mg/kg of body weight per day. Using the incidence of kidney tumours in male mice from this study, quantitative risk estimates have been calculated, yielding a slope factor[1] of 4.8×10^{-3} [mg/kg of body weight per day]$^{-1}$ and a calculated dose of 2.1 µg/kg of body weight per day for a risk level of 10^{-5} (IRIS, 1993). A slope factor of 4.2×10^{-3} [mg/kg of body weight per day]$^{-1}$ (2.4 µg/kg of body weight per day for a 10^{-5} risk) was derived based on the incidence of large intestine carcinomas in the male rat. IARC (1991, 1999) has classified BDCM in Group 2B (possibly carcinogenic to humans).

DBCM and bromoform were studied in long-term bioassays. In a 2-year corn oil gavage study, DBCM induced hepatic tumours in female mice, but not in rats, at a dose of 100 mg/kg of body weight per day (NTP, 1985). In previous evaluations, it has been suggested that the corn oil vehicle may play a role in the induction of tumours in female mice (WHO, 1996). A small increase in tumours of the large intestine in rats was observed in the bromoform study at a dose of 200 mg/kg of body weight per day. No neoplastic effects were associated with exposure of mice to chloroform (NTP, 1989a). The slope factors based on these tumours are 6.5×10^{-3} [mg/kg of body weight per day]$^{-1}$ for DBCM or 1.5 µg/kg of body weight per day for 10^{-5} risk (IRIS, 1992) and 1.3×10^{-3} [mg/kg of body weight per day]$^{-1}$ or 7.7 µg/kg of body weight per day for 10^{-5} risk for bromoform (IRIS, 1991).

---

[1] Slope factors given here do not incorporate a surface area to body weight correction.

These two brominated THMs are weakly mutagenic in a number of assays, and they were by far the most mutagenic DBPs of the class in the GST-mediated assay system (DeMarini et al., 1997; Pegram et al., 1997). Because they are the most lipophilic THMs, additional concerns about whether corn oil may have affected their bioavailability in the long-term studies should be considered. A NOAEL for DBCM of 30 mg/kg of body weight per day has been established in a 13-week corn oil gavage study, based on the absence of histopathological effects in the liver of rats (NTP, 1985). A TDI for DBCM of 30 µg/kg of body weight was derived based on the NOAEL for liver toxicity of 30 mg/kg of body weight per day and an uncertainty factor of 1000 (10 each for inter- and intraspecies variation and 10 for the short duration of the study and possible carcinogenicity). IARC (1991, 1999) has classified DBCM in Group 3 (not classifiable as to its carcinogenicity to humans).

A NOAEL for bromoform of 25 mg/kg of body weight per day can be derived on the basis of the absence of liver lesions in rats after 13 weeks of dosing by corn oil gavage (NTP, 1989a). A TDI for bromoform of 25 µg/kg of body weight was derived based on this NOAEL for liver toxicity and an uncertainty factor of 1000 (10 each for inter- and intraspecies variation and 10 for the short duration of the study and possible carcinogenicity). IARC (1991, 1999) has classified bromoform in Group 3 (not classifiable as to its carcinogenicity to humans).

6.1.1.5 Haloacetic acids

The induction of mutations by DCA is very improbable at the low doses that would be encountered in chlorinated drinking-water. The available data indicate that DCA differentially affects the replication rates of normal hepatocytes and hepatocytes that have been initiated (Pereira & Phelps, 1996). The dose–response relationships are complex, with DCA initially stimulating division of normal hepatocytes. However, at the lower chronic doses used in animal studies (but still very high relative to those that would be derived from drinking-water), the replication rate of normal hepatocytes is eventually sharply inhibited. This indicates that normal hepatocytes eventually down-regulate those pathways that are sensitive to stimulation by DCA. However, the effects in altered cells, particularly those that express high amounts of a protein that is immunoreactive to a c-Jun antibody, do not seem to be able to down-regulate this response (Stauber & Bull, 1997). Thus, the rates of replication in the pre-neoplastic lesions with this phenotype are very high at the doses that cause DCA tumours to develop with a very low latency. Preliminary data suggest that this continued alteration in cell birth and death rates is also necessary for the tumours to progress to malignancy (Bull et al., 1990). This interpretation is supported by studies that employ initiation/promotion designs as well (Pereira, 1996).

Based upon the above considerations, it is suggested that the currently available cancer risk estimates for DCA be modified by incorporation of newly developing information on its comparative metabolism and modes of action to formulate a biologically based dose–response model. These data are not available at this time, but they should become available within the next 2–3 years.

The effects of DCA appear to be closely associated with doses that induce hepatomegaly and glycogen accumulation in mice. The LOAEL for these effects in an 8-week study in mice was 0.5 g/litre, corresponding to approximately 100 mg/kg of body weight per day, and the NOAEL was 0.2 g/litre, or approximately 40 mg/kg of body weight per day (Kato-Weinstein et al., 1998). A TDI of 40 µg/kg of body weight has been calculated by applying an uncertainty factor of 1000 to this NOAEL (10 each for inter- and intraspecies variation and 10 for the short duration of the study and possible carcinogenicity). IARC (1995) has classified DCA in Group 3 (not classifiable as to its carcinogenicity to humans).

TCA is one of the weakest activators of the PPAR known (Issemann & Green, 1990). It appears to be only marginally active as a peroxisome proliferator, even in rats (DeAngelo et al., 1989). Furthermore, treatment of rats with high levels of TCA in drinking-water does not induce liver tumours (DeAngelo et al., 1997). These data strongly suggest that TCA presents little carcinogenic hazard to humans at the low concentrations found in drinking-water.

From a broader toxicological perspective, the developmental effects of TCA are the end-point of concern (Smith et al., 1989a; Saillenfait et al., 1995). Animals appear to tolerate concentrations of

TCA in drinking-water of 0.5 g/litre (approximately 50 mg/kg of body weight per day) with little or no signs of adverse effect. At 2 g/litre, the only sign of adverse effect appears to be hepatomegaly. The hepatomegaly is not observed in mice at doses of 0.35 g of TCA per litre in drinking-water, estimated to be equivalent to 40 mg/kg of body weight per day (Pereira, 1996).

In a study by Smith et al. (1989a), soft tissue anomalies were observed at approximately 3 times the rate in controls at the lowest dose administered of 330 mg/kg of body weight per day. At this dose, the anomalies were mild and would clearly be in the range where hepatomegaly (and carcinogenic effects) would occur. Considering the fact that the PPAR interacts with cell signalling mechanisms that can affect normal developmental processes, a common mechanism underlying hepatomegaly and the carcinogenic and developmental effects of this compound should be considered.

The TDI for TCA is based on a NOAEL estimated to be 40 mg/kg of body weight per day for hepatic toxicity in a long-term study in mice (Pereira, 1996). Application of an uncertainty factor of 1000 to the estimated NOAEL (10 each for inter- and intraspecies variation and 10 for possible carcinogenicity) gives a TDI of 40 µg/kg of body weight. IARC (1995) has classified TCA in Group 3 (not classifiable as to its carcinogenicity to humans).

Data on the carcinogenicity of brominated acetic acids are too preliminary to be useful in risk characterization. Data available in abstract form suggest, however, that the doses required to induce hepatocarcinogenic responses in mice are not dissimilar to those of the chlorinated acetic acids (Bull & DeAngelo, 1995). In addition to the mechanisms involved in DCA- and TCA-induced cancer, it is possible that increased oxidative stress secondary to their metabolism might contribute to their effects (Austin et al., 1996; Parrish et al., 1996).

There are a significant number of data on the effects of DBA on male reproduction. No effects were observed in rats at doses of 2 mg/kg of body weight per day for 79 days, whereas an increased retention of step 19 spermatids was observed at 10 mg/kg of body weight per day. Higher doses led to progressively more severe effects, including marked atrophy of the seminiferous tubules at 250 mg/kg of body weight per day, which was not reversed 6 months after treatment was suspended (Linder et al., 1997b). A TDI of 20 µg/kg of body weight was determined by allocating an uncertainty factor of 100 (10 each for inter- and intraspecies variation) to the NOAEL of 2 mg/kg of body weight per day.

6.1.1.6   Chloral hydrate

In a 2-year study, chloral hydrate at 1 g/litre of drinking-water (166 mg/kg of body weight per day) induced liver tumours in male mice (Daniel et al., 1992a). Lower doses have not been evaluated. Chloral hydrate has been shown to induce chromosomal anomalies in several *in vitro* tests but has been largely negative when evaluated *in vivo* (IARC, 1995). It is probable that the liver tumours induced by chloral hydrate involve its metabolism to TCA and/or DCA. As discussed previously, these compounds are considered to act as tumour promoters. IARC (1995) has classified chloral hydrate in Group 3 (not classifiable as to its carcinogenicity to humans).

Chloral hydrate administered to rats for 90 days in drinking-water induced hepatocellular necrosis at concentrations of 1200 mg/litre and above, with no effect being observed at 600 mg/litre (approximately 60 mg/kg of body weight per day) (Daniel et al., 1992b). Hepato-megaly was observed in male mice at doses of 144 mg/kg of body weight per day administered by gavage for 14 days. No effect was observed at 14.4 mg/kg of body weight per day in the 14-day study, but mild hepatomegaly was observed when chloral hydrate was administered in drinking-water at 70 mg/litre (16 mg/kg of body weight per day) in a 90-day follow-up study (Sanders et al., 1982). An uncertainty factor of 1000 (10 each for inter- and intraspecies variation and 10 for the use of a LOAEL instead of a NOAEL) applied to this value gives a TDI of 16 µg/kg of body weight.

6.1.1.7   Haloacetonitriles

Without appropriate human data or an animal study that involves a substantial portion of an experimental animal's lifetime, there is no generally accepted basis for estimating carcinogenic risk from the HANs.

Data developed in subchronic studies provided some indication of NOAELs for the general toxicity of DCAN and DBAN. NOAELs of 8 and 23 mg/kg of body weight per day were identified in 90-day studies in rats for DCAN and DBAN, respectively, based on decreased body weights at the next higher doses of 33 and 45 mg/kg of body weight per day, respectively (Hayes et al., 1986).

A Working Group for the WHO *Guidelines for drinking-water quality* considered DCAN and DBAN (WHO, 1993). This Working Group determined a TDI of 15 µg/kg of body weight for DCAN based on a NOAEL of 15 mg/kg of body weight per day in a reproductive toxicity study in rats (Smith et al., 1989b) and incorporating an uncertainty factor of 1000 (10 each for intra- and interspecies variation and 10 for the severity of effects). Reproductive and developmental effects were observed with DBAN only at doses that exceeded those established for general toxicity (about 45 mg/kg of body weight per day) (Smith et al., 1987). A TDI of 23 µg/kg of body weight was calculated for DBAN based on the NOAEL of 23 mg/kg of body weight per day in the 90-day study in rats (Hayes et al., 1986) and incorporating an uncertainty factor of 1000 (10 each for intra- and interspecies variation and 10 for the short duration of the study). There are no new data that indicate that these TDIs should be changed.

LOAELs for TCAN were identified at 7.5 mg/kg of body weight per day for embryotoxicity and 15 mg/kg of body weight per day for developmental effects in rats (Smith et al., 1988). However, later studies suggest that these responses were dependent upon the vehicle used (Christ et al., 1996). No TDI can be established for TCAN.

There are no data useful for risk characterization purposes for other members of the HANs.

6.1.1.8   MX

The mutagen MX has recently been studied in a long-term study in rats in which some carcinogenic responses were observed (Komulainen et al., 1997). These data indicate that MX induces thyroid and bile duct tumours. An increased incidence of thyroid tumours was seen at the lowest dose of MX administered (0.4 mg/kg of body weight per day). The induction of thyroid tumours with high-dose chemicals has long been associated with halogenated compounds. The induction of thyroid follicular tumours could involve modifications in thyroid function or mutagenic mode of action. A dose-related increase in the incidence of cholangiomas and cholangiocarcinomas was also observed, beginning at the low dose in female rats, with a more modest response in male rats. The increase in cholangiomas and cholangio-carcinomas in female rats was utilized to derive a slope factor for cancer. The 95% upper confidence limit for a 10^{-5} lifetime risk based on the linearized multistage model was calculated to be 0.06 μg/kg of body weight per day.

6.1.1.9   Chlorite

The primary and most consistent finding arising from exposure to chlorite is oxidative stress resulting in changes in the red blood cells (Heffernan et al., 1979a; Harrington et al., 1995a). This end-point is seen in laboratory animals and, by analogy with chlorate, in humans exposed to high doses in poisoning incidents. There are sufficient data available to estimate a TDI for humans exposed to chlorite, including chronic toxicity studies and a two-generation reproductive toxicity study. Studies in human volunteers for up to 12 weeks did not identify any effect on blood parameters at the highest dose tested, 36 μg/kg of body weight per day (Lubbers & Bianchine, 1984; Lubbers et al., 1984a). Because these studies do not identify an effect level, they are not informative for establishing a margin of safety.

In a two-generation study in rats, a NOAEL of 2.9 mg/kg of body weight per day was identified based on lower auditory startle ampli-tude, decreased absolute brain weight in the F_1 and F_2 generations and altered liver weights in two generations (CMA, 1997). Application of an uncertainty factor of 100 to this NOAEL (10 each for inter- and intraspecies variation) gives a TDI of 30 μg/kg of body weight. This TDI is supported by the human volunteer studies.

6.1.1.10   Chlorate

Like chlorite, the primary concern with chlorate is oxidative dam-age to red blood cells. Also like chlorite, 0.036 mg/kg of body weight per day of chlorate for 12 weeks did not result in any adverse effect in human volunteers (Lubbers et al., 1981). Although the database for chlorate is less extensive than that for chlorite, a recent well conducted 90-day study in rats is available, which identified a NOAEL of 30 mg/kg of body weight per day based on thyroid gland colloid depletion at the next higher dose of 100 mg/kg of body weight per day (McCauley et al., 1995). A TDI is not derived because a long-term study is in progress, which should provide more information on chronic exposure to chlorate.

6.1.1.11 Bromate

Bromate is an active oxidant in biological systems and has been shown to cause an increase in renal tumours, peritoneal mesotheliomas and thyroid follicular cell tumours in rats and, to a lesser extent, hamsters, and only a small increase in kidney tumours in mice. The lowest dose at which an increased incidence of renal tumours was observed in rats was 6 mg/kg of body weight per day (DeAngelo et al., 1998).

Bromate has also been shown to give positive results for chromosomal aberrations in mammalian cells *in vitro* and *in vivo* but not in bacterial assays for point mutation. An increasing body of evidence, supported by the genotoxicity data, suggests that bromate acts by generating oxygen radicals in the cell.

In the WHO *Guidelines for drinking-water quality*, the linearized multistage model was applied to the incidence of renal tumours in a 2-year carcinogenicity study in rats (Kurokowa et al., 1986a), although it was noted that if the mechanism of tumour induction is oxidative damage in the kidney, application of the low-dose cancer model may not be appropriate. The calculated upper 95% confidence interval for a 10^{-5} risk was 0.1 μg/kg of body weight per day (WHO, 1993).

The no-effect level for the formation of renal cell tumours in rats is 1.3 mg/kg of body weight per day (Kurokowa et al., 1986a). If this is used as a point of departure from linearity and if an uncertainty factor of 1000 (10 each for inter- and intraspecies variation and 10 for possible carcinogenicity) is applied, a TDI of 1 μg/kg of body weight can be calculated. This compares with the value of 0.1 μg/kg of body weight per day associated with an excess lifetime cancer risk of 10^{-5}.

At present, there are insufficient data to allow a decision as to whether bromate-induced tumours are a result of cytotoxicity and reparative hyperplasia or a genotoxic effect. IARC (1986, 1987) has assigned potassium bromate to Group 2B: the agent is possibly carcinogenic to humans.

6.1.2 *Epidemiological studies*

Epidemiological studies must be carefully evaluated to ensure that observed associations are not due to bias and that the design is appropriate for an assessment of a possible causal relationship. Causality can be evaluated when there is sufficient evidence from several well designed and well conducted studies in different geographic areas. Supporting toxicological and pharmacological data are also important. It is especially difficult to interpret epidemiological data from ecological studies of disinfected drinking-water, and these results are used primarily to help develop hypotheses for further study.

Results of analytical epidemiological studies are insufficient to support a causal relationship for any of the observed associations. It is especially difficult to interpret the results of currently published analytical studies because of incomplete information about exposures to specific water contaminants that might confound or modify the risk. Because inadequate attention has been paid to assessing water contaminant exposures in epidemiological studies, it is not possible to properly evaluate increased relative risks that were reported. Risks may be due to other water contaminants or to other factors for which chlorinated drinking-water or THMs may serve as a surrogate.

6.2 Characterization of exposure

6.2.1 *Occurrence of disinfectants and disinfectant by-products*

Disinfectant doses of several milligrams per litre are typically employed, corresponding to doses necessary to inactivate microorganisms (primary disinfection) or to maintain a distribution system residual (secondary disinfection). A necessary ingredient for an exposure assessment is DBP occurrence data. Unfortunately, there are few published international studies that go beyond case-study or regional data.

Occurrence data suggest, on average, an exposure in chlorinated drinking-water to total THMs of about 35–50 µg/litre, with chloroform and BDCM being the first and second most dominant species. Exposure to total HAAs can be approximated by a total HAA concentration (sum of five species) corresponding to about one-half of the total THM concentration (although this ratio can vary significantly); DCA and TCA are the first and second most dominant species. In waters with a high bromide to TOC ratio and/or a high bromide to chlorine ratio, greater formation of brominated THMs and HAAs can be expected. When a hypochlorite solution (versus chlorine gas) is used, chlorate may also occur in the hypochlorite solution and be found in chlorinated water.

DBP exposure in chloraminated water is a function of the mode of chloramination, with the sequence of chlorine followed by ammonia leading to the formation of (lower levels of) chlorine DBPs (i.e., THMs and HAAs) during the free-chlorine period; however, the suppression of chloroform and TCA formation is not paralleled by a proportional reduction in DCA formation.

All factors being equal, bromide concentration and ozone dose are the best predictors of bromate formation during ozonation, with about a 50% conversion of bromide to bromate. A study of different European water utilities showed bromate levels in water leaving operating water treatment plants of less than the detection limit (2 µg/litre) up to 16 µg/litre. The brominated organic DBPs formed upon ozonation generally occur at low levels. The formation of chlorite can be estimated by a simple percentage (50–70%) of the applied chlorine dioxide dose.

6.2.2 Uncertainties of water quality data

A toxicological study attempts to extrapolate a laboratory (controlled) animal response to a potential human response; one possible outcome is the estimation of cancer risk factors. An epidemiological study attempts to link human health effects (e.g., cancer) to a causative agent or agents (e.g., a DBP) and requires an exposure assessment.

The chemical risks associated with disinfected drinking-water are potentially based on several routes of exposure: (i) ingestion of DBPs in drinking-water; (ii) ingestion of chemical disinfectants in drinking-water and the concomitant formation of DBPs in the stomach; and (iii) inhalation of volatile DBPs during showering. Although the *in vivo* formation of DBPs and the inhalation of volatile DBPs may be of potential health concern, the following discussion is based on the premise that the ingestion of DBPs present in drinking-water poses the most significant chemical health risk.

Human exposure is a function of both DBP concentration and exposure time. More specifically, human health effects are a function of exposure to complex mixtures of DBPs (e.g., THMs versus HAAs, chlorinated versus brominated species) that can change seasonally/temporally (e.g., as a function of temperature and nature and concentration of NOM) and spatially (i.e., throughout a distribution system). Each individual chemical disinfectant can form a mixture of DBPs; combinations of chemical disinfectants can form even more complex mixtures. Upon their formation, most DBPs are stable, but some may undergo transformation by, for example, hydrolysis. In the absence of DBP data, surrogates such as chlorine dose (or chlorine demand), TOC (or UVA_{254}) or bromide can be used to indirectly estimate exposure. While TOC serves as a good surrogate for organic DBP precursors, UVA_{254} provides additional insight into NOM characteristics, which can vary geographically. Two key water quality variables, pH and bromide, have been identified as significantly affecting the type and concentrations of DBPs that are produced.

An exposure assessment should first attempt to define the individual types of DBPs and resultant mixtures likely to form as well as their time-dependent concentrations, as affected by their stability and transport through a distribution system. For epidemiological studies, some historical databases exist for disinfectant (e.g., chlorine) doses, possibly DBP precursor (e.g., TOC) concentrations, and possibly total THM (and in some cases, THM species) concentrations. In contrast to THMs, which have been monitored over longer time frames because of regulatory scrutiny, monitoring data for HAAs (and HAA species), bromate and chlorite are much more recent and hence sparse. However, DBP models can be used to simulate missing or past data (e.g., concentrations of HAAs can be predicted using data on THM concentrations). Another important consideration is documentation of past changes in water treatment practice.

6.2.3 Uncertainties of epidemiological data

Even in well designed and well conducted analytical studies, relatively poor exposure assessments were conducted. In most studies, duration of exposure to disinfected drinking-water and the water source were considered. These exposures were estimated from residential histories and water utility or government records. In only a few studies was an attempt made to estimate a study participant's water consumption and exposure to either total THMs or individual THM species. In only one study was an attempt made to estimate exposures to other DBPs. In evaluating some potential risks, i.e., adverse outcomes of pregnancy, that may be associated with relatively short term exposures to volatile by-products, it may be important to consider the inhalation as well as the ingestion route of exposure from drinking-water. In some studies, an effort was made to estimate both by-product levels in drinking-water for etiologically relevant time periods and cumulative exposures. Appropriate models and sensitivity analysis such as Monte Carlo simulation can be used to help estimate these exposures for relevant periods.

A major uncertainty surrounds the interpretation of the observed associations, as exposures to a relatively few water contaminants have been considered. With the current data, it is difficult to evaluate how unmeasured DBPs or other water contaminants may have affected the observed relative risk estimates.

More studies have considered bladder cancer than any other cancer. The authors of the most recently reported results for bladder cancer risks caution against a simple interpretation of the observed associations. The epidemiological evidence for an increased relative risk of bladder cancer is not consistent — different risks are reported for smokers and non-smokers, for men and women, and for high and low water consumption. Risks may differ among various geographic areas because the DBP mix may be different or other water contaminants are also present. More comprehensive water quality data must be collected or simulated to improve exposure assessments for epidemiological studies.

7. RISK CONCLUSIONS AND COMPARISONS

Chlorination of drinking-water has been a cornerstone of efforts to prevent the spread of waterborne disease for almost a century (Craun et al., 1993). It is important to retain chlorination as an inexpensive and efficacious process unless a clear public health concern arises to eliminate it. It is uncertain that alternative chemical disinfectants reduce these estimated risks significantly (Bull & Kopfler, 1991).

Identifying the safest way of producing drinking-water requires more conclusive toxicological or epidemiological evidence than is available today. It is important to recognize that there is a sizeable set of data already present on this issue and that resolution of this problem will not simply come from an expansion of that database. The focus must be elevated from questions of individual by-products and routine toxicological testing to a much more systematic approach towards the resolution of these larger issues.

7.1 Epidemiological studies

The epidemiological associations between chlorinated drinking-water and human cancer have been subjected to several recent reviews, and the conclusions remain controversial. The small to medium relative risks for all the tumour sites studied (relative risks or odds ratios almost always less than 2) and uncertainty related to the magnitude and type of human exposures make it difficult to conclude that real risks result from the ingestion of chlorinated drinking-water.

7.2 Toxicological studies

Toxicological studies are best suited for developing information on individual by-products or known combinations of by-products. The deficiencies in the present toxicological database are outlined below.

7.2.1 Diversity of by-products

Significant qualitative and quantitative differences in the toxicological properties of DBPs have been demonstrated, depending upon whether they have some bromine substitution. Among the THMs,

BDCM is of particular interest because it produces tumours in both rats and mice at several sites (NTP, 1987). Moreover, its potency calculated under the assumptions of the linearized multistage model is an order of magnitude greater than that of chloroform (Bull & Kopfler, 1991). DBCM produced liver tumours only in mice (NTP, 1985), but bromoform produced colon tumours in rats (NTP, 1989a). The fact that both BDCM and bromoform given in corn oil vehicle induce colon cancer in animals is of interest because of the epidemiological associations seen with colo-rectal tumours and consumption of chlorinated water.

As with the THMs, however, a full complement of brominated and mixed bromochlorinated acetates are produced with the chlorination of drinking-water. These compounds have received little attention. While the chlorinated HAAs appear to be without significant genotoxic activity, the brominated HAAs appear to induce oxidative damage to DNA. Increases in the 8-OH-dG levels in hepatic DNA were observed with both acutely administered oral doses (Austin et al., 1996) and more prolonged exposures in drinking-water (Parrish et al., 1996). This activity increased with the degree of bromine substitution. Therefore, it cannot be concluded that the brominated HAAs are the mechanistic equivalents of the chlorinated HAAs.

Association of mutagenic activity with the chlorination of drinking-water was first observed by Cheh et al. (1980). While some of the major DBPs are mutagenic, they are much too weak as mutagens to account for this activity. By far the largest individual contributor to this activity is the compound referred to as MX. This compound has been variously reported to account for up to 57% of the mutagenic activity produced in the chlorination of drinking-water (Meier et al., 1985a,b; Hemming et al., 1986; Kronberg & Vartiainen, 1988). MX has recently been shown to be a carcinogen in rats (Komulainen et al., 1997). As with other classes of DBPs, brominated analogues and structurally related compounds that could be of importance are produced in the chlorination of drinking-water (Daniel et al., 1991b; Suzuki & Nakanishi, 1995).

7.2.2 *Diversity of modes of action*

It is important to recognize that the ways in which DBPs induce cancer are quite different. All of the modern work that has come forward on chloroform (Larson et al., 1994a,b, 1996) would strongly undermine the hypothesis that chloroform is contributing to the cancers observed in epidemiological studies. These toxicological results make a convincing case that tumorigenic responses in both the mouse liver and rat kidney are dependent upon necrosis and reparative hyperplasia. There is no basis for associating this type of target organ damage with the consumption of chlorinated drinking-water. On the other hand, brominated THMs are mutagenic (Zeiger, 1990; Pegram et al., 1997). It is generally assumed that mutagenic carcinogens will produce linear dose–response relationships at low doses, as mutagenesis is generally considered to be an irreversible and cumulative effect.

In the HAA class, significant differences in mode of action have been demonstrated for DCA and TCA. Despite the close structural resemblance of DCA and TCA and their common target organ (liver cancer induction), it is becoming clear that the mechanisms by which they act are different. TCA is a peroxisome proliferator, and the tumour phenotype and genotype seen in mice are consistent with this being the mode of action by which it acts. However, DCA clearly produced tumours at doses below those that are required for peroxisome pro-liferation (DeAngelo et al., 1989, 1996; Daniel et al., 1992a; Richmond et al., 1995). The tumour phenotypes that DCA and TCA produce in mice are very different (Pereira, 1996; Pereira & Phelps, 1996; Stauber & Bull, 1997). From a risk assessment standpoint, however, one would question whether either DCA or TCA, alone, is likely to present signi-ficant cancer risk to humans at the low levels found in drinking-water. Neither compound appears to influence the carcinogenic process by a mutagenic mechanism (Stauber & Bull, 1997; Harrington-Brock et al., 1998; Stauber et al., 1998). Although different mechanisms appear to be involved, the mode of action for both compounds appears to be tumour promotion. In experiments of short duration, they tend to increase replication rates of normal hepatocytes; with more extended exposures or very high doses, however, they tend to depress replication rates (Carter et al., 1995; Stauber & Bull, 1997). There is evidence to suggest that the depression of cell replication is paralleled by depressed rates of apoptosis (Snyder et al., 1995).

It is noteworthy that there is little support in the animal data for certain target organs that are prominently associated with chlorinated drinking-water in epidemiological studies (e.g., bladder cancer). There-fore, the possibility has to be left open that the carcinogenic effect of

DBPs may be dependent on genetically determined characteristics of a target organ (or tissue) that make it more susceptible than the same organ in test animals. This problem can be resolved only by conducting toxicological studies in the appropriate human tissues and by developing much stronger epidemiological associations to guide these studies.

The epidemiological studies can contribute to the resolution of the problem by (i) better identifying the drinking-water conditions that are associated with bladder or colo-rectal cancer, (ii) focusing on those characteristics of susceptibility that may increase the sensitivity at these target sites, and (iii) determining if interactions between biomarkers of susceptibility at these sites contribute to the epidemiological associations with disinfection of drinking-water. These "tasks" need to be accomplished sequentially. If epidemiological studies can provide insights into the first two tasks, then the experimental scientists can work much more profitably with epidemiologists to address the third task.

7.2.3 *Reproductive, developmental and neurotoxic effects*

Much of this review has focused on questions related to chemical carcinogenesis, in part because that is where the bulk of the experimental data are found. There are other toxicological effects associated with some DBPs that could be of importance. Recently published epidemiological data (Waller et al., 1998) suggest the possibility that increased spontaneous abortion rates may be related to DBPs in drinking-water.

Reproductive effects in females have been principally embryolethality and fetal resorptions associated with the HANs (Smith et al., 1988, 1989b). The dihaloacetates, DCA and DBA, have both been associated with effects on male reproduction, marked primarily by degeneration of the testicular epithelium (Toth et al., 1992; Linder et al., 1994a,b). Some effects on reproductive performance are noted at doses of DBA as low as 10 mg/kg of body weight per day. Dogs display testicular degeneration when administered doses of DCA of this same magnitude (Cicmanec et al., 1991).

7.3 Risks associated with mixtures of disinfectant by-products

Disinfected drinking-water is a very complex mixture of chemicals, most of which have not been identified. Studies on individual DBPs may not represent the risk posed by the mixture. Research on complex mixtures was recently reviewed by ILSI (1998). Studies of simple combinations of chemicals provided positive results, but only at concentrations so much greater than those that occur in drinking-water as to be irrelevant. Studies utilizing complex mixtures of chemicals as they could be isolated from water or produced by chlorinating high concentrations of humic or fulvic acids produce little convincing evidence of adverse effect. A variety of methodological issues prevent our being too comfortable with that conclusion (ILSI, 1998). Moreover, the effort never developed to the point that the diverse qualities of water in various parts of the country could be taken into account.

To be efficient, toxicological research needs to have a focus, and the research performed to solve this problem must be hypothesis-driven. This means that hypotheses of interactions would be based on knowledge of the toxic properties of individual by-products and would be subjected to experimental test. This can be much more efficient than designing complex multifactorial studies of all possible combinations of by-products produced by a disinfectant. An additional nuance would be to develop hypotheses as explicit tests of epidemiological findings. This would ensure that resources are appropriately directed and would provide a research agenda that would progress in a predictive way. At some stage, a hypothesis loses credibility or becomes recognized as being as close to "truth" as can be achieved experimentally.

Similarly, epidemiological studies must begin to focus on what is known about the toxicology of individual DBPs. Testing of hypotheses about certain adverse health effects should begin with some understanding of which DBPs are known to produce an effect of interest in experimental systems. Epidemiologists then need to focus on those mechanisms of toxicity and interactions that are likely to be important at low doses (i.e., those that can be logically extrapolated to dose levels encountered from drinking disinfected drinking-water). Finally, information of this type should be used to develop new parameters that can be incorporated into the design of epidemiological studies.

8. CONCLUSIONS AND RECOMMENDATIONS

Disinfection is unquestionably the most important step in the treatment of water for drinking-water supplies. The microbial quality of drinking-water should not be compromised because of concern over the potential long-term effects of disinfectants and DBPs. The risk of illness and death resulting from exposure to pathogens in drinking-water is very much greater than the risks from disinfectants and DBPs. Where local circumstances require that a choice be made between microbiological limits or limits for disinfectants and DBPs, the microbiological quality must always take precedence. Efficient disinfection must *never* be compromised.

The microbiological quality of drinking-water is of paramount importance and must receive priority over any other considerations in relation to drinking-water treatment. However, the use of any chemical disinfectant results in the formation of by-products that themselves may be of health significance. A thorough understanding of how these DBPs form and the factors that control their formation is valuable in achieving a successful balance between satisfactory inactivation of pathogens and the minimization of DBP formation. The microbiological quality of drinking-water should always receive priority over the minimization of DBPs.

Where it is possible, without compromising the microbiological quality of drinking-water, steps should be taken to minimize the concentrations of DBPs produced by the disinfectant(s) in use. Strategies to minimize exposure to DBPs should focus on the elimination of precursors through source water protection. Not only is this often the most efficient method of reducing DBP concentrations, but it will also assist in improving the microbiological quality of the water. Where treatment is required, DBP control strategies should emphasize DBP organic precursor (TOC) removal.

8.1 Chemistry

Chlorine and alternative chemical disinfectants (ozone, chlorine dioxide and chloramine) all lead to the formation of DBPs. However, between disinfectants or combinations thereof, there are differences in

DBP groups, species and mixtures that may affect human health. Key water quality determinants of DBPs include TOC, bromide and pH. Based on the current knowledge of both occurrence and health effects, the DBPs of most concern include total THMs and THM species, total HAAs and HAA species, bromate and chlorite.

8.2 Toxicology

None of the chlorination by-products studied to date is a potent carcinogen at concentrations normally found in drinking-water.

The toxicology of the DBPs suggests that the likelihood of adverse effects is not significantly different between the described disinfectant options.

Toxicological information on mode and mechanism of action of disinfectants and their by-products is the major limitation for understanding the potential health risks at low doses.

8.3 Epidemiology

Epidemiological studies have not identified an increased risk of cardiovascular disease associated with chlorinated or chloraminated drinking-water.

The hypothesis of a causal relationship between consumption of chlorination by-products and the increased relative risk of any cancer remains an open question. There is insufficient epidemiological evidence to support a causal relationship between bladder cancer and exposures to chlorinated drinking-water, THMs, chloroform or other THM species. The epidemiological evidence is inconclusive and equivocal for an association between colon cancer and long duration of exposure to chlorinated drinking-water, THMs or chloroform. There is insufficient epidemiological information to properly interpret the observed risks for rectal cancer and the risks for other cancers observed in single analytical studies.

The results of currently published studies do not provide convincing evidence that chlorinated water or THMs cause adverse pregnancy outcomes.

9. RESEARCH NEEDS

9.1 Chemistry of disinfectants and disinfectant by-products

There is a need to consider the requirements of developing and developed countries. While future research needs are articulated below, technology transfer is important in implementing past research into practice. The disinfection practice common to all countries is chlorination; thus, chlorine DBPs should be the primary focus.

- There is a need for a study to develop more DBP occurrence data from an international perspective; such an effort should also compile information on DBP precursors (TOC and bromide).

- Because of the expertise required to measure certain DBPs (e.g., HAAs) and the deficiencies of historical databases, there is a need to develop improved models for predicting DBP formation and precursor removal, allowing the use of DBPs (e.g., chloroform) or surrogates (e.g., TOC) that are more simple to measure. These models can also be used to predict the formation of DBPs from the use of a particular disinfectant and the factors that control the appearance and formation of these DBPs, thus allowing appropriate control strategies to be developed and better assessment of exposure.

- Although HAAs have been monitored for several years, this monitoring effort has been based on measurements of the sum of five or six species. There is a need to develop more information on the occurrence of the nine species of HAAs.

- For analytical reasons, non-polar organic by-products (measurable by GC) and ionic by-products (measurable by IC) have received more attention. There is a need to develop analytical methods for polar by-products and to define their occurrence.

- A significant percentage of TOX remains unaccounted for by specific halogenated DBPs; there is a need to identify these compounds.

- Given the health effects data on bromate and the anticipated higher ozone doses that will be required to inactivate *Cryptosporidium*, more data are needed on bromate formation in low-bromide waters when high ozone doses are used.

- More information is needed on the composition of NOM to assist in determining the type and extent of DBP formation that can be expected in a given water and how well treatment processes will achieve precursor removal.

- There is a need to develop a better understanding of how water quality parameters affect the extent of bromine incorporation into DBPs.

- To assist small water supply systems in minimizing DBP formation, there is a need to develop simple, easily operated treatment systems for the removal of NOM from source waters.

9.2 Toxicology

- Toxicological research needs to be focused to be effective. One approach to accomplish this is to design experiments to determine if a biological basis can be established for the epidemiological findings.

- Further toxicological characterization of the effects of DBPs at low doses is needed. These studies should be directed at understanding the mechanisms that are operative at these doses in humans.

- There are at least three areas that need the attention of both toxicologists and epidemiologists: risks posed by brominated by-products, how risks are modified by pH, and risks posed by the use of a disinfectant as an oxidizing agent during drinking-water treatment.

- A relatively small fraction of DBPs has received substantive toxicological study. Future studies should be directed at those by-products that occur with high frequency and at relatively high concentrations.

- Little attention has been paid to those individuals in a population who possess sensitivities to particular chemicals and/or modes of action because of genetic and lifestyle factors. An example is major polymorphic differences in enzymes that metabolize DBPs.

- Humans are exposed to complex mixtures of disinfectants and DBPs. It is becoming apparent that chemicals with like mechanisms interact in an additive way at low concentrations. Little information exists on the potential non-additive interaction of chemicals with different mechanisms.

9.3   Epidemiology

- Additional studies to evaluate cancer risks should be analytical and should include a more comprehensive assessment of drinking-water exposures, especially for DBPs, for etiologically relevant time periods. The interpretation of the results from currently conducted studies of both cancer and adverse pregnancy outcomes suffers from lack of knowledge about exposures to other DBPs and other water contaminants. It may be possible to assess additional water exposures for study participants in several recently conducted studies of cancer and reproductive risks. If this can be done, a better estimate of exposure to water contaminants and DBPs will be available for additional analyses of risks in these study populations. Depending on the results of these reanalyses, the need for additional studies of possible cancer risks can be better evaluated.

- It is important to improve the quality of future epidemiological studies with adequate and appropriate exposure information. This underscores the need to include in the planning and conduct of epidemiological studies individuals who are knowledgeable about DBP chemistry.

- Additional studies are needed to better assess the importance of the observed association between DBPs and early miscarriage or neural tube defects. Research should continue on possible reproductive and developmental effects associated with drinking-water disinfection.

- The most important research need is to improve the assessment of drinking-water exposures for epidemiological studies. There is a need for improved models that can be used to estimate exposures to various specific by-products and mixtures of by-products. There is also a need to collect more complete information about individual water consumption and activity patterns that may influence exposure assessments. Better and more complete exposure information will improve the sensitivity of epidemiological studies.

10. PREVIOUS EVALUATIONS BY INTERNATIONAL BODIES

A number of disinfectants and DBPs have been considered by IARC. On the basis of the available published data, the most recent classification of these chemicals is as follows:

Disinfectants

Hypochlorite salts: Group 3 (1991)

Disinfectant by-products

Trihalomethanes
    Bromodichloromethane: Group 2B (1999)
    Dibromochloromethane: Group 3 (1999)
    Bromoform: Group 3 (1999)
Haloacetic acids
    Dichloroacetic acid: Group 3 (1995)
    Trichloroacetic acid: Group 3 (1995)
Haloacetaldehyde
    Chloral and chloral hydrate: Group 3 (1995)
Haloacetonitriles
    Bromochloroacetonitrile: Group 3 (1999)
    Chloroacetonitrile: Group 3 (1999)
    Dibromoacetonitrile: Group 3 (1999)
    Dichloroacetonitrile: Group 3 (1999)
    Trichloroacetonitrile: Group 3 (1999)
Other disinfectant by-products
    Potassium bromate: Group 2B (1987)
    Sodium chlorite: Group 3 (1991)

In addition, IARC has classified chlorinated drinking-water in Group 3 (1991).

Disinfectants and DBPs were evaluated in the *Guidelines for drinking-water quality*, and the following guideline values recommended (WHO, 1993, 1996, 1998):

Disinfectants

Chlorine (hypochlorous acid and hypochlorite): 5 mg/litre (1993)
Monochloramine: 3 mg/litre (1993)

Disinfectant by-products

Trihalomethanes
Bromodichloromethane: 60 μg/litre for an excess lifetime cancer risk of 10^{-5} (1993)
Dibromochloromethane: 100 μg/litre (1993)
Bromoform: 100 μg/litre (1993)
Chloroform: 200 μg/litre (1998)
Haloacetic acids
Dichloroacetic acid: 50 μg/litre (provisional) (1993)
Trichloroacetic acid: 100 μg/litre (provisional) (1993)
Haloacetaldehyde
Chloral hydrate: 10 μg/litre (provisional) (1993)
Haloacetonitriles
Dibromoacetonitrile: 100 μg/litre (provisional) (1993)
Dichloroacetonitrile: 90 μg/litre (provisional) (1993)
Trichloroacetonitrile: 1 μg/litre (provisional) (1993)
Other disinfectant by-products
Bromate: 25 μg/litre (provisional) for an excess lifetime cancer risk of 7×10^{-5} (1993)
Chlorite: 200 μg/litre (provisional) (1993)
Cyanogen chloride (as cyanide): 70 μg/litre (1993)
Formaldehyde: 900 μg/litre (1993)
2,4,6-Trichlorophenol: 200 μg/litre for an excess lifetime cancer risk of 10^{-5} (1993)

JECFA (FAO/WHO, 1993) evaluated potassium bromate and concluded that it was genotoxic and carcinogenic.

The International Programme on Chemical Safety (IPCS) published an evaluation of chloroform in its Environmental Health Criteria Monograph series (WHO, 1994).

The IPCS Concise International Chemical Assessment Document (CICAD) on chloral hydrate (in press) considers the dose level of 16 mg/kg in the study of Sanderson et al. (1982) to be a NOAEL rather than a LOAEL (as in the present document), and therefore uses studies in humans as the basis of a tolerable intake. On the basis of a LOAEL of 11 mg/kg, and using an uncertainty factor of 10 for intraspecies variation and 10 for conversion of LOAEL to NOAEL, the CICAD derived a tolerable intake of 0.1 mg/kg.

REFERENCES

Abbas R & Fisher JW (1997) A physiologically-based pharmacokinetic model for trichloroethylene and its metabolites, chloral hydrate, trichloroacetate, dichloroacetate, trichloroethanol and tri-chloroethanol glucuronide in B6C3F$_1$ mice. Toxicol Appl Pharmacol, 147: 15-30.

Abbas RR, Seckel CS, Kidney JK, & Fisher JW (1996) Pharmacokinetic analysis of chloral hydrate and its metabolism in B6C3F$_1$ mice. Drug Metab Dispos, 24: 1340-1346.

Abdel-Rahman MS, Couri D, & Bull RJ (1980) Kinetics of ClO_2 and effects of ClO_2, ClO_2^-, and ClO_3^- in drinking water on blood glutathione and hemolysis in rat and chicken. J Environ Pathol Toxicol, 3: 431-449.

Abdel-Rahman MS, Berardi MR, & Bull RJ (1982a) Effect of chlorine and monochloramine in drinking water on the developing rat fetus. J Appl Toxicol, 2(3): 156.

Abdel-Rahman MS, Couri D, & Bull RJ (1982b) Metabolism and pharmacokinetics of alternate drinking water disinfectants. Environ Health Perspect, 46: 19-23.

Abdel-Rahman MS, Waldron DM, & Bull RJ (1983) A comparative kinetics study of mono-chloramine and hypochlorous acid in rat. J Appl Toxicol, 3: 175-179.

Abdel-Rahman MS, Couri D, & Bull RJ (1984a) Toxicity of chlorine dioxide in drinking water. J Am Coll Toxicol, 3: 277-284.

Abdel-Rahman MS, Couri D, & Bull RJ (1984b) The kinetics of chlorite and chlorate in the rat. J Am Coll Toxicol, 3: 261-267.

Acharya S, Mehta K, Rodrigues S, Pereira J, Krishnan S, & Rao CV (1995) Administration of subtoxic doses of t-butyl alcohol and trichloroacetic acid to male Wistar rats to study the interactive toxicity. Toxicol Lett, 80: 97-104.

Ade P, Guastadisegni C, Testai E, & Vittozzi L (1994) Multiple activation of chloroform in kidney microsomes from male and female DBA/2J mice. J Biochem Toxicol, 9: 289-295.

Adler ID (1993) Synopsis of the in vivo results obtained with the 10 known or suspected aneugens tested in the CEC collaborative study. Mutat Res, 287(1): 131-137.

Agarwal AK & Mehendele HM (1983) Absence of potentiation of bromoform hepatotoxicity and lethality by chlordecone. Toxicol Lett, 15: 251-257.

Ahmed AE, Soliman SA, Loh JP, & Hussein GI (1989) Studies on the mechanism of haloacetonitriles toxicity: Inhibition of rat hepatic glutathione-S-transferases in vitro. Toxicol Appl Pharmacol, 100: 271-279.

Ahmed AE, Jacob S, & Loh JP (1991) Studies on the mechanism of haloacetonitriles toxicity: quantitative whole body autoradiographic distribution of [2-^{14}C]chloroacetonitrile in rats. Toxicology, 67: 279-302.

Aida Y, Takada K, Uchida O, Yasuhara K, Kurokawa Y, & Tobe M (1992a) Toxicities of microencapsulated tribromomethane, dibromochloromethane and bromodichloromethane admin-istered in the diet to Wistar rats for one month. J Toxicol Sci, 17: 119-133.

Aida Y, Yasuhara K, Takada K, Kurokawa Y, & Tobe M (1992b) Chronic toxicity of micro-encapsulated bromodichloromethane administered in the diet to Wistar rats. J Toxicol Sci, **17**: 51-68, [Erratum] 17:167.

Aieta EM & Berg JD (1986) A review of chlorine dioxide in drinking water treatment. J Am Water Works Assoc, **78**(6): 62-72.

Alavanja M, Goldstein I, & Susser M (1978) Case-control study of gastrointestinal and urinary tract cancer mortality and drinking water chlorination. In: Jolley RL, Gorchev H, & Hamilton DH ed. Water chlorination: Environmental impact and health effects. Ann Arbor, Michigan, Ann Arbor Science Publishers, vol 2, pp 395-409.

Allen JW, Collins BW, & Evansky PA (1994) Spermatid micronucleus analyses of trichloroethylene and chloral hydrate effects in mice. Mutat Res, **323**(1-2): 81-88.

Almeyda J & Levantine A (1972) Cutaneous reactions to barbiturates, chloral hydrate and its derivatives. Br J Dermatol, **86**: 313-316.

Ames RG & Stratton JW (1987) Effect of chlorine dioxide water disinfection on hematologic and serum parameters of renal dialysis. Arch Environ Health, **42**(5): 280-285.

Ammann P, Laethem CL, & Kedderis GL (1998) Chloroform-induced cytolethality in freshly isolated male B6C3F₁ mouse and F344 rat hepatocytes. Toxicol Appl Pharmacol, **149**(2): 217-225.

Amy G, Chadik PA, & Chowdhury ZK (1987) Developing models for predicting THM formation potential and kinetics. J Am Water Works Assoc, **79**(7): 89-96.

Amy G, Siddiqui M, Ozekin K, & Westerhoff P (1993) Threshold levels for bromate ion formation in drinking water. In: Proceedings of the International Water Supply Association Workshop, Paris. Boston, Massachusetts, Blackwell Scientific Publications, pp 169-180.

Amy G, Siddiqui M, Zhai W, & Debroux J (1994) Survey on bromide in drinking water and impacts on DBP formation. Denver, Colorado, American Water Works Association (Report No. 90662).

Amy G, Siddiqui M, Ozekin K, Zhu HW, & Wang C (1998) Empirically-based models for predicting chlorination and ozonation by-products: Trihalomethanes, haloacetic acids, chloral hydrate, and bromate. Cincinnati, Ohio, US Environmental Protection Agency (EPA-815-R-98-005).

Anders MW, Stevens JL, Sprague RW, Shaath Z, & Ahmed AE (1978) Metabolism of haloforms to carbon monoxide. II. *In vivo* studies. Drug Metab Dispos, **6**: 556-560.

Andrews SA & Ferguson MJ (1995) Minimizing DBP formation while ensuring *Giardia* control. In: Minear RA & Amy GL ed. Disinfection by-products in water treatment. Chelsea, Michigan, Lewis Publishers, Inc.

Andrews SA, Huch PM, Chute AJ, Bolton JR, & Anderson WA (1996) UV oxidation for drinking water-feasibility studies for addressing specific water quality issues. In: Proceedings of the Water Quality Technology Conference, New Orleans, LA. Denver, Colorado, American Water Works Association.

Angel P & Karin M (1991) The role of Jun, Fos, and the AP-1 complex in cell proliferation and transformation. Biochim Biophys Acta, **1072**: 126-157.

Anna CH, Maronpot RR, Pereira MA, Foley JF, Malarkey DE, & Anderson MW (1994) Ras proto-oncogene activation in dichloroacetic-, trichloroethylene- and tetrachloroethylene-induced liver tumors in B6C3F$_1$ mice. Carcinogenesis, **15**: 2255-2261.

APHA (American Public Health Association) (1995) Standard methods for the examination of water and wastewater, 19th ed. Washington, DC, American Public Health Association/American Water Works Association/Water Pollution Control Federation.

Aschengrau A, Zierler S, & Cohen A (1989) Quality of community drinking water and the occurrence of spontaneous abortions. Arch Environ Health, **44**(5): 283-290.

Aschengrau A, Zierler S, & Cohen A (1993) Quality of community drinking water and the occurrence of late adverse pregnancy outcomes. Arch Environ Health, **48**(2): 105-114.

Ashby J, Mohammed R, & Callander RD (1987) N-Chloropiperidine and calcium hypochlorite: Possible examples of toxicity-dependent clastogenicity, in vitro. Mutat Res, **189**: 59-68.

Austin EW & Bull RJ (1997) The effect of pretreatment with dichloroacetate and trichloroacetate on the metabolism of bromodichloroacetate. J Toxicol Environ Health, **52**: 367-383.

Austin EW, Okita JR, Okita RT, Larson JL, & Bull RJ (1995) Modification of lipoperoxidative effects of dichloroacetate and trichloroacetate is associated with peroxisome proliferation. Toxicology, **97**: 59-69.

Austin EW, Parrish JM, Kinder DH, & Bull RJ (1996) Lipid peroxidation and formation of 8-hydroxydeoxyguanosine from acute doses of halogenated acetic acids. Fundam Appl Toxicol, **31**: 77-82.

AWWARF (1991) Disinfection by-products database and model project. Denver, Colorado, American Water Works Association Research Foundation.

Bailar JC (1995) The practice of meta-analysis. J Clin Epidemiol, **48**(1): 149-157.

Bailey PS (1978) Ozonation in organic chemistry. New York, London, Academic Press.

Balster RL & Borzelleca JF (1982) Behavioral toxicity of trihalomethane contaminants of drinking water in mice. Environ Health Perspect, **46**: 127-136.

Banerji AP & Fernandes AO (1996) Field bean protease inhibitor mitigates the sister-chromatid exchanges induced by bromoform and depresses the spontaneous sister-chromatid exchange frequency of human lymphocytes in vitro. Mutat Res, **360**: 29-35.

Bean JA, Isacson P, Hausler WJ, & Kohler J (1982) Drinking water and cancer incidence in Iowa I. Trends and incidence by source of drinking water and size of municipality. Am J Epidemiol, **116**(6): 912-923.

Bempong MA & Scully FE Jr (1985) Mutagenicity and clastogenicity of N-chloropiperidine. J Environ Pathol Toxicol, **6**: 241-251.

Bempong MA, Montgomery C, & Scully FE Jr (1980) Mutagenic activity of N-chloropiperidine. J Environ Pathol Toxicol, **4**: 345-354.

Bercz JP & Bawa R (1986) Iodination of nutrients in the presence of chlorine based disinfectants used in drinking water treatment. Toxicol Lett, **34**(2-3): 141-147.

Bercz JP, Jones L, Garner L, Murray D, Ludwig A, & Boston J (1982) Subchronic toxicity of chlorine dioxide and related compounds in drinking water in the nonhuman primate. Environ Health Perspect, **46**: 47-55.

Bercz JP, Jones LL, Harrington RM, Bawa R, & Condie L (1986) Mechanistic aspects of ingested chlorine dioxide on thyroid function: Impact of oxidants on iodide metabolism. Environ Health Perspect, **69**: 249-255.

Bersin RM, Wolfe C, Kwasman M, Lau D, Klinski C, Tanaka K, Khorrami, P, Henderson GN, De Marco T, & Chatterjee K (1994) Improved hemodynamic function and mechanical efficiency in congestive heart failure with sodium dichloroacetate. J Am Coll Cardiol, **23**: 1617-1624.

Bhat HK, Kanz MF, Campbell GA, & Ansari GAS (1991) Ninety day toxicity study of chloroacetic acids in rats. Fundam Appl Toxicol, **17**: 240-253.

Bhunya SP & Behera BC (1987) Relative genotoxicity of trichloroacetic acid (TCA) as revealed by different cytogenetic assays: Bone marrow chromosome aberration, micronucleus and sperm-head abnormality in the mouse. Mutat Res, **188**: 215-221.

Bignami M, Conti G, Conti L, Crebelli R, Misuraca F, Puglia AM, Randazzo R, Sciandrello G, & Carere A (1980) Mutagenicity of halogenated aliphatic hydrocarbons in *Salmonella typhimurium, Streptomyces coelicolor* and *Aspergillus nidulans*. Chem-Biol Interact, **30**: 9-23.

Blackshear PJ, Holloway PA, & Alberti KM (1974) The metabolic effects of sodium dichloroacetate in the starved rat. Biochem J, **142**: 279-286.

Blazak WF, Meier JR, Stewart BE, Blachman DC, & Deahl JT (1988) Activity of 1,1,1- and 1,1,3-trichloroacetones in a chromosomal aberration assay in CHO cells and the micronucleus and spermhead abnormality assays in mice. Mutat Res, **206**: 431-438.

Bloxham CA, Wright N, & Hoult JG (1979) Self-poisoning by sodium chlorate: Some unusual features. Clin Toxicol, **15**: 185-188.

Bolyard M & Fair PS (1992) Occurrence of chlorate in hypochlorite solutions used for drinking water treatment. Environ Sci Technol, **26**(8): 1663-1665.

Bolyard M, Fair PS, & Hautman DP (1993) Sources of chlorate ion in U.S. drinking water. J Am Water Works Assoc, **85**: 81-88.

Borzelleca JF & Carchman RA (1982) Effects of selected organic drinking water contaminants on male reproduction. Research Triangle Park, North Carolina, US Environmental Protection Agency (EPA 600/1-82-009; NTIS PB82-259847).

Bove FJ, Fulcomer MC, Koltz JB, Esmart J, Dufficy EM, & Zagraniski RT (1992a) Report on phase IV-A: public drinking water contamination and birthweight fetal deaths, and birth defects, a cross-sectional study. Trenton, New Jersey, New Jersey Department of Health.

Bove FJ, Fulcomer MC, Koltz JB, Esmart J, Dufficy EM, Zagraniski RT, & Savrin JE (1992b) Report on phase IV-B: public drinking water contamination and birthweight and selected birth defects, a case-control study. Trenton, New Jersey, New Jersey Department of Health.

Bove FJ, Fulcomer MC, Klotz JB, Esmart J, Dufficy EM, & Savrin JE (1995) Public drinking water contamination and birth outcomes. Am J Epidemiol, **141**(9): 850-862.

Bowman FJ, Borzelleca JF, & Munson AE (1978) The toxicity of some halomethanes in mice. Toxicol Appl Pharmacol, **44**: 213-215.

Brennan RJ & Schiestl RH (1998) Chloroform and carbon tetrachloride induce intra-chromosomal recombination and oxidative free radicals in *Saccharomyces cerevisiae*. Mutat Res, **397**(2): 271-278.

Brenniman GR, Vasilomanolakis-Lagos J, Amsel J, Namekata T, & Wolff AH (1980) Case-control study of cancer deaths in Illinois communities served by chlorinated or nonchlorinated water. In: Jolley RL, Brungs WA, Cumming RB, & Jacobs VA ed. Water chlorination: Environmental impact and health effects. Ann Arbor, Michigan, Ann Arbor Science Publishers, Inc., vol 3, pp 1/043-1/057.

Bronzetti G, Galli A, Corsi C, Cundari E, Del Carratore R, Nieri R, & Paolini M (1984) Genetic and biochemical investigation on chloral hydrate *in vitro* and *in vivo*. Mutat Res, **141**: 19-22.

Brown DM, Langley PF, Smith D, & Taylor DC (1974) Metabolism of chloroform - 1. The metabolism of [^{14}C]chloroform by different species. Xenobiotica, **4**: 151-163.

Brown-Woodman PD, Hayes LC, Huq F, Herlihy C, Picker K, & Webster WS (1998) *In vitro* assessment of the effect of halogenated hydrocarbons: Chloroform, dichloromethane, and dibromoethane on embryonic development of the rat. Teratology, **57**(6): 321-333.

Bruchet A, Costentin E, Legrand MF, & Malleviale J (1992) Influence of the chlorination of natural nitrogenous organic compounds on tastes and odours in finished drinking waters. Water Sci Technol, **25**(2): 323-333.

Brunborg G, Holme JA, Soderlund EJ, & Dybing E (1990) Organ-specific genotoxic effects of chemicals: The use of alkaline elution to detect DNA damage in various organs of *in vivo* exposed animals. Prog Clin Biol RES, **340D**: 43-52.

Brunborg G, Holme JA, Soderlund EJ, Hongslo JK, Vartiainen T, Lotjonen S, & Becher G (1991) Genotoxic effects of the drinking water mutagen 3-chloro-4-(dichloromethyl)-5-hydroxy-2[5H]-furanone (MX) in mammalian cells *in vitro* and in rats *in vivo*. Mutat Res, **260**: 55-64.

Bruschi SA & Bull RJ (1993) *In vitro* cytotoxicity of mono-, di- and trichloroacetate and its modulation by peroxisome proliferation. Fundam Appl Toxicol, **21**: 366-375.

Brusick D (1986) Genotoxic effects in cultured mammalian cells produced by low pH treatment conditions and increased ion concentrations. Environ Mutagen, **8**: 879-886.

Bull RJ (1980) Health effects of alternate disinfectants and their reaction products. J Am Water Works Assoc, **72**: 299-303.

Bull RJ (1982a) Health effects of drinking water disinfectants and disinfectant by-products. Environ Sci Technol, **16**: 554A-559A.

Bull RJ (1982b) Toxicological problems associated with alternative methods of disinfection. J Am Water Works Assoc, **74**: 642-648.

Bull RJ (1992) Toxicology of drinking water disinfection. In: Lippman M ed. Environmental toxicants: Human exposures and their health effects. New York, Van Nostrand Reinhold, pp 184-230.

Bull RJ (1993) Toxicology of disinfectants and disinfectant by-products. In: Craun GF ed. Safety of water disinfection: Balancing chemical and microbial risks. Washington, DC, ILSI Press, pp 239-256.

Bull RJ & DeAngelo AB (1995) Carcinogenic properties of brominated haloacetates - Disinfection by-products in drinking water: Critical issues in health effects research. Washington, DC, International Life Sciences Institute, p 29.

Bull RJ & Robinson M (1985) Carcinogenic activity of haloacetonitrile and haloacetone derivatives in the mouse skin and lung. In: Jolley RL, Bull RJ, & Davis WP ed. Water chlorination: Chemistry, environmental impact and health effects. Chelsea, Michigan, Lewis Publishers, Inc., vol 5, pp 221-236.

Bull RJ & Kopfler FC (1991) Health effects of disinfectants and disinfection by-products. Denver, Colorado, American Water Works Association Research Foundation and American Water Works Association.

Bull RJ, Meier JR, Robinson M, Ringhand HP, Laurie RD, & Stober JA (1985) Evaluation of mutagenic and carcinogenic properties of brominated and chlorinated haloacetonitriles: By-products of chlorination. Fundam Appl Toxicol, **5**: 1065-1074.

Bull RJ, Sanchez IM, Nelson MA, Larson JL, & Lansing AL (1990) Liver tumor induction in B6C3F$_1$ mice by dichloroacetate and trichloroacetate. Toxicology, **63**: 341-359.

Bull RJ, Templin M, Larson JL, & Stevens DK (1993) The role of dichloroacetate in the hepatocarcinogenicity of trichloroethylene. Toxicol Lett, **68**: 203-211.

Bull RJ, Birnbaum LS, Cantor KP, Rose JB, Butterworth BE, Pegram R, & Tuomisto J (1995) Water chlorination: Essential process or cancer hazard? Fundam Appl Toxicol, **28**: 155-166.

Burton-Fanning FW (1901) Poisoning by bromoform. Br Med J, **18 May**: 1202-1203.

Butler TC (1948) The metabolic fate of chloral hydrate. J Pharmacol Exp Ther, **92**: 49-58.

Butler TC (1949) Reduction and oxidation of chloral hydrate by isolated tissues *in vitro*. J Pharmacol Exp Ther, **95**: 360-362.

Butterworth BE, Templin MV, Constan AA, Sprankle CS, Wong BA, Pluta LJ, Everitt JI, & Recio L (1998) Long-term mutagenicity studies with chloroform and dimethylnitrosamine in female *lacI* transgenic B6C3F$_1$ mice. Environ Mol Mutagen, **31**(3): 248-256.

Cabana BE & Gessner PK (1970) The kinetics of chloral hydrate metabolism in mice and the effect thereon of ethanol. J Pharmaocol Exp Ther, **174**: 260-275.

Canada (1993) Guidelines for Canadian drinking water quality. Ottawa, Ontario, Health Canada, Health Protection Branch.

Cantor KP (1997) Drinking water and cancer. Cancer Causes Control, **8**(3): 292-308.

Cantor KP, Hoover R, & Hartge P (1985) Drinking water source and bladder cancer: A case-control study. In: Jolley RL, Bull RJ, & Davis WP ed. Water chlorination: Chemistry, environmental impact, and health effects. Chelsea, Michigan, Lewis Publishers, Inc., vol 5, pp 145-152.

Cantor KP, Hoover R, & Hartge P (1987) Bladder cancer, drinking water source, and tap water consumption: A case-control study. J Natl Cancer Inst, **79**(1): 1269-1279.

Cantor KP, Hoover R, & Hartge P (1990) Bladder cancer, tap water consumption, and drinking water source. In: Jolley RL, Condie LW, & Johnson JD ed. Water chlorination: Chemistry, environmental impact, and health effects. Chelsea, Michigan, Lewis Publishers, Inc., vol 6, pp 411-419.

Cantor KP, Lynch CF, & Hildesheim M (1995) Chlorinated drinking water and risk of bladder, colon, and rectal cancers: A case-control study in Iowa. In: Disinfection by-products in drinking water: Critical issues in health effects research. Washington, DC, International Life Sciences Institute, p 133.

Cantor KP, Lynch CF, & Hildesheim M (1996) Chlorinated drinking water and risk of glioma: a case-control study in Iowa, USA. Epidemiology, **7**(suppl 4): S83.

Cantor KP, Lynch CF, Hildesheim ME, Dosemeci M, Lubin J, Alavanja M, & Craun G (1998) Drinking water source and chlorination byproducts: Risk of bladder cancer. Epidemiology, **9**(1): 21-28.

Carlo GL & Mettlin CJ (1980) Cancer incidence and trihalomethane concentrations in a public drinking water system. Am J Public Health, **70**: 523-525.

Carlson M & Hardy D (1998) Controlling DBPs with monochloramine. Effect of water quality conditions on controlling disinfection by-products with chloramines. J Am Water Works Assoc, **90**(2): 95-106.

Carlton BD, Bartlett A, Basaran AH, Colling K, Osis I, & Smith MK (1986) Reproductive effects of alternative disinfectants. Environ Health Perspect, **69**: 237-241.

Carlton BD, Habash DL, Basaran AH, George EL, & Smith MK (1987) Sodium chlorite administration in Long-Evans rats: Reproductive and endocrine effects. Environ Res, **42**: 238-245.

Carlton BD, Basaran AH, Mezza LE, George EL, & Smith MK (1991) Reproductive effects in Long-Evans rats exposed to chlorine dioxide. Environ Res, **56**: 170-177.

Carraro F, Klein S, Rosenblatt JI, & Wolfe RR (1989) The effect of dichloroacetate on lactate concentration in exercising humans. J Appl Physiol, **66**: 591-597.

Carter JH, Carter HW, & DeAngelo AB (1995) Biochemical, pathologic and morphometric alterations induced in male B6C3F$_1$ mouse liver by short-term exposure to dichloroacetic acid. Toxicol Lett, **81**: 55-71.

Cattley RC, DeLuca J, Elcombe C, Fenner-Crisp P, Lake BG, Marsman DS, Pastoor TA, Popp JA, Robinson DE, Schwetz B, Tugwood J, & Wahli W (1998) Do peroxisome proliferating compounds pose a hepatocarcinogenic hazard to humans? Regul Toxicol Pharmacol, **27**: 47-60.

Cavanagh JE, Weinberg HS, Gold A, Sangalah R, Marbury D, & Glaze WH (1992) Ozonation by-products: identification of bromohydrins from the ozonation of natural waters with enhanced bromide levels. Environ Sci Technol, **26**(8): 1658-1662.

Chang J-HS, Vogt CR, Sun GY, & Sun AY (1981) Effects of acute administration of chlorinated water on liver lipids. Lipids, **16**: 336-340.

Chang LW, Daniel FB, & DeAngelo AB (1992) Analysis of DNA strand breaks induced in rodent liver *in vivo*, hepatocytes in primary culture, and a human cell line by chlorinated acetic acids and chlorinated acetaldehydes. Environ Mol Mutagen, **20**: 277-288.

Cheh AM, Skochdopole J, Koski P, & Cole L (1980) Nonvolatile mutagens in drinking water: Production by chlorination and destruction by sulfite. Science, **207**: 90-92.

Chipman JK, Davies JE, Parson JL, Mair J, O'Neil G, & Fawell JK (1998) DNA oxidation by potassium bromate: a direct mechanism or linked to lipid peroxidation? Toxicology, **126**(2): 93-102.

Cho DH, Hong JT, Chin K, Cho TS, & Lee BM (1993) Organotropic formation and disappearance of 8-hydroxydeoxyguanosine in the kidney of Sprague-Dawley rats exposed to Adriamycin and KBrO$_3$. Cancer Lett, **74**: 141-145.

Chow BM & Roberts PV (1981) Halogenated by-product formation by chlorine dioxide and chlorine. J Environ Eng Div, **107**: 609-618.

Christ SA, Read EJ, Stober JA, & Smith MK (1996) Developmental effects of trichloroacetonitrile administered in corn oil to pregnant Long-Evans rats. J Toxicol Environ Health, **47**: 233-247.

Christman RF, Norwood DS, Millington DS, & Johnson JD (1983) Identity and yields of major halogenated products of aquatic fulvic acid chlorination. Environ Sci Technol, **17**: 625-628.

Chu I, Secours VE, Marino I, & Villeneuve DC (1980) The acute toxicity of four trihalomethanes in male and female rats. Toxicol Appl Pharmacol, **5**: 351-353.

Chu I, Villeneuve DC, Secours VE, Becking GC, & Valli VE (1982) Toxicity of trihalomethanes: I. The acute and subacute toxicity of chloroform, bromodichloromethane, chlorodibromomethane, and bromoform in rats. J Environ Sci Health, **B17**: 205-224.

Cicmanec JL, Condie LW, Olson GR, & Wang SR (1991) 90-day toxicity study of dichloracetate in dogs. Fundam Appl Toxicol, **17**: 376-389.

Clark RM, Adams JQ, & Kyjins BW (1994) DBP control in drinking water: cost and performance. J Environ Eng, **120**(4): 759-771.

Claude J, Kunze E, & Frentzel-Beyne R (1986) Life-style and occupational risk factors in cancer of the lower urinary tract. Am J Epidemiol, **124**: 578.

Claus TH & Pilkis SJ (1977) Effect of dichloroacetate and glucagon on the incorporation of labeled substrates into glucose and on pyruvate dehydrogenase in hepatocytes from fed and starved rats. Arch Biochem Biophys, **182**: 52-63.

CMA (1997) Sodium chlorite: drinking water rat two-generation reproductive toxicity study. Washington, DC, Chemical Manufacturers Association (Quintiles Report CMA/17/96).

Cole WJ, Mitchell RG, & Salamonsen RF (1975) Isolation, characterization and quantitation of chloral hydrate as a transient metabolite of trichloroethylene in man using electron capture gas chromatography and mass fragmentography. J Pharm Pharmacol, **27**: 167-171.

Coleman WE, Munch JW, Kaylor WH, Streicher RP, Ringhand HP, & Meier JR (1984) Gas chromatography/mass spectroscopy analysis of mutagenic extracts of aqueous chlorinated humic acid. A comparison of the byproducts to drinking water contaminants. Environ Sci Technol, **18**: 674-681.

Coleman WE, Munch JW, & Kopfler FC (1992) Ozonation/post-chlorination of humic acids: a model for predicting drinking water DBPs. J Ozone Sci Eng, **14**: 349-355.

Condie LW, Smallwood CL, & Laurie RD (1983) Comparative renal and hepatotoxicity of halomethanes: bromodichloromethane, bromoform, chloroform, dibromochloromethane and methylene chloride. Drug Chem Toxicol, **6**: 563-578.

Connor MJ & Gillings D (1974) An empiric study of ecological inference. Am J Public Health, **74**: 555-559.

Connor PM, Moore GS, Calabrese EJ, & Howe GR (1985) The renal effects of sodium chlorite in the drinking water of C57L/J male mice. J Environ Pathol Toxicol Oncol, **6**: 253-260.

Conolly RB & Butterworth BE (1995) Biologically based dose response model for hepatic toxicity: a mechanistically based replacement for traditional estimates of noncancer risk. Toxicol Lett, **82**: 901-906.

Cooper WJ, Meyer LM, Bofill CC, & Cordal E (1983) Quantitative effects of bromine on the formation and distribution of trihalomethanes in groundwater with a high organic content. In: Jolley RL, Brungs WA, Cotruvo JA, Cumming RB, Mattice JS, & Jacobs VA ed. Water chlorination: Environmental impacts and health effects - Book 1: Chemistry and water treatment. Ann Arbor, Michigan, Ann Arbor Science Publishers, vol 4, pp 285-296.

Cooper WJ, Zika RG, & Steinhauer MS (1985) Bromide-oxidant interactions and THM formation: a literature review. J Am Water Works Assoc, **77**(4): 116-121.

Corley RA, Mendrala AL, Smith FA, Staats DA, Gargas ML, Conolly RB, Andersen ME, & Reitz RH (1990) Development of a physiologically based pharmacokinetic model for chloroform. Toxicol Appl Pharmacol, **103**: 512-527.

Cosby NC & Dukelow WR (1992) Toxicology of maternally ingested trichloroethylene (TCE) on embryonal and fetal development in mice and of TCE metabolites on *in vitro* fertilization. Fundam Appl Toxicol, **19**: 268-274.

Cotter JL, Fader RC, Lilley C, & Herndon DN (1985) Chemical parameters, antimicrobial activities, and tissue toxicity of 0.1 and 0.5% sodium hypochlorite solutions. Antimicrob Agents Chemother, **28**: 118-122.

Coude FX, Saudubray JM, DeMaugre F, Marsac C, Leroux JP, & Charpentier C (1978) Dichloroacetate as treatment for congenital lactic acidosis. N Engl J Med, **299**: 1365-1366.

Couri D & Abdel-Rahman MS (1980) Effect of chlorine dioxide and metabolites on glutathione dependent system in rat, mouse and chicken blood. J Environ Pathol Toxicol, **3**: 451-460.

Couri D, Miller CH, Bull RJ, Delphia JM, & Ammar EM (1982a) Assessment of maternal toxicity, embryotoxicity and teratogenic potential of sodium chlorite in Sprague-Dawley rats. Environ Health Perspect, **46**: 25-29.

Couri D, Abdel-Rahman MS, & Bull RJ (1982b) Toxicological effects of chlorine dioxide, chlorite and chlorate. Environ Health Perspect, **46**: 13-17.

Cove DJ (1976) Chlorate toxicity in *Aspergillus nidulans*: Studies of mutants altered in nitrate assimilation. Mol Gen Genet, **146**: 147-159.

Crabb DW & Harris RA (1979) Mechanism responsible for the hypoglycemic actions of dichloroacetate and 2-chloropropionate. Arch Biochem Biophys, **198**: 145-152.

Crabb DW, Yount EA, & Harris RA (1981) The metabolic effects of dichloroacetate. Metabolism, **30**: 1024-1039.

Cragle DL, Shy CM, Struba RJ, & Stiff EJ (1985) A case-control study of colon cancer and water chlorination in North Carolina. In: Jolley RL, Bull RJ, & Davis WP ed. Water chlorination: Chemistry, environmental impact, and health effects. Chelsea, Michigan, Lewis Publishers, Inc., vol 5, pp 153-159.

Craun GF (1985) Epidemiologic studies of organic micro-pollutants in drinking water. Sci Total Environ, **47**: 461.

Craun GF (1991) Epidemiologic studies of organic micropollutants in drinking water. In: Hutzinger O ed. The handbook of environmental chemistry - Volume 5A: Water pollution. Berlin, Heidelberg, New York, Springer-Verlag, p 1-44.

Craun GF, Clark RM, Doull J, Grabow W, Marsh GM, Okun DA, Sobsey MD, & Symons JM (1993) In: Craun GF ed. Safety of water disinfection: Balancing chemical and microbial risks - Conference conclusions. Washington, DC, ILSI Press, pp 657-667.

Crebelli R, Conti G, Conti L, & Carere A (1985) Mutagenicity of trichloroethylene, trichloroethanol and chloral hydrate in *Aspergillus nidulans*. Mutat Res, **155**: 105-111.

Crozes G, White P, & Marshall M (1995) Enhanced coagulation: its effects on NOM removal and chemical costs. J Am Water Works Assoc, **87**(1): 78-89.

Crump KS, Hoel D, Langley H, & Peto R (1976) Fundamental carcinogenic processes and their implications to low dose risk assessment. Cancer Res, **36**: 2973, 2979-2357.

Crump KS & Guess HA (1982) Drinking water and cancer: Review of recent epidemiological findings and assessment of risks. Annu Rev Public Health, **3**: 339.

Cucinell SA, Odessky L, Weiss M, & Dayton PG (1966) The effect of chloral hydrate on bis-hydroxycoumarin metabolism. J Am Med Assoc, **197**: 366-368.

Curry SH, Chu P-I, Baumgartner TG, & Stacpoole PW (1985) Plasma concentrations and metabolic effects of intravenous sodium dichloroacetate. Clin Pharmacol Ther, **37**: 89-93.

Curry SH, Lorenz A, Chu P-I, Limacher M, & Stacpoole PW (1991) Disposition and pharmacodynamics of dichloroacetate (DCA) and oxalate following oral DCA doses. Biopharm Drugs Dispos, **12**(5): 375-390.

Cunliffe DA (1991) Bactericidal nitrification in chloraminated water supplies. App Environ Microbiol, **57**(11): 3399-3402.

Dalhamn T (1957) Chlorine dioxide: Toxicity in animal experiments and industrial risks. Arch. Ind Health, **15**: 101-107.

Daniel FB, Schenck KM, Mattox JK, Lin EL, Haas DL, & Pereira MA (1986) Genotoxic properties of haloacetonitriles: Drinking water by-products of chlorine disinfection. Fundam Appl Toxicol, **6**: 447-453.

Daniel FB, Robinson M, Condie LW, & York RG (1990a) Ninety-day oral toxicity study of dibromochloromethane in Sprague-Dawley rats. Drug Chem Toxicol, **13**: 135-154.

Daniel FB, Condie LW, Robinson M, Stober JA, York RG, Olson GR, & Wang S-R (1990b) Comparative 90-day subchronic toxicity studies on three drinking water disinfectants, chlorine, monochloramine and chlorine dioxide, in the Sprague-Dawley rats. J Am Water Works Assoc, **82**: 61-69.

Daniel FB, Ringhand HP, Robinson M, Stober JA, Olson GR, & Page NP (1991a) Comparative subchronic toxicity of chlorine and monochloramine in the B6C3F$_1$ mouse. J Am Water Works Assoc, **83**: 68-75.

Daniel FB, Olson GR, & Stober JA (1991b) Induction of gastrointestinal tract nuclear anomalies in B6C3F$_1$ mice by 3-chloro-4-(dichloromethyl)-5-hydroxy-2(5H)-furanone and 3,4-(dichloro)-5-hydroxy-2(5H)-furanone. Environ Mol Mutagen, **17**: 32-39.

Daniel FB, DeAngelo AB, Stober JA, Olson GR, & Page NP (1992a) Hepatocarcinogenicity of chloral hydrate, 2-chloroacetaldehyde, and dichloroacetic acid in male B6C3F$_1$ mouse. Fundam Appl Toxicol, **19**: 159-168.

Daniel FB, Robinson M, Stober JA, Page NP, & Olson GR (1992b) Ninety-day toxicity study of chloral hydrate in the Sprague-Dawley rat. Drug Chem Toxicol, **15**: 217-232.

Daniel FB, Robinson M, Stober JA, Olson GR, & Page NR (1993a) Toxicity of 1,1,1-trichloro-2-propanone in Sprague-Dawley rats. J Toxicol Environ Health, **39**: 383-393.

Daniel FB, Meier JR, & DeAngelo AB (1993b) Advances in research on carcinogenic and genotoxic by-products of chlorine disinfection: Chlorinated hydroxyfuranones and chlorinated acetic acids. Ann Ist Super Sanita, **29**: 279-291.

Das R & Blanc PD (1993) Chlorine gas exposure and the lung: A review. Toxicol Ind Health, **9**: 439-455.

Davis ME (1990) Subacute toxicity of trichloroacetic acid in male and female rats. Toxicology, **63**: 63-72.

DeAngelo AB, Daniel FB, McMillan L, Wernsing P, & Savage RE (1989) Species and strain sensitivity to the induction of peroxisome proliferation by chloroacetic acids. Toxicol Appl Pharmacol, **101**: 285-298.

DeAngelo AB, Daniel FB, Stober JA, & Olson GR (1991) The carcinogenicity of dichloroacetic acid in the male B6C3F₁ mouse. Fundam Appl Toxicol, **16**: 337-347.

DeAngelo AB, Daniel FB, Most BM, & Olson GR (1996) The carcinogenicity of dichloroacetic acid in the male Fischer 344 rat. Toxicology, **114**: 207-221.

DeAngelo AB, Daniel FB, Most BM, & Olson GR (1997) Failure of monochloroacetic acid and trichloroactic acid administered in the drinking water to produce liver cancer in male F344/N rats. J Toxicol Environ Health, **52**: 425-445.

DeAngelo AB, George MH, Kilburn SR, Moore TM, & Wolf DC (1998) Carcinogenicity of potassium bromate administered in the drinking water to male B6C3F₁ mice and F344/N rats. Toxicol Pathol, **26**(5): 587-594.

De Biasi A, Sbraccia M, Keizer J, Testai E, & Vittozzi L (1992) The regioselective binding of CHCl₃ reactive intermediates to microsomal phospholipids. Chem-Biol Interact, **85**: 229-242.

de Groot H & Noll T (1989) Halomethane hepatotoxicity: Induction of lipid peroxidation and inactivation of cytochrome P-450 in rat liver microsomes under low oxygen partial pressures. Toxicol Appl Pharmacol, **97**: 530-537.

De Leer EW, Damste JS, Erkelens C, & de Galan L (1985) Identification of intermediates leading to chloroform and C-4 diacids in the chlorination of humic acid. Environ Sci Technol, **19**: 512-522.

De Leer EW, Bagerman T, van Schaik P, Zuydeweg CWS, & de Galan L (1986) Chlorination of ω-cyanoalkanoic acids in aqueous medium. Environ Sci Technol, **20**(12): 1218-1223.

Dechert S & Dekant W (1996) The possible role of *S*-chloromethylglutathione in the genotoxicity of dichloromethane. Toxicologist, **30**: 93 (abstract).

Delehanty JM, Imai N, & Liang CS (1992) Effects of dichloroacetate on hemodynamic responses to dynamic exercise in dogs. J Appl Physiol, **72**: 515-520.

DeMarini DM, Perry E, & Shelton ML (1994) Dichloroacetic acid and related compounds: Induction of prophage in *E. coli* and mutagenicity and mutation spectra in *Salmonella* TA100. Mutagenesis, **9**: 429-437.

DeMarini DM, Abu-Sharkra A, Felton CF, Patterson KS, & Shelton ML (1995) Mutation spectra in *Salmonella* of chlorinated, chloraminated, or ozonated drinking water extracts: Comparison to MX. Environ Mol Mutagen, **26**: 270-285.

DeMarini DM, Shelton ML, Warren SH, Ross TM, Shim JY, Richard AM, & Pegram RA (1997) Glutathione *S*-transferase-mediated induction of GC to AT transitions by halomethanes in *Salmonella*. Environ Mol Mutagen, 30: 440-447.

Dick D, Ng KM, Sauder DN, & Chu I (1995) *In vitro* and *in vivo* percutaneous absorption of ^{14}C-chloroform in humans. Hum Exp Toxicol, 14: 260-265.

Dix KJ, Kedderis GL, & Borghoff SJ (1997) Vehicle-dependent oral absorption and target tissue dosimetry of chloroform in male rats and female mice. Toxicol Lett, 91: 197-209.

Dlyamandoglu V & Selleck RE (1992) Reactions and products of chloramination. Environ Sci Technol, 26(4): 808.

Douglas GR, Nestmann ER, McKague AB, San RHC, Lee EG, Liu-Lee VW, & Kobel DJ (1985) Determination of potential hazads from pulp and paper mills: Mutagenicity and chemical analysis. In: Stich HF ed. Carcinogens and mutagens in the environment - Volume 5: The workplace. Boca Raton, Florida, CRC Press, Inc., pp 151-166.

Doyle TJ, Zheng W, Cerhan JR, Hong CP, Sellars TA, Kushi LH, & Folsom AR (1997) The association of drinking water source and chlorination by-products with cancer incidence among postmenopausal women in Iowa: a prospective cohort study. Am J Public Health, 87(7): 1168-1176.

Druckrey H (1968) [Chlorinated drinking water, toxicity tests involving seven generations of rats.] Food Cosmet Toxicol, 6: 147-154.

Drugan JK, Khosravi-Far R, White MA, Der CJ, Sung YJ, Hwang YW, & Campbell SL (1996) Ras interaction with two distinct binding domains of Raf-1 may be required for Ras transformation. J Biol Chem, 271: 233-237.

Dwelle EH (1903) Fatal bromoform poisoning. J Am Med Assoc, 41: 1540.

Eaton JW, Kolpin CF, & Swofford HS (1973) Chlorinated urban water: a cause of dialysis induced hemolytic anemia. Science, 181: 463-464.

Engerholm BA & Amy GL (1983) A predictive model for chloroform formation with chlorination of humic substances. Water Res, 17: 1797.

Enzer M & Whittington FM (1983) The actions of dichloroacetic acid on blood glucose, liver glycogen and fatty acid synthesis in obese-hyperglycemic (ob/ob) and lean mice. Horm Metab Res, 15: 225-229.

Epstein DL, Nolen GA, Randall JL, Christ SA, Read EJ, Stober JA, & Smith MK (1992) Cardiopathic effects of dichloroacetate in the fetal Long-Evans rat. Teratology, 46: 225-235.

Exon JH, Koller LD, O'Reilly CA, & Bercz JP (1987) Immunotoxicologic evaluation of chlorine-based drinking water disinfectants, sodium hypochlorite and monochloramine. Toxicology, 44: 257-269.

Eyre RJ, Stevens DK, Parker JC, & Bull RJ (1995) Acid-labile adducts to protein can be used as indicators of the cysteine S-conjugate pathway of trichloroethene metabolism. J Toxicol Environ Health, 46: 443-464.

FAO/WHO (1989) Toxicological evaluations of certain food additives and contaminants prepared by the thirty-third meeting of the Joint FAO/WHO Expert Committee on Food Additives. Geneva, World Health Organization, pp 25-36 (WHO Food Additives Series 24).

FAO/WHO (1993) Toxicological evaluations of certain food additives and contaminants prepared by the thirty-ninth meeting of the Joint FAO/WHO Expert Committee on Food Additives. Geneva, World Health Organization (WHO Food Additives Series 30).

Farber B & Abramow A (1985) Acute laryngeal edema due to chloral hydrate. Isr J Med Sci, **21**: 858-859.

Fawell JK (1990) The fate and significance of mutagenic by-products of chlorination *in vivo*. Marlow, Buckinghamshire, Foundation for Water Research.

Fayad NM (1993) Seasonal variations of THMs in Saudi Arabian drinking water. J Am Water Works Assoc, **85**: 46-50.

Fekadu K, Parzefall W, Kronberg L, Franzen R, Schulte-Hermann R, & Knasmuller S (1994) Induction of genotoxic effects by chlorohydroxyfuranones, byproducts of water disinfection, in *E. coli* K-12 cells recovered from various organs of mice. Environ Mol Mutagen, **24**: 317-324.

Feng TH (1966) Behaviour of organic chloramines in disinfection. J Water Pollut Control Fed, **38**(4): 614-628.

Ferguson LR, Morcombe P, &Triggs CN (1993) The size of cytokinesis-blocked micronuclei in human peripheral blood lymphocytes as a measure of aneuploidy induction by Set A compounds in the EEC trial. Mutat Res, **287**(1): 101-112.

Ferreira-Gonzalez A, DeAngelo AB, Nasim S, & Garrett CT (1995) Ras oncogene activation during hepatocarcinogenesis in B6C3F$_1$ male mice by dichloroacetic and trichloroacetic acids. Carcinogenesis, **16**: 495-500.

Fidler IJ (1977) Depression of macrophages in mice drinking hyperchlorinated water. Nature (Lond), **270**: 735-736.

Fidler IJ, Barnes Z, Fogler WE, Kirsh R, Bugelski P, & Poste G (1982) Involvement of macrophages in the eradication of established metastasis following intravenous injection of liposomes containing macrophage activators. Cancer Res, **42**: 496-501.

Fisher N, Hutchinson JB, Berry R, Hardy J, Ginocchio AV, & Waite V (1979) Long-term toxicity and carcinogenicity studies of the bread improver potassium bromate: 1. Studies in rats. Food Cosmet Toxicol, **17**(1): 33-39.

Fisher JW, Whittaker TA, Taylor DH, Clewell HJ, & Andersen ME (1989) Physiologically-based pharmacokinetic modeling of the pregnant rat: A multiroute exposure model for trichloroethylene and its metabolite, trichloroacetic acid. Toxicol Appl Pharmacol, **99**: 395-414.

Fisher JW, Gargas ML, Allen BC, & Andersen ME (1991) Physiologically based pharmacokinetic modelling with trichloroethylene and its metabolite, trichloroacetic acid, in the rat and mouse. Toxicol Appl Pharmacol, **109**: 183-195.

Flaten TP (1992) Chlorination of drinking water and cancer incidence in Norway. Int J Epidemiol, **21**: 6-15.

Fleischacker SJ & Randtke SJ (1983) Formation of organic chlorine in public water supplies. J Am Water Works Assoc, **75**(3): 132-138.

Fox AW, Sullivan BW, Buffini JD, Neichin ML, Nicora R, Hoehler FK, O'Rourke R, & Stoltz RR (1996) Reduction of serum lactate by dichloroacetate, and human pharmacokinetic-pharmaco-dynamic relationships. J Pharmacol Exp Ther, **279**: 686-693.

Fox TR, Schumann AM, Watanabe PG, Yano BL, Maher VM, & McCormick JJ (1990) Mutational analysis of the H-ras oncogene in spontaneous C57BL/6 × C3H/He mouse liver tumors and tumors induced with genotoxic and nongenotoxic hepatocarcinogens. Cancer Res, **50**: 4014-4019.

Fox AW, Yang X, Murli H, Lawlor TE, Cifone MA, & Reno FE (1996) Absence of mutagenic effects of sodium dichloroacetate. Fundam Appl Toxicol, **32**: 87-95.

Freedman MD, Cantor KP, Lee NL, Chen L, Lei H, Ruhl CE, & Wang SS (1997) Bladder cancer and drinking water: a population-based case-control study in Washington County, Maryland (United States). Cancer Causes Control, **8**: 738-744.

French AS, Copeland CB, Andrews DL, Williams WC, Riddle MM, & Luebke RW (1998) Evaluation of the potential immunotoxicity of chlorinated drinking water in mice. Toxicology, **125**: 53-58.

French AS, Copeland DB, Andrews DL, Williams WC, Riddle MM, & Luebke RW (1999) Evaluation of the potential immunotoxicity of bromodichloromethane in rats and mice. J Toxicol Environ Health, **56**(5): 297-310.

Fu L-J, Johnson EM, & Newman LM (1990) Prediction of the development toxicity hazard potential of halogenated drinking water disinfection by-products tested by the *in vitro* hydra assay. Regul Toxicol Pharmacol, **11**: 213-219.

Fujie K, Aoki T, & Wada M (1990) Acute and subacute cytogenetic effects of the trihalomethanes on rat bone marrow cells *in vivo*. Mutat Res, **242**: 111-119.

Fujie K, Aoki T, Ito Y, & Maeda S (1993) Sister-chromatid exchanges induced by trihalomethanes in rat erythroblastic cells and their suppression by crude catechin extracted from green tea. Mutat Res, **300**: 241-246.

Furnus CC, Ulrich MA, Terreros MC, & Dulout FN (1990) The induction of aneuploidy in cultured Chinese hamster cells by propionaldehyde and chloral hydrate. Mutagenesis, 5: 323-326.

Fuscoe JC, Afshari AJ, George MH, DeAngelo AB, Tice RR, Salman R, & Allen JW (1996) *In vivo* genotoxicity of dichloroacetic acid: Evaluation with the mouse peripheral blood micronucleus assay and the single cell gel assay. Environ Mol Mutagen, **27**: 1-9.

Galal-Gorchev H & Morris JC (1965) Formation and stability of bromamide, bromimide and nitrogen tribromide in aqueous solution. Inorg Chem, 4(6): 899-905.

Gao P & Pegram RA (1992) *In vitro* hepatic microsomal lipid and protein binding by metabolically activated bromodichloromethane. Toxicologist, **12**: 421.

Gao P, Thorton-Manning JR, & Pegram RA (1996) Protective effects of glutathione on bromodichloromethane *in vivo* toxicity and *in vitro* macromolecular binding in Fischer 344 rats. J Toxicol Environ Health, **49**: 149-159.

Garrett ER & Lambert HJ (1973) Pharmacokinetics of trichloroethanol and metabolites and interconversions among variously referenced pharmacokinetic parameters. J Pharm Sci, **62**: 550-572.

Gemma S, Faccioli S, Chieco P, Sbraccia M, Testai E, & Vittozzi L (1996) *In vivo* $CHCl_3$ bioactivation, toxicokinetics, toxicity, and induced compensatory cell proliferation in B6C3F$_1$ male mice. Toxicol Appl Pharmacol, **141**: 394-402.

Gessner PK & Cabana BE (1970) A study of the interaction of the hypnotic effects and of the toxic effects of chloral hydrate and ethanol. J Pharmacol Exp Ther, **174**: 247-259.

Giller S, Le Curieux F, Gauthier L, Erb F, & Marzin D (1995) Genotoxicity assay of chloral hydrate and chloropicrine. Mutat Res, **348**: 147-152.

Giller S, Le Curieux F, Erb F, & Marzin D (1997) Comparative genotoxicity of halogenated acetic acids found in drinking water. Mutagenesis, **12**: 321-328.

Gilli G (1990) Water disinfection: Relationship between ozone and aldehyde production. J Ozone Sci Eng, **12**: 116-125.

Gilman AG, Rall TW, Neis AS, & Taylor P (1991) Goodman and Gilman's pharmacological basis of therapeutics, 8th ed. New York, Pergamon Press, pp 364-365.

Ginwalla AS & Mikita MA (1992) Reaction products of Suwannee River fulvic acid with chloramine: characterization of products via 15-N NMR. Environ Sci Technol, **26**(6): 1148-1150.

Glaze WH, Weinberg HS, & Cavanagh JE (1993) Evaluating the formation of brominated DBPs during ozonation. J Am Water Works Assoc, **85**: 96-103.

Goldberg SJ, Lebowitz MD, & Graver EJ (1990) An association of human congenital cardiac malformations and drinking water contaminants. J Am Coll Cardiol, **16**: 155-164.

Golden RJ, Holm SE, Robinson DE, Julkunen PH, & Reese EA (1997) Chloroform mode of action: Implications for cancer risk assessment. Regul Toxicol Pharmacol, **26**(2): 142-145.

Goldsworthy TL & Popp JA (1987) Chlorinated hydrocarbon-induced peroxisomal enzyme activity in relation to species and organ carcinogenicity. Toxicol Appl Pharmacol, **88**: 225-233.

Gonzalez-Leon A, Schultz IR, & Bull RJ (1997) Pharmacokinetics and metabolism of dichloro-acetate in the F344 rat after prolonged administration in drinking water. Toxicol Appl Pharmacol, **146**(2): 189-195.

Gordon G (1993) The chemical aspects of bromate control in ozonated drinking water containing bromide ion. In: Proceedings of the International Water Supply Association Workshop, Paris. Boston, Massachusetts, Blackwell Scientific Publications, pp 41-49.

Gordon G & Emmert GL. (1996) Bromate ion formation in water when chlorine dioxide is photolyzed in the presence of bromide ion. In: Proceedings of the Water Quality Technology Conference, New Orleans, LA. Denver, Colorado, American Water Works Association.

Gordon G & Rosenblatt A (1996) Gaseous, chlorine-free chlorine dioxide for drinking water. In: Proceedings of the Water Quality Technology Conference, New Orleans, LA. Denver, Colorado, American Water Works Association.

Gordon WP, Soderlund EJ, Holme JA, Nelson SD, Iyer L, Rivedal E, & Dybing E (1985) The genotoxicity of 2-bromoacrolein and 2,3-dibromopropanal. Carcinogenesis, 6: 705-709.

Gordon G, Slootmaekers B, Tachiyashiki S, & Wood DW (1990) Minimizing chlorite ion and chlorate ion in water treated with chlorine dioxide. J Am Water Works Assoc, 82(4): 160-165.

Gordon G, Adam L, & Bubnis B (1995) Minimizing chlorate ion formation. J Am Water Works Assoc, 87(6): 97-106.

Gordon G, Adams LC, Bubnis BP, Kuo C, Cushing RS, & Sakaji RH (1997) Predicting liquid bleach decomposition. J Am Water Works Assoc, 89(4): 142-149.

Gottlieb MS, Carr JK, & Morris DT (1981) Cancer and drinking water in Louisiana: Colon and rectal. Int J Epidemiol, 10: 117-125.

Gottlieb MS, Carr JK, & Clarkson JR (1982) Drinking water and cancer in Louisiana: A retrospective mortality study. Am J Epidemiol, 116: 652-667.

Gray ET, Margerum DW, & Huffman RP (1979) Chloramine equilibria and the kinetics of disproportionation in aqueous solution. In: Brinkman FE & Bellama JM ed. Organometals and organometalloids, occurrence and fate in the environment. Washington, DC, American Chemical Society, pp 264-277 (ACS Symposium Series No. 82).

Green T & Hathway DE (1978) Interactions of vinyl chloride with rat-liver *in vivo*. Chem-Biol Interact, 22: 211-224.

Greenland S (1987) Quantitative methods in the review of epidemiologic literature. Epidemiol Rev, 9: 1-30.

Greenland S (1994) Invited commentary - A critical look at some popular meta-analytic methods. Am J Epidemiol, 140: 290-296.

Greenland S & Robins J (1994a) Invited commentary - Ecologic studies: Biases, misconceptions, and counterexamples. Am J Epidemiol, 139(8): 747-760.

Greenland S & Robins J (1994b) Accepting the limits of ecologic studies. Am J Epidemiol, 139(8): 769-771

Guastadisegni C, Balduzzi M, & Vittozzi L (1996) Preliminary characterization of phospholipid adducts formed by [^{14}C]-CHCl$_3$ reactive intermediates in hepatocyte suspensions. J Biochem Toxicol, 11: 21-25.

Guastadisegni C, Guidoni L, Balduzzi M, Viti V, Di Consiglio E, & Vitozzi L (1998) Characterization of a phospholipid adduct formed in Sprague Dawley rats by chloroform metabolism: NMR studies. J Biochem Mol Toxicol, 12(2): 93-102.

Haberer K (1994) [Survey of disinfectants use and occurrence of disinfectant by-products in German waterworks.] Wasser Abwasser, 135: 409-417 (in German).

Haessler R, Davis RF, Wolff RA, Kuzume K, Shangraw R, & Van Winkle DM (1996) Dichloro-acetate reduces plasma lactate levels but does not reduce infarct size in rabbit myocardium. Shock, 5: 66-71.

Halestrap AP (1975) The mitochondrial pyruvate carrier: Kinetics and specificity for substrates and inhibitors. Biochem J, 148: 85-96.

Halestrap AP (1978) Pyruvate and ketone-body transport across the mitochondrial membrane: Exchange properties, pH-dependence, and mechanism of the carrier. Biochem J, 172: 377-387.

Haller JF & Northgraves WW (1955) Chlorine dioxide and safety. TAPPI, 38: 199-202.

Hara A, Yamamoto H, Deyashiki Y, Nakayama T, Oritani H, & Sawada H (1991) Aldehyde dismutation catalyzed by pulmonary carbonyl reductase: kinetic studies of chloral hydrate metabolism to trichloroacetic acid and trichloroethanol. Biochim Biophys Acta, 1075: 61-67.

Harada K, Ichiyama T, Ikeda H, Ishihara T, & Yoshida K (1997) An autopsy case of acute chloroform intoxication after intermittent inhalation for years. Nippon Hoigaku Zasshi, 51(4): 319-323.

Harrington RM, Shertzer HG, & Bercz JP (1985) Effects of chlorine dioxide on the absorption and distribution of dietary iodide in the rat. Fundam Appl Toxicol, 5: 672-678.

Harrington RM, Shertzer HG, & Bercz JP (1986) Effects of chlorine dioxide on thyroid function in the African green monkey and the rat. J Toxicol Environ Health, 19: 235-242.

Harrington RM, Romano RR, Gates D, & Ridgway P (1995a) Subchronic toxicity of sodium chlorite in the rat. J Am Coll Toxicol, 14: 21-33.

Harrington RM, Romano RR, & Irvine L (1995b) Developmental toxicity of sodium chlorite in the rabbit. J Am Coll Toxicol, 14: 108-118.

Harrington-Brock K, Doerr CL, & Moore M (1995) Mutagenicity and clastogenicity of 3-chloro-4-(dichloromethyl)-5-hydroxy-2(5H)-furanone (MX) in L5178y/TK$^{+/-}$-3.7.2C mouse lymphoma cells. Mutat Res, 348: 105-110.

Harrington-Brock K, Doerr CL, & Moore MM (1998) Mutagenicity of three disinfection by-products: di- and trichloroacetic acid and chloral hydrate in L5178Y/TK$^{+/-}$-3.7.2C mouse lymphoma cells. Mutat Res, 413: 265-276.

Harris RH (1974) Implications of cancer-causing substances in Mississippi River water. Washington, DC, Environmental Defense Fund.

Hasegawa R, Takahashi M, & Kobulo T (1986) Carcinogenicity study of sodium hypochlorite in F344 rats. Food Chem Toxicol, 24: 1295-1302.

Hautman DP & Bolyard M (1993) Using ion chromatography to analyze inorganic disinfection by-products. J Am Water Works Assoc, 85(10): 88-93.

Hayashi M, Kishi M, Sofuni T, & Ishidate M (1988) Micronucleus tests in mice on 39 food additives and eight miscellaneous chemicals. Food Chem Toxicol, 26: 487-500.

Hayashi M, Sutou S, Shimada H, Sato S, Sasaki YF, & Wakata A (1989) Difference between intraperitoneal and oral gavage application in the micronucleus test. Mutat Res, 223: 329-344.

Hayatsu H, Hoshimo H, & Kawazoe Y (1971) Potential carcinogenicity of sodium hypochlorite. Nature (Lond), 233: 495.

Hayes JR, Condie LW, & Borzelleca JF (1986) Toxicology of haloacetonitriles. Environ Health Perspect, 69: 183-202.

Heffernan WP, Guion C, & Bull RJ (1979a) Oxidative damage to the erythrocyte induced by sodium chlorite, *in vivo*. J Environ Pathol Toxicol, 2: 1487-1499.

Heffernan WP, Guion C, & Bull RJ (1979b) Oxidative damage to the erythrocyte induced by sodium chlorite, *in vitro*. J Environ Pathol Toxicol, 2: 1501-1510.

Hegi ME, Fox TR, Belinsky SA, Devereux TR, & Anderson MW (1993) Analysis of activated protooncogenes in B6C3F$_1$ mouse liver tumors induced by ciprofibrate, a potent peroxisome proliferator. Carcinogenesis, 14: 145-149.

Heiskanen K, Lindstrom-Seppa P, Haataja L, Vaittinen SL, Vartiainen T, & Komulainen H (1995) Altered enzyme activities of xenobiotic biotransformation in kidneys after subchronic administration of 3-chloro-4-(dichloromethyl)-5-hydroxy-2(5H) furanone (MX) to rats. Toxicology, 100: 121-128.

Helliwell M & Nunn J (1979) Mortality in sodium chlorate poisoning. Br Med J, **April 28**(6171): 1119.

Helma C, Kronberg L, Ma TH, & Knasmuller S (1995) Genotoxic effects of the chlorinated hydroxyfuranones 3-chloro-4-(dichloromethyl)-5-hydroxy-2[5H]-furanone and 3,4-dichloro-5-hydroxy-2[5H]-furanone in *Tradescantia* micronucleus assays. Mutat Res, 346: 181-186.

Hemming J, Holmbom B, Reunanen M, & Tikkanen L (1986) Determination of the strong mutagen 3-chloro-4-(dichloromethyl)-5-hydroxy-2(5H)-furanone in chlorinated drinking and humic waters. Chemosphere, 5: 549-556.

Herbert V, Gardner A, & Colman N (1980) Mutagenicity of dichloroacetate, an ingredient of some formulations of pangamic acid (trade-named "vitamin B$_{15}$"). Am J Clin Nutr, 33: 1179-1182.

Herren-Freund SL, Pereira MA, Khoury MD, & Olson G (1987) The carcinogenicity of trichloroethylene and its metabolites, trichloroacetic acid and dichloroacetic acid, in mouse liver. Toxicol Appl Pharmacol, 90: 183-189.

Hewitt WR, Brown EM, & Plaa GL (1983) Acetone-induced potentiation of trihalomethane toxicity in male rats. Toxicol Lett, 16: 285-296.

Heywood R, Sortwell RJ, Kelly PJ, & Street AE (1972) Toxicity of sodium chlorate to the dog. Vet Rec, **90**: 416-418.

Heywood R, Sortwell RJ, Noel PR, Street AE, Prentice DE, Roe FJ, Wadsworth PF, Worden AN, & Van Abbe NJ (1979) Safety evaluation of toothpaste containing chloroform. III. Long-term study in beagle dogs. J Environ Pathol Toxicol, **2**: 835-851.

Hildesheim ME, Cantor KP, Lynch CF, Dosemeci M, Lubin J, Alavanja M, & Craun G (1998) Drinking water source and chlorination byproducts: risk of colon and rectal cancers. Epidemiology, **9**(1): 28-36.

Hill AB (1965) Environment and disease: Association or causation? Proc R Soc Med, **58**: 295-300.

Hirsch IA & Zauder HL (1986) Chloral hydrate: A potential cause of arrhythmias. Anesth Analg, **65**: 691-692.

Hobara T, Kobayashi H, Kawamoto T, Iwamoto S, & Sakai T (1987) Extrahepatic metabolism of chloral hydrate, trichloroethanol and trichloroacetic acid in dogs. Pharmacol Toxicol, **61**: 58-62.

Hoehn RC, Dietrich AM, Farmer WS, Orr MP, Lee RG, Aieta EM, Wood DW, & Gordon G (1990) Household odours associated with the use of chlorine dioxide. J Am Water Works Assoc, **82**(4): 166-172.

Hogan MD, Chi PY, Hoel DG, & Mitchell TJ (1979) Association between chloroform levels in finished drinking water supplies and various site-specific cancer mortality rates. J Environ Pathol Toxicol, **2**: 873-887.

Hoigne J & Bader H (1994) Kinetics of reactions of chlorine dioxide in water - I. Rate constants for inorganic and organic compounds. Water Res, **28**(1): 45-56.

Hoigne J, Bader H, Haag WR, & Staehelin J (1985) Rate constants of reactions of ozone with organic and inorganic compounds in water: III. Inorganic compounds and radicals. Water Res, **19**(8): 993-1004.

Holmbom BR, Voss RH, Mortimer RD, & Wong A (1984) Fractionation, isolation and characterization of Ames mutagenic compounds in kraft chlorination effluents. Environ Sci Technol, **18**: 333-337.

Horth H, Fawell JK, James CP, & Young WF (1991) The fate of the chlorination-derived mutagen MX *in vivo*. Marlow, Buckinghamshire, Foundation for Water Research.

Howe GR, Burch JD, & Miller AB (1977) Artificial sweeteners and human bladder cancer. Lancet, **2**: 578-581.

Hoz S, Basch H, Wolk JL, Rappoport Z, & Goldberg M (1991) Calculated double bond stabilization by bromine and chlorine: Relevance to the k_B/k_{Cl} element effect. J Org Chem, **56**: 5424-5426.

Huebner W & Jung F (1941) [About the theory of chlorate intoxication.] Schweiz Med Wochenschr, **71**: 247-250 (in German).

Hussein GI & Ahmed AE (1987) Studies on the mechanism of haloacetonitrile acute toxicity: Establishment of toxic doses and target organs of toxicity in rats. Toxicologist, **7**: 148.

Hutton PH & Chung FI (1992) Simulating THM formation potential in Sacramento Delta. J Water Res Planning Manage, **118**(5): 513-542 (Parts I & II).

Hyttinen JM & Jansson K (1995) PM2 DNA damage induced by 3-chloro-4-(dichloromethyl)-5-hydroxy-2(5H)-furanone (MX). Mutat Res, **348**: 183-186.

Hyttinen JM, Myohanen S, & Jansson K (1996) Kinds of mutations induced by 3-chloro-4-(dichloromethyl)-5-hydroxy-2(5H)-furanone (MX) in the hprt gene of Chinese hamster ovary cells. Carcinogenesis, **17**: 1179-1181.

IARC (1986) Potassium bromate. In: Some naturally occurring and synthetic food components, furocoumarins and ultraviolet radiation. Lyon, International Agency for Research on Cancer, pp 207-220 (IARC Monographs on the Evaluation of the Carcinogenic Risk of Chemicals to Humans, Volume 40).

IARC (1987) Overall evaluations of carcinogenicity: An updating of IARC Monographs 1 to 42. Lyon, International Agency for Research on Cancer (IARC Monographs on the Evaluation of the Carcinogenic Risk of Chemicals to Humans, Supplement 7).

IARC (1991) Chlorinated drinking-water; chlorination by-products; some other halogenated compounds; cobalt and cobalt compounds. Lyon, International Agency for Research on Cancer (IARC Monographs on the Evaluation of the Carcinogenic Risk of Chemicals to Humans, Volume 52).

IARC (1995) Dry cleaning, some chlorinated solvents and other industrial chemicals. Lyon, International Agency for Research on Cancer (IARC Monographs on the Evaluation of Carcinogenic Risks to Humans, Volume 63).

IARC (1999) Re-evaluation of some organic chemicals, hydrazine and hydrogen peroxide. Lyon, International Agency for Research on Cancer (IARC Monographs on the Evaluation of Carcinogenic Risks to Humans, Volume 71).

Ijsselmuiden CB, Gaydos C, Feighner B, Novakoski WL, Serwadda D, Caris V, & Comstock GW (1992) Cancer of the pancreas and drinking water: A population-based case-control study in Washington County, Maryland. Am J Epidemiol, **136**: 836-842.

ILSI (1995) Disinfection by-products in drinking water: Critical issues in health effects research - Proceedings of a workshop, Chapel Hill, NC, 23-25 October 1995. Washington, DC, International Life Sciences Institute.

ILSI (1997) An evaluation of EPA's proposed guidelines for carcinogen risk assessment using chloroform and dichloroacetate as case studies: Report of an expert panel. Washington, DC, International Life Sciences Institute.

ILSI (1998) The toxicity and risk assessment of complex mixtures in drinking water. Washington, DC, International Life Sciences Institute.

INERIS (1996) Study of acute toxicity of chlorite dioxide administered to rats by vapour inhalation: Determination of the 50% lethal concentration (LC_{50}/4 hrs). Paris, Elf Atochem SA.

IPCS (1994) Environmental health criteria 163: Chloroform. Geneva, World Health Organization, International Programme on Chemical Safety.

IRIS (1991) Integrated risk information system - Bromoform. Washington, DC, US Environmental Protection Agency.

IRIS (1992) Integrated risk information system - Dibromochloromethane. Washington, DC, US Environmental Protection Agency.

IRIS (1993) Integrated risk information system - Bromodichloromethane. Washington, DC, US Environmental Protection Agency.

Isaac RA & Morris JC (1983) Transfer of active chlorine from chloramine to nitrogenous organic compounds. Environ Sci Technol, 17: 738-742.

Ishidate M (1987) Data book of chromosomal aberrations *in vitro*. Tokyo, Life-Science Information Center, p 383.

Ishidate M, Sofuni T, Yoshikawa K, & Hayashi M (1982) Studies on the mutagenicity of low boiling organohalogen compounds. Tokyo, Medical and Dental University (Unpublished intraagency report to the National Institute of Hygienic Sciences, Tokyo).

Ishidate M, Sofuni T, Yoshikawa K, Hayashi M, Nohmi T, Sawada M, & Matsuoka A (1984) Primary mutagenicity screening of food additives currently used in Japan. Food Chem Toxicol, 22: 623-636.

Ishiguro Y, Santodonato J, & Neal MW (1988) Mutagenic potency of chlorofuranones and related compounds in *Salmonella*. Environ Mol Mutagen, 11: 225-234.

Islam MS, Zhao L, Zhou J, Dong L, McDougal JN, & Flynn GL (1996) Systemic uptake and clearance of chloroform by hairless rats following dermal exposure: I. Brief exposure to aqueous solutions. Risk Anal, 16: 349-357.

Issemann I & Green S (1990) Activation of a member of the steroid hormone receptor superfamily by peroxisome proliferators. Nature (Lond), 347: 645-650.

Jacobsen JS, Perkins CP, Callahan JT, Sambamurti K, & Humayun HZ (1989) Mechanisms of mutagenesis by chloroacetaldehyde. Genetics, 121: 213-222.

Jamison KC, Larson JL, Butterworth BE, Harden R, Skinner BL, & Wolf DC (1996) A non-bile duct origin for intestinal crypt-like ducts with periductular fibrosis induced in livers of F344 rats by chloroform inhalation. Carcinogenesis, 17: 675-682.

Jansson K & Hyttinen JM (1994) Induction of gene mutation in mammalian cells by 3-chloro-4-(dichloromethyl)-5-hydroxy-2(5H)-furanone (MX), a chlorine disinfection by-product in drinking water. Mutat Res, 322: 129-132.

Jansson K, Maki-Paakkanen J, Vaittinen SL, Vartiainen T, Komulainen H, & Tuomisto J (1993) Cytogenetic effects of 3-chloro-4-(dichloromethyl)-5-hydroxy-2(5H)-furanone (MX) in rat peripheral lymphocytes *in vitro* and *in vivo*. Mutat Res, 229: 25-28.

Jansson K, Hyttinen JM, Niittykoski M, & Maki-Paakkanen J (1995) Mutagenicity *in vitro* of 3,4-dichloro-5-hydroxy-2(5H)-furanone (mucochloric acid), a chlorine disinfection by-product in drinking water. Environ Mol Mutagen, 25: 284-287.

Jensen OM, Wahrendorf J, Knudsen JB, & Sorensen BL (1986) The Copenhagen case-control study of bladder cancer: II. Effect of coffee and other beverages. Int J Cancer, **37**: 651.

Johnson JD & Jensen JN (1986) THM and TOX formation: routes, rates and precursors. J Am Water Works Assoc, **78**(4): 156-162.

Jones PS, Savory R, Barratt P, Bell AR, Gray TJ, Jenkins NA, Gilbert DJ, Copeland NG, & Bell DR (1995) Chromosomal localisation, inducibility, tissue-specific expression and strain differences in three murine peroxisome-proliferator-activated-receptor genes. Eur J Biochem, **233**: 219-226.

Jow L & Mukherjee R (1995) The human peroxisome proliferator-activated receptor (PPAR) subtype NUC1 represses the activation of hPPAR and thyroid hormone receptors. J Biol Chem, **270**: 3836-3840.

Jung F (1947) [About the theory of chlorate intoxication III.] Arch Exp Pathol Pharmakol, **204**: 157-165 (in German).

Jung F (1965) [On the reaction of methemoglobin with potassium chlorate.] Acta Biol Med Ger, **15**: 554-568 (in German).

Kanitz S, Franco Y, Patrone V, & Caltabellotta (1996) Association between drinking water disinfection and somatic parameters at birth. Environ Health Perspect, **104**(5): 516-520.

Kaplan HL, Forney RB, Hughes FW, Jain NC, & Crim D (1967) Chloral hydrate and alcohol metabolism in human subjects. J Forensic Sci, **12**: 295-304.

Kaplan HL, Jain NC, Forney RB, & Richards AB (1969) Chloral hydrate-ethanol interactions in the mouse and dog. Toxicol Appl Pharmacol, **14**: 127-137.

Kasai H, Nishimura S, Kurokawa Y, & Hayashi Y (1987) Oral administration of the renal carcinogen, potassium bromate, specifically produces 8-hydroxydeoxyguanosine in rat target organ DNA. Carcinogenesis, **8**: 1959-1961.

Katayama Y & Welsh FA (1989) Effect of dichloroacetate on regional energy metabolites and pyruvate dehydrogenase activity during ischemia and reperfusion in gerbil brain. J Neurochem, **52**: 1817-1822.

Kato-Weinstein J, Lingohr MK, Orner GA, Thrall BD, & Bull RJ (1998) Effects of dichloroacetate treatment on carbohydrate metabolism in B6C3F$_1$ mice. Toxicology, **130**(2-3): 141-154.

Katz R, Tai CN, Deiner RM, McConnell RF, & Semonick DE (1981) Dichloroacetate, sodium: 3-month oral toxicity studies in rats and dogs. Toxicol Appl Pharmacol, **57**: 273-287.

Kavanaugh MC, Trussell AR, Cromer J, & Trussell RR (1980) An empirical kinetic model of THM formation: application to meet the proposed THM standards. J Am Water Works Assoc, **72**(10): 578-582.

Kawamoto T, Hobara T, Kobayashi H, Iwamoto S, Sakai T, Takano T, & Miyazaki Y (1987) The metabolic ratio as a function of chloral hydrate dose and intracellular redox as a function of chloral hydrate dose and intracellular redox state in the perfused rat liver. Pharmacol Toxicol, **60**: 325-329.

Kawachi T, Komatsu T, Kada T, Ishidate M, Sasaki M, Sugiyami T, Tazima Y, & Williams GM ed. (1980) In: The predictive value of short-term screening tests in carcinogenicity evaluation. Amsterdam, Oxford, New York, Elsevier Science Publishers, pp 253-267.

Keegan TE, Simmons JE, & Pegram RA (1998) NOAEL and LOAEL determinations of acute hepatoxicity for chloroform and bromodichloromethane delivered in an aqueous vehicle to F344 rats. J Toxicol Environ Health, 55(1): 65-75.

Keller DA & Heck HD (1988) Mechanistic studies on chloral toxicity: relationship to trichloroethylene carcinogenesis. Toxicol Lett, 42: 183-191.

Ketcha MM, Stevens DK, Warren DA, Bishop CT, & Brashear WT (1996) Conversion of trichloro-acetic acid to dichloroacetic acid in biological samples. J Anal Toxicol, 20: 236-241.

Kevekordes S, Porzig J, Gebel T, & Dunkelberg H (1998) [Mutagenicity of mixtures of halogenated aliphatic hydrocrabons and polycyclic aromatic hydrocarbons in the Ames test with TA98 and TA100.] Zent.bl Hyg U.weltmed, 200(5-6): 531-531 (in German).

Kimura S, Osaka H, Saitou K, Ohtuki N, Kobayashi T, & Nezu A (1995) Improvement of lesions shown on MRI and CT scan by administration of dichloroacetate in patients with Leigh syndrome. J Neurol Sci, 134: 103-107.

King WD & Marrett LD (1996) Case-control study of bladder cancer and chlorination by-products in treated water. Cancer Causes Control, 7(6): 596-604.

Kirmeyer GJ, Foust GW, Pierson GC, & Simmler JJ (1993) Optimizing chloramine treatment. Denver, Colorado, American Water Works Association Research Foundation.

Kirmeyer GJ, Foust GW, Pierson GC, & Simmler JJ (1995) Occurrence of nitrification in chloraminated water systems. Denver, Colorado, American Water Works Association Research Foundation.

Kitchin KT & Brown JL (1994) Dose-response relationship for rat liver DNA damage caused by 49 rodent carcinogens. Toxicology, 88: 31-49.

Klinefelter GR, Suarez JD, Roberts NL, & DeAngelo AB (1995) Preliminary screening for the potential of drinking water disinfection byproducts to alter male reproduction. Reprod Toxicol, 9: 571-578.

Klotz J & Pyrch L (1998) Neural tube defects and drinking water disinfection. Epidemiology, 10(4): 383-390.

Klotz J, Pyrch L, Haltmeier P, Trimbath L, & Weisel C (1996) Neural tube defects and chlorination by-products in drinking water. Epidemiology, 7(suppl 4): S63 (abstract).

Knasmuller S, Zohrer E, Kronberg L, Kundi M, Franzen R, & Schulte-Hermann R (1996) Mutational spectra of Salmonella typhimurium revertants induced by chlorohydroxyfuranones, byproducts of chlorine disinfection of drinking water. Chem Res Toxicol, 9: 374-381.

Knecht KT & Mason RP (1991) The detection of halocarbon-derived radical adducts in bile and liver of rats. Drug Metab Dispos, 19: 325-331.

Koch B, Crofts EW, Schimpff WK, & Davis MK (1988) Analysis of halogenated DBPs by capillary chromatography. In: Proceedings of the Water Quality Technology Conference, St Louis, MO. Denver, Colorado, American Water Works Association.

Koch B, Krasner SW, Sclimenti MJ, & Schimpff WK (1991) Predicting the formation of DBPs by the simulated distribution system. J Am Water Works Assoc, **83**(10): 62-70.

Koch-Weser J, Sellers EM, Udall JA, Griner PF, & Rickles FR (1971) Chloral hydrate and warfarin therapy. Ann Intern Med, **75**(1): 141-142.

Koepke UC, Coon JM, & Triolo AJ (1974) Effect of paraoxon on the hypnotic action of chloral hydrate. Toxicol Appl Pharmacol, **30**: 36-51.

Koivusalo M, Jaakkola JJ, Vartiainen T, Hakulinen T, Karjalainen S, Pukkala E, & Tuomisto J (1994a) Drinking water mutagenicity in past exposure assessment of the studies on drinking water and cancer: Application and evaluation in Finland. Environ Res, **64**: 90-101.

Koivusalo M, Jaakkola JJ, Vartiainen T, & Hakulinen S (1994b) Drinking water mutagenicity and gastrointestinal and urinary tract cancers: An ecological study in Finland. Am J Public Health, **84**: 1223-1228.

Koivusalo M, Vartiainen T, Hakulinen S, Pukkala E, & Jaakkola JJ (1995) Drinking water mutagenicity and leukemia, lymphomas, and cancers of the liver, pancreas and soft tissue. Arch Environ Health, **50**: 269-276.

Koivusalo M, Pukkala E, Vartiainen T, Jaakkola JJ, Hakulinen S, & Tuomisto J (1996) Drinking water chlorination and cancer - a cohort study in Finland. Epidemiology, 7(suppl 4): S82 (abstract).

Koivusalo M, Pukkala E, Vartiainen T, Jaakkola JJ, Hakulinen S, & Tuomisto J (1997) Drinking water chlorination and cancer - a historical cohort study in Finland. Cancer Causes Control, **8**: 192-200.

Komulainen H, Vaittinen SL, Vartiainen T, Lotjonen S, Paronen P, & Tuomisto J (1992) Pharmacokinetics in rat of 3-chloro-4-(dichloromethyl)-5-hydroxy-2(5H)-furanone (MX), a drinking water mutagen, after a single dose. Pharmacol Toxicol, **70**: 424-428.

Komulainen H, Huuskonen H, Kosma VM, Lotjonen S, & Vartiainen T (1994) Toxic effects and excretion in urine of 3-chloro-4-(dichloromethyl)-5-hydroxy-2(5H)-furanone (MX) in the rat after a single oral dose. Arch Toxicol, **68**: 398-400.

Komulainen H, Kosma VM, & Vaittinen S (1997) Carcinogenicity of the drinking water mutagen 3-chloro-4-(dichloromethyl)-5-hydroxy-2(5H)-furanone (MX). J Natl Cancer Inst, **89**: 848-856.

Koransky W (1952) [A contribution to the theory of chlorate oxidation.] Arch Exp Pathol Pharmakol, **215S**: 483-491 (in German).

Korz V & Gattermann R (1997) Behavioral alterations in male golden hamsters exposed to chlorodibromomethane. Pharmacol Biochem Behav, **58**(3): 643-647.

Kraft J & van Eldik R (1989) Kinetics and mechanisms of the iron (III)-catalyzed autooxidation of sulfur(IV) oxides in aqueous solution. Inorg Chem, **28**(12): 2297-2315.

Kramer MD, Lynch CF, Isacson P, & Hanson JW (1992) The association of waterborne chloroform with intrauterine growth retardation. Epidemiology, 3: 407-413.

Krasner SW, McGuire MJ, Jacangelo JG, Patania NL, Reagan KM, & Aieta ME (1989) The occurrence of disinfection by-products in US drinking water. J Am Water Works Assoc, 81(8): 41-53.

Krasner SW, Glaze WH, Weinberg HS, Daniel PA, & Najm IN (1993) Formation and control of bromate during ozonation of waters containing bromide. J Am Water Works Assoc, 85: 73-81.

Krasner SW, Scliminti MJ, & Chin R (1995) The impact of TOC and bromide on chlorination by-product formation: Disinfection by-products in water treatment. Boca Raton, Florida, CRC Press, Inc.

Kringstad KP, Ljungquist PO, de Sousa F, & Stromberg LM (1981) Identification and mutagenic properties of some chlorinated aliphatic compounds in the spent liquor from kraft pulp chlorination. Environ Sci Technol, 15: 562-566.

Krishna S, Agbenyega T, Angus BJ, Bedu-Addo G, Ofori-Amanfo G, Henderson G, Szwandt IS, O'Brien R, & Stacpoole PW (1995) Pharmacokinetics and pharmacodynamics of dichloroacetate in children with lactic acidosis due to severe malaria. Q J Med, 88: 341-349.

Kristiansen NK, Froshaug M, Aune KT, & Becher G (1994) Identification of halogenated compounds in chlorinated seawater and drinking water produced offshore using *n*-pentane extraction and open-loop stripping technique. Environ Sci Technol, 28: 1669-1673.

Kroll RB, Robinson GD, & Chung JH (1994a) Characterization of trihalomethane (THM)-induced renal dysfunction in the rat: I. Effects of THM on glomerular filtration and renal concentrating ability. Arch Environ Contam Toxicol, 27: 1-4.

Kroll RB, Robinson GD, & Chung JH (1994b) Characterization of trihalomethane (THM)-induced renal dysfunction in the rat: I. Relative potency of THMs in promoting renal dysfunction. Arch Environ Contam Toxicol, 27: 5-7.

Kronberg L & Vartiainen T (1988) Ames mutagenicity and concentration of the strong mutagen 3-chloro-4-(dichloromethyl)-5-hydroxy-2(5H)-furanone and its geometric isomer (E)-2-chloro-3-(dichloromethyl)-4-oxo-butenoic acid in chlorine-treated tap water. Mutat Res, 206: 177-182.

Kronberg L, Holmbon B, Reunanen M, & Tikkanen L (1988) Identification and quantification of the Ames mutagenic compound 3-chloro-4-(dichloromethyl)-5-hydroxy-2(5H)-furanone and of its geometric isomer (E)-2-chloro-3-(dichloromethyl)-4-oxobutenoic acid in chlorine treated humic water and drinking water extracts. Environ Sci Technol, 22(9): 1097-1103.

Kronberg L, Karlsson S, & Sjoholm R (1993) Formation of ethenocarbaldehyde derivatives of adenosine and cytidine in reactions with mucochloric acid. Chem Res Toxicol, 6: 495-499.

Kruithof JC & Meijers RT (1993) Presence and formation of bromate ion in Dutch drinking water treatment. In: Proceedings of the International Water Supply Association Workshop, Paris. Boston, Massachusetts, Blackwell Scientific Publications, pp 125-133.

Kurlemann G, Paetzke I, Moller H, Masur H, Schuierer G, Weglage J, & Koch HG (1995) Therapy of complex I deficiency: Peripheral neuropathy during dichloroacetate therapy. Eur J Pediatr, **154**: 928-932.

Kurokawa Y, Hayashi Y, Maekawa A, Takahashi M, Kokubo T, & Odashima S (1983) Carcinogenicity of potassium bromate administered orally to F344 rats. J Natl Cancer Inst, **71**: 965-972.

Kurokawa Y, Takamura N, Matsushima Y, Imazawa T, & Hayashi Y (1984) Studies on the promoting and complete carcinogenic activities of some oxidizing chemicals in skin carcinogenesis. Cancer Lett, **24**: 299-304.

Kurokawa Y, Imazawa T, Matsushima M, Takamura N, & Hayashi Y (1985a) Lack of promoting effect of sodium chlorate and potassium chlorate in two-stage rat renal carcinogenesis. J Am Coll Toxicol, **4**: 331-337.

Kurokawa Y, Aoki S, Imazawa T, Hayashi Y, Matsushima Y, & Takamura N (1985b) Dose-related enhancing effect of potassium bromate on renal tumorigenesis in rats initiated with N-ethyl-N-hydroxyethyl-nitrosamine. Jpn J Cancer Res (Gann), **76**: 583-589.

Kurokawa Y, Aoki S, Matsushima Y, Takamura N, Imazawa T, & Hayashi Y (1986a) Dose-response studies on the carcinogenicity of potassium bromate in F344 rats after long-term oral exposure. J Natl Cancer Inst, **77**: 977-982.

Kurokawa Y, Takayama S, Konishi Y, Hiasa Y, Asahina S, Takahashi M, Maekawa A, & Hayashi Y (1986b) Long-term *in vivo* carcinogenicity tests of potassium bromate, sodium hypochlorite, and sodium chlorite conducted in Japan. Environ Health Perspect, **69**: 221-235.

Kurokawa Y, Matsushima Y, Takamura N, Imazawa T, & Hayashi Y (1987a) Relationship between the duration of treatment and the incidence of renal cell tumors in male F344 rats administered potassium bromate. Jpn J Cancer Res (Gann), **78**: 358-364.

Kurokawa Y, Takamura N, Matsuoka C, Imazawa T, Matsushima Y, Onodera H, & Hayashi Y (1987b) Comparative studies on lipid peroxidation in the kidney of rats, mice, and hamsters and on the effect of cysteine, glutathione, and diethyl maleate treatment on mortality and nephrotoxicity after administration of potassium bromate. J Am Coll Toxicol, **6**: 489-501.

Kurokawa Y, Maekawa A, Takahashi M, & Hayashi Y (1990) Toxicity and carcinogenicity of potassium bromate - A new renal carcinogen. Environ Health Perspect, **87**: 309-335.

Kuwahara T, Ikehara Y, Kanatsu K, Doi T, Nagai H, Nakayashiki H, Tamura T, & Kawai C (1984) Two cases of potassium bromate poisoning requiring long-term hemodialysis therapy for irreversible tubular damage. Nephron, **37**: 278-280.

Lacey JH & Randle PJ (1978) Inhibition of lactate gluconeogenesis in rat kidney by dichloroacetate. Biochem J, **170**: 551-560.

Lake BG (1995) Peroxisome proliferation: current mechanisms relating to non-genotoxic carcinogenesis. Toxicol Lett, **82/83**: 673-681.

LaLonde RT & Xie S (1992) A study of inactivation reactions of *N*-acetylcysteine with mucochloric acid, a mutagenic product of the chlorination of humic substances in water. Chem Res Toxicol, 5: 618-624.

LaLonde RT & Xie S (1993) Glutathione and *N*-acetylcysteine inactivations of mutagenic 2(5H)-furanones from the chlorination of humics in water. Chem Res Toxicol, 6: 445-451.

LaLonde RT, Cook GP, Perakyla H, & Dence CW (1991a) Effect on mutagenicity of the stepwise removal of hydroxyl group and chlorine atoms from 3-chloro-4-(dichloromethyl)-5-hydroxy-2(5H)-furanone: ^{13}C NMR chemical shifts as determinants of mutagenicity. Chem Res Toxicol, 4: 35-40.

LaLonde RT, Cook GP, Perakyla H, & Bu L (1991b) Structure-activity relationships of bacterial mutagens related to 3-chloro-4-(dichloromethyl)-5-hydroxy-2(5H)-furanone: An emphasis on the effect of stepwise removal of chlorine from the dichloromethyl group. Chem Res Toxicol, 4: 540-545.

LaLonde RT, Leo H, Perakyla H, Dence CW, & Farrell RP (1992) Associations of the bacterial mutagenicity of halogenated 2(5H)-furanones with their MNDO-PM3 computed properties and mode of reactivity with sodium borohydride. Chem Res Toxicol, 5: 392-400.

Lambert GH, Muraskas J, Anderson CL, & Myers TF (1990) Direct hyperbilirubinemia associated with chloral hydrate administration in the newborn. Pediatrics, 86: 277-281.

Lange AL & Kawczynski E (1978) Controlling organics: the Contra Costa County Water District experience. J Am Water Works Assoc, 70(11): 63.

Laptook AR & Rosenfeld CR (1984) Chloral hydrate toxicity in a preterm infant. Pediatr Pharmacol, 4: 161-165.

Larson JL & Bull RJ (1992) Metabolism and lipoperoxidative activity of trichloroacetate and dichloroacetate in rats and mice. Toxicol Appl Pharmacol, 115: 268-277.

Larson RA & Rockwell AL (1979) Chloroform and chlorophenol production by decarboxylation of natural acids during aqueous chlorination. Environ Sci Technol, 13(3): 325-329.

Larson JL, Wolf DC, & Butterworth BE (1994a) Induced cytolethality and regenerative cell proliferation in the livers and kidneys of male B6C3F$_1$ mice given chloroform by gavage. Fundam Appl Toxicol, 23: 537-543.

Larson JL, Wolf DC, & Butterworth BE (1994b) Induced cytotoxicity and cell proliferation in the hepatocarcinogenicity of chloroform in female B6C3F$_1$ mice: Comparison of administration by gavage in corn oil vs. ad libitum in drinking water. Fundam Appl Toxicol, 22(1): 90-102.

Larson JL, Wolf DC, & Butterworth BE (1995a) Induced regenerative cell proliferation in livers and kidneys of male F-344 rats given chloroform in corn oil by gavage or ad libitum in drinking water. Toxicology, 95: 73-86.

Larson JL, Wolf DC, Mery S, Morgan KT, & Butterworth BE (1995b) Toxicity and cell proliferation in the liver, kidneys, and nasal passages of female F-344 rats induced by chloroform administered by gavage. Food Chem Toxicol, 33: 443-456.

Larson JL, Templin MV, Wolf DC, Jamison KC, Leininger JR, Mery S, Morgan KT, Wong BA, Conolly RB, & Butterworth BE (1996) A 90-day chloroform inhalation study in female and male B6C3F₁ mice: implications for cancer risk assessment. Fundam Appl Toxicol, 30: 118-137.

Laurie RD, Bercz JP, Wessendarp TK, & Condie LW (1986) Studies of the toxic interactions of disinfection by-products. Environ Health Perspect, 69: 203-207.

Lawrence WH, Dillingham EO, Turner JE, & Autian J (1972) Toxicity profile of chloroacetaldehyde. J Pharm Sci, 61: 19-25.

Lawrence CE, Taylor PR, Trock BJ, & Reilly AA (1984) Trihalomethanes in drinking water and human colorectal cancer. J Natl Cancer Inst, 72: 563-568.

Leavitt SA, DeAngelo AB, George MH, & Ross JA (1997) Assessment of the mutagenicity of dichloroacetic acid in *lacI* transgenic B6C3F₁ mice. Carcinogenesis, 18: 2101-2106.

LeBel GL, Benoit FM, & Williams DT (1995) Variation of chlorinated DBPs in water from treatment plants using three different disinfection processes. In: Proceedings of the Conference on Water Quality Technology, New Orleans, LA.

Le Curieux F, Gauthier L, Erb F, & Marzin D (1995) The use of the SOS chromotest, the Ames-fluctuation test and the newt micronucleus test to study the genotoxicity of four trihalomethanes. Mutagenesis, 10: 333-341.

Lee SS, Pineau T, Drago J, Lee EJ, Owens JW, Kroetz DL, Fernandez-Salguero PM, Westphal H, & Gonzalez FJ (1995) Targeted disruption of the isoform of the peroxisome proliferator-activated receptor gene in mice results in abolishment of the pleiotropic effects of peroxisome proliferators. Mol Cell Biol, 15: 3012-3022.

Legube B, Bourbigot M, Bruchet A, Deguin A, Montiel A, & Matia L (1993) Bromide ion/bromate ion survey on different European water utilities. In: Proceedings of the International Water Supply Association Workshop, Paris. Boston, Massachusetts, Blackwell Scientific Publications.

Leuschner J & Leuschner F (1991) Evaluation of the mutagenicity of chloral hydrate *in vitro* and *in vivo*. Drug Res, 41: 1101-1103.

Lewandowski ED & White LT (1995) Pyruvate dehydrogenase influences postischemic heart function. Circulation, 91: 2071-2079.

Lichtenberg R, Zeller WP, Gatson R, & Hurley RM (1989) Clinical and laboratory observations: Bromate poisoning. J. Pediatr, 114: 891-894.

Lilly PD, Simmons JE, & Pegram RA (1994) Dose-dependent vehicle differences in the acute toxicity of bromodichloromethane. Fundam Appl Toxicol, 23: 132-140.

Lilly PD, Simmons JE, & Pegram RA (1996) Effect of subchronic corn oil gavage on the acute toxicity of orally administered bromodichloromethane. Toxicol Lett, 87: 93-102.

Lilly PD, Ross TM, & Pegram RA (1997a) Trihalomethane comparative toxicity: Acute renal and hepatic toxicity of chloroform and bromodichloromethane following aqueous gavage. Fundam Appl Toxicol, 40: 101-110.

Lilly PD, Andersen ME, Ross TM, & Pegram RA (1997b) Physiologically based estimation of *in vivo* rates of bromodichloromethane metabolism. J Toxicol, **124**: 141-152.

Lilly PD, Andersen ME, Ross TM, & Pegram RA (1998) A physiologically based pharmacokinetic description of the oral uptake, tissue dosimetry and rates of metabolism of bromodichloromethane in the male rat. Toxicol Appl Pharmacol, **150**: 205-217.

Lin EL, Daniel FB, Herren-Freund SL, & Pereira MA (1986) Haloacetonitriles: Metabolism, geno-toxicity, and tumor-initiating activity. Environ Health Perspect, **69**: 67-71.

Lin EL, Reddy TV, & Daniel FB (1992) Macromolecular adduction by trichloroacetonitrile in the Fischer 344 rat following oral gavage. Cancer Lett, **62**: 1-9.

Lin EL, Mattox JK, & Daniel FB (1993) Tissue distribution, excretion, and urinary metabolites of dichloroacetic acid in the male Fischer 344 rat. J Toxicol Environ Health, **38**: 19-32.

Linder RE, Strader LF, Slott VL, & Suarez JD (1992) Endpoints of spermatoxicity in the rat after short duration exposures to fourteen reproductive toxicants. Reprod Toxicol, **6**: 491-505.

Linder RE, Klinefelter GR, Strader LF, Suarez JD, & Dyer CJ (1994a) Acute spermatogenic effects of bromoacetic acids. Fundam Appl Toxicol, **22**: 422-430.

Linder RE, Klinefelter GR, Strader LF, Suarez JD, Roberts NL, & Dyer CJ (1994b) Spermato-toxicity of dibromoacetic acid in rats after 14 daily exposures. Reprod Toxicol, **8**: 251-259.

Linder RE, Klinefelter GR, Strader LF, Narotosky MG, Suarez JD, Roberts NL, & Perreault SD (1995) Dibromoacetic acid affects reproductive competence and sperm quality in the male rat. Fundam Appl Toxicol, **28**: 9-17.

Linder RE, Klinefelter GR, Strader LF, Suarez JD, & Roberts NL (1997a) Spermatoxicity of dichloroacetic acid. Reprod Toxicol, **11**: 681-688.

Linder RE, Klinefelter GR, Strader LF, Veeramachaneni DR, Roberts NL, & Suarez JD (1997b) Histopathological changes in the testes of rats exposed to dibromoacetic acid. Reprod Toxicol, **11**: 47-56.

Lindstrom AB, Pleil JD, & Berkoff DC (1997) Alveolar breath sampling and analysis to assess trihalomethane exposures during competitive swimming training. Environ Health Perspect, **105**(6): 636-642.

Lipscomb JC, Mahle DA, Brashear WT, & Barton HA (1995) Dichloroacetic acid: Metabolism in cytosol. Drug Metab Dispos, **23**: 1202-1205.

Lock EA, Gyte A, Widdowson P, Simpson M, & Wyatt I (1995) Chloropropionic acid-induced alterations in glucose metabolic status: possible relevance to cerebellar cell necrosis. Arch Toxicol, **69**: 640-643.

Lopaschuk GD & Saddik M (1992) The relative contribution of glucose and fatty acids to ATP production in hearts reperfused following ischemia. Mol Cell Biochem, **116**: 111-116.

Loveday KS, Anderson BE, Resnick MA, & Zeiger E (1990) Chromosome aberration and sister chromatid exchange tests in Chinese hamster ovary cells *in vitro*: V. Results with 46 chemicals. Environ Mol Mutagen, **16**: 272-303.

Lubbers JR & Bianchine JR (1984) Effects of the acute rising dose administration of chlorine dioxide, chlorate and chlorite to normal healthy adult male volunteers. J Exp Pathol Toxicol Oncol, **5**: 215-228.

Lubbers JR, Chauhan S, & Bianchine JR (1981) Controlled clinical evaluations of chlorine dioxide, chlorite and chlorate in man. Fundam Appl Toxicol, **1**: 334-338.

Lubbers JR, Chauan S, & Bianchine R (1982) Controlled clinical evaluations of chlorine dioxide, chlorite, and chlorite in man. Environ Health Perspect, **46**: 57-62.

Lubbers JR, Chauhan S, Miller JK, & Bianchine JR (1984a) The effects of chronic administration of chlorine dioxide, chlorite and chlorate to normal healthy adult male volunteers. J Exp Pathol Toxicol Oncol, **5**: 229-238.

Lubbers JR, Chauhan S, Miller JK, & Bianchine JR (1984b) The effects of chronic administration of chlorite to glucose-6-phosphate dehydrogenase deficient healthy adult male volunteers. J Environ Pathol Toxicol Oncol, **5**: 239-242.

Lue JN, Johnson CE, & Edwards DL (1988) Drug experience: Bromate poisoning from ingestion of professional hair-care neutralizer. Clin Pharm, **7**: 66-70.

Lukas G, Vyas KH, Brindle SD, Le Sher AR, & Wagner WE (1980) Biological disposition of sodium dichloroacetate in animals and humans after intravenous administration. J Pharm Sci, **69**: 419-421.

Lukasewycz MT, Bieringer CM, Liukkonen RJ, Fitzsimmons ME, Corcoran HF, Sechoing L, & Carlson RM (1989) Analysis of inorganic and organic chloramines: derivatization with 2-mercapto-benzothiazole. Environ Sci Technol, **23**(2): 196-199.

Luknitskii FI (1975) The chemistry of chloral. Chem Rev, **75**: 82-94.

Lykins BW & Clark RM (1988) GAC for removing THMs. Washington, DC, US Environmental Protection Agency (EPA 600/9-88/004).

Lynch AM & Parry JM (1993) The cytochalasin-B micronucleus/kinetochore assay *in vitro*: Studies with 10 suspected aneugens. Mutat Res, **287**(1): 71-86.

Lynch CF, Woolson RF, O'Gorman T, & Cantor KP (1989) Chlorinated drinking water and bladder cancer: effect of misclassification on risk estimates. Arch Environ Health, **44**: 252-259.

Lynch CF, VanLier S, & Cantor KP (1990) A case-control study of multiple cancer sites and water chlorination in Iowa. In: Jolley RL, Condie LW, & Johnson JD ed. Water chlorination: Chemistry, environmental impact and health effects. Chelsea, Michigan, Lewis Publishers, Inc., vol 6, p 387.

McCabe LJ (1975) Association between halogenated methanes in drinking water and mortality (NORS data). Cincinnati, Ohio, US Environmental Protection Agency, Water Quality Division, 4 pp.

McCauley PT, Robinson M, Daniel FB, & Olson GR (1995) The effects of subchronic chlorate exposure in Sprague-Dawley rats. Drug Chem Toxicol, **18**: 185-199.

McGeehin M, Reif J, Becker J, & Mangione E (1993) A case-control study of bladder cancer and water disinfection in Colorado. Am J Epidemiol, **138**(7): 492-501 (Abstract 127).

McGregor DB, Brown AG, Howgate S, McBride D, Riach C, & Caspary WJ (1991) Responses of the L5178Y mouse lymphoma cell forward mutation assay: V. 27 coded chemicals. Environ Mol Mutagen, **17**: 96-219.

McGuire MJ & Meadow RG (1988) AWWARF trihalomethane survey. J Am Water Works Assoc, **80**(1): 61-68.

Mackay JM, Fox V, Griffiths K, Fox DA, Howard CA, Coutts C, Wyatt I, & Styles JA (1995) Trichloroacetic acid: investigation into the mechanism of chromosomal damage in the *in vitro* human lymphocyte cytogenetic assay and the mouse bone marrow micronucleus test. Carcinogenesis, **16**(5): 1127-1133.

McVeigh JJ & Lopaschuk GD (1990) Dichloroacetate stimulation of glucose oxidation improves recovery of ischemic rat hearts. Am J Physiol, **259**: H1079-H1085.

Mailhes JB, Aardema MJ, & Marchetti F (1993) Investigation of aneuploidy induction in mouse oocytes following exposure to vinblastine-sulfate, pyrimethamine, diethylstilbestrol, or chloral hydrate. Environ Mol Mutagen, **22**(2): 107-114.

Maki-Paakkanen & Jansson K (1995) Cytogenetic effects in the peripheral lymphocytes and kidney cells of rats exposed to 3-chloro-4-(dichloromethyl)-5-hydroxy-2(5H)-furanone (MX) orally on three consecutive days. Mutat Res, **343**: 151-156.

Man KC & Brosnan JT (1982) Inhibition of medium and short-chain fatty acid oxidation in rat heart mitochondria by dichloroacetate. Metabolism, **31**: 744-748.

Marcus PM, Savitz DA, Millikan RC, & Morgenstern H (1998) Female breast cancer and trihalomethanes in drinking water in North Carolina. Epidemiology, **9**(2): 156-160.

Maronpot RR, Fox T, Malarkey DE, & Goldsworthy TL (1995) Mutations in the ras proto-oncogene: clues to etiology and molecular pathogenesis of mouse liver tumors. Toxicology, **101**: 125-156.

Marshall EK & Owens AH (1954) Absorption, excretion, and metabolic fate of chloral hydrate and trichloroethanol. Bull Johns Hopkins Hosp, **95**: 1-18.

Mather GG, Exon JH, & Koller LD (1990) Subchronic 90 day toxicity of dichloroacetic and trichloroacetic acid in rats. Toxicology, **64**: 71-80.

Mathews JM, Troxler PS, & Jeffcoat AR (1990) Metabolism and distribution of bromodichloromethane in rats after single and multiple oral doses. J Toxicol Environ Health, **30**: 15-22.

Matsuoka A, Hayashi M, & Ishidate M (1979) Chromosomal aberration tests on 29 chemicals combined with S9 mix *in vitro*. Mutat Res, **66**: 277-290.

Mayers DJ, Hindmarsh KW, Sankaran K, Gorecki DK, & Kasian GF (1991) Chloral hydrate disposition following single-dose administration to critically ill neonates and children. Dev Pharmacol Ther, **16**: 71-77.

Meier JR (1988) Genotoxic activity of organic chemicals in drinking water. Mutat Res, **196**: 211-245.

Meier JR, Lingg RD, & Bull RJ (1983) Formation of mutagens following chlorination of humic acid: A model for mutagen formation during drinking water. Mutat Res, **118**: 25-41.

Meier JR, Ringhand HP, Coleman WE, Munch JW, Streicher RP, Kaylor WH, & Schenk KM (1985a) Identification of mutagenic compounds formed during chlorination of humic acid. Mutat Res, **157**: 111-122.

Meier JR, Bull RJ, Stober JA, & Cimino MC (1985b) Evaluation of chemicals used for drinking water disinfection for production of chromosomal damage and sperm-head abnormalities in mice. Environ Mutagen, **7**: 201-211.

Meier JR, Ringhand HP, Coleman WE, & Schenck KM (1986) Mutagenic by-products from chlorination of humic acid Environ Health Perspect, **69**: 101-107.

Meier JR, Knohl RB, Coleman WE, Ringhand HP, Munch JW, Kaylor WH, Streicher RP, & Kopfler FC (1987a) Studies on the potent bacterial mutagen, 3-chloro-4-(dichloromethyl)-5-hydroxy-2(5H)-furanone: aqueous stability, XAD recovery and analytical determination in drinking water and in chlorinated humic acid solutions. Mutat Res, **189**: 363-373.

Meier JR, Blazek WF, & Knohl RB (1987b) Mutagenic and clastogenic properties of 3-chloro-4-(dichloromethyl)-5-hydroxy-2(5H)-furanone: A potent bacterial mutagen in drinking water. Environ Mol Mutagen, **10**: 411-424.

Meier JR, Monarca S, Patterson KS, Villarini M, Daniel FB, Moretti M, & Pasquini R (1996) Urine mutagenicity and biochemical effects of the drinking water mutagen, 3-chloro-4-(dichloromethyl)-5-hydroxy-2(5H)-furanone (MX) following repeated oral administration to mice and rats. Toxicology, **110**: 59-70.

Mel HC, Jolly WL, & Latimer W (1953) The heat and free energy of formation of bromate ion. J Am Chem Soc, **75**: 3827.

Melnick RL, Kohn MC, Dunnick JK, & Leininger KR (1998) Regenerative hyperplasia is not required for liver tumor induction in female B6C3F$_1$ mice exposed to trihalomethanes. Toxicol Appl Pharmacol, **148**(1): 133-136.

Mengele K, Schwarzmeier J, Schmidt P, & Moser K (1969) [Clinical features and investigations of the erythrocyte metabolism in case of intoxication with sodium chlorate.] Int J Clin Pharmacol, **2**: 120-125 (in German).

Merdink JL, Gonzalez-Leon A, Bull RJ, & Schultz IR (1998) The extent of dichloroacetate formation from trichloroethylene, chloral hydrate, trichloroacetate and trichloroethanol in B6C3F$_1$. Toxicol Sci, **45**(1): 33-41.

Merdink JL, Stenner RD, Stevens DK, Parker JC, & Bull RJ (1999) Effect of enterohepatic circulation on the pharmacokinetics of chloral hydrate in F344 rats. J Toxicol Environ Health, **57**(5): 357-368.

Merlet N, Thibaud H, & Dore M (1985) Chloropicrin formation during oxidative treatment in the preparation of drinking water. Sci Total Environ, **47**: 223-228.

Merrick BA, Smallwood CL, Meier JR, McKean DL, Kaylor WH, & Condie LW (1987) Chemical reactivity, cytotoxicity, and mutagenicity of chloropropanones. Toxicol Appl Pharmacol, **91**: 46-54.

Merrick BA, Meier JR, Smallwood CL, McKean DL, & Condie LW (1990) Biochemical mechanisms of *in vitro* chloropropanone toxicity. In: Jolley RL, Condie LW, & Johnson JD ed. Water chlorination: Chemistry, environmental impact and health effects. Ann Arbor, Michigan, Lewis Publishers, Inc., vol 6, pp 329-339.

Michael GE, Miday RK, Bercz JP, Miller RG, Greathouse DG, Kraemer DF, & Lucas JB (1981) Chlorine dioxide water disinfection: A prospective epidemiological study. Arch Environ Health, **36**: 20-27.

Miller WJ & Uden PC (1983) Characterization of nonvolatile aqueous chlorination products of humic substances. Environ Sci Technol, **17**(3): 150-152.

Miller LH, Brownstein MH, & Hyman AB (1966) Fixed eruption due to chloral hydrate. Arch Dermatol, **94**: 60-61.

Miltner RJ, Shukairy HM, & Summers RS (1992) Disinfection by-product formation and control by ozonation and biotreatment. J Am Water Works Assoc, **84**(11): 53-62.

Mink FL, Coleman WE, Munch JW, Kaylor WH, & Ringhand HP (1983) *In vivo* formation of halogenated reaction products following peroral sodium hypochlorite. Bull Environ Contam Toxicol, **30**: 394-399.

Mink FL, Brown TJ, & Rickabaugh J (1986) Absorption, distribution and excretion of ^{14}C-trihalomethanes in mice and rats. Bull Environ Contam Toxicol, **37**: 752-758.

MMWR (1991) Chlorine gas toxicity from mixture of bleach with other cleaning products - California. Morb Mortal Wkly Rep, **40**(36): 619-621.

Mobley SA, Taylor DH, Laurie RD, & Pfohl RJ (1990) Chlorine dioxide depresses T_3 uptake and delays development of locomotor activity in young rats. In: Jolley RL, Condie LW, & Johnson JD ed. Water chlorination: Chemistry, environmental impact and health effects. Ann Arbor, Michigan, Lewis Publishers, Inc., vol 6, pp 347-360.

Monson RR (1980) Occupational epidemiology. Boca Raton, Florida, CRC Press, Inc., p 88.

Montgomery Watson, Inc. (1993) Disinfection/DBP database for the negotiated regulation. Denver, Colorado, American Water Works Association.

Moore GS & Calabrese EJ (1980) The effects of chlorine dioxide and sodium chlorite on erythrocytes of A/J and C57BL/J mice. J Environ Pathol Toxicol, **4**: 513-524.

Moore GS & Calabrese EJ (1982) Toxicological effects of chlorite in the mouse. Environ Health Perspect, **46**: 31-37.

Moore BB & Sherman M (1991) Chronic reactive airway disease following acute chlorine gas exposure in an asymptomatic atopic patient. Chest, **100**: 855-856.

Moore GS, Tuthill RW, & Polakoff DW (1979a) A statistical model for predicting chloroform levels in chlorinated surface water supplies. J Am Water Works Assoc, **71**: 37-45.

Moore GW, Swift LL, Rabinowitz DR, Crofford OB, Oates JA, & Stacpoole PW (1979b) Reduction of serum cholesterol in two patients with homozygous familial hypercholesterolemia by dichloroacetate. Atherosclerosis, **33**: 285-293.

Moore GS, Calabrese EJ, & McGee M (1980a) Health effects of monochloramine in drinking water. J Environ Sci Health, **A15**: 239-258.

Moore GS, Calabrese EJ, & Leonard DA (1980b) Effects of chlorite exposure on conception rate and litters of A/J mice. Bull Environ Contam Toxicol, **25**: 689-696.

Moore GS, Calabrese EJ, & Forti A (1984) The lack of nephrotoxicity in the rat by sodium chlorite, a possible byproduct of chlorine dioxide disinfection in drinking water. J Environ Sci Health, **A19**: 643-661.

Moore TC, DeAngelo AB, & Pegram RA (1994) Renal toxicity of bromodichloromethane and bromoform administered chronically to rats and mice in drinking water. Toxicologist, **14**: 281 (abstract).

Morimoto K & Koizumi A (1983) Trihalomethanes induce sister chromatid exchanges in human lymphocytes *in vitro* and mouse bone marrow cells *in vivo*. Environ Res, **32**: 72-79.

Morris JC, Ram N, Baum B, & Wajon E (1980) Formation and significance of *N*-chloro compounds in water supplies. Washington, DC, US Environmental Protection Agency (EPA 600/2-80-031).

Morris RD, Audet AM, & Angelillo IF (1992) Chlorination, chlorination by-products and cancer: a meta-analysis. Am J Public Health, **82**: 955-963.

Morrow NM & Minear RA (1987) Use of regression models to link raw water characteristics to THM concentration in drinking water. Water Res, **21**: 41.

Müller G, Spassovski M, & Henschler D (1974) Metabolism of trichloroethylene in man: II. Pharmacokinetics of metabolites. Arch Toxicol, **32**: 283-295.

Muller SP, Wolna P, Wunscher U, & Pankow D (1997) Cardiotoxicity of chlorodibromomethane and trichloromethane in rats and isolated rat cardiac myocytes. Arch Toxicol, **71**(12): 766-777.

Mullins PA & Proudlock RJ (1990) Assessment of nuclear anomalies in mice after administration of MX. Medmenham, United Kingdom, Water Research Centre (Report prepared by the Huntingdon Research Centre, United Kingdom).

Munson AE, Sain LE, Sanders VM, Kauffman BM, White KL, Page DG, Barnes DW, & Borzelleca JF (1982) Toxicology of organic water contaminants: trichloromethane, bromodichloromethane, dibromochloromethane and tribromomethane. Environ Health Perspect, **46**: 117-126.

Murphy PA (1993) Quantifying chemical risk from epidemiology studies: Application to the disinfectant by-product issue. In: Craun GF ed. Safety of water disinfection: Balancing chemical and microbial risks. Washington, DC, ILSI Press, pp 373-387.

Murphy PA & Craun GF (1990) A review of previous studies reporting associations between drinking water disinfection and cancer. In: Jolley RL, Condie LW, & Johnson JD ed. Water chlorination: Chemistry, environmental impact and health effects. Chelsea, Michigan, Lewis Publishers, Inc., vol 6, p 361.

Musil J, Knotek A, Chalupa J, & Schmidt P (1964) Toxicologic aspects of chlorine dioxide application for the treatment of water containing phenols. Scientific papers from Institute of Chemical Technology, Prague. Technol Water, 8: 327-345.

Nakajima M, Kitazawa M, Oba K, Kitagawa Y, & Toyoda Y (1989) Effect of route of administration in the micronucleus test with potassium bromate. Mutat Res, 223: 399-402.

Nakajima T, Elovaara E, Okino T, Gelboin HV, Klockars M, Riihimaki V, Aoyama T, & Vainio H (1995) Different contributions of cytochrome P450 2E1 and P450 2B1/2 to chloroform hepato-toxicity in rat. Toxicol Appl Pharmacol, 133: 215-222.

Narotsky MG, Hamby BT, Mitchell DS, & Kavlock RJ (1993) Bromoform requires a longer exposure period than carbon tetrachloride to induce pregnancy loss in F-344 rats. Toxicologist, 13: 255.

Narotsky MG, Pegram RA, & Kavlock RJ (1997) Effect of dosing vehicle on the developmental toxicity of bromodichloromethane and carbon tetrachloride in rats. Fundam Appl Toxicol, 40: 30-36.

NAS (1980) Committee on Drinking Water - Drinking water and health. Washington, DC, National Academy of Sciences, National Academy Press, vol 3, 415 pp.

NAS (1986) Committee on Drinking Water - Drinking water and health. Washington, DC, National Academy of Sciences, National Academy Press, vol 6, 457 pp.

Natarajan AT, Duivenvoorden WC, Meijers M, & Zwanenburg TS (1993) Induction of mitotic aneuploidy using Chinese hamster primary embryonic cells: Test results of 10 chemicals. Mutat Res, 287(1): 47-56.

National Center for Environmental Assessment (NCEA) (1998) NCEA position paper regarding risk assessment use of the results from the published study. Am J Public Health, 82: 955-963.

Nelson MA & Bull RJ (1988) Induction of strand breaks in DNA by trichloroethylene and metabolites in rat and mouse liver *in vivo*. Toxicol Appl Pharmacol, 94: 45-54.

Nelson MA, Lansing AJ, Sanchez IM, Bull RJ, & Springer DL (1989) Dichloroacetic acid and trichloroacetic acid-induced DNA strand breaks are independent of peroxisome proliferation. Toxicology, 58: 239-248.

Nelson MA, Sanchez IM, Bull RJ, & Sylvester SR (1990) Increased expression of c-myc and c-H-ras in dichloroacetate and trichloroacetate-induced liver tumors in B6C3F$_1$ mice. Toxicology, 64: 47-57.

Nestmann ER, Chu I, Kowbel DJ, & Matula TI (1980) Short-lived mutagen in *Salmonella* produced by reaction of trichloroacetic acid and dimethyl sulphoxide. Can J Genet Cytol, **22**(1): 35-40.

Neutra RR & Ostro B (1992) An evaluation of the role of epidemiology in assessing current and future disinfection technologies for drinking water. Sci Total Environ, **127**: 91-138.

Ni YC, Wong TY, Lloyd RV, Heinze TM, Shelton S, Casciano D, Kadlubar FF, & Fu PP (1996) Mouse liver microsomal metabolism of chloral hydrate, trichloroacetic acid, and trichloroethanol leading to induction of lipid peroxidation via a free radical mechanism. Drug Metab Dispos, **24**: 81-90.

Nicholl TA, Lopaschuk GD, & McNeill JH (1991) Effects of free fatty acids and dichloroacetate on isolated working diabetic heart. Am J Physiol, **261**: H1053-H1059.

Nieminski EC, Chaudhuri S, & Lamoreaux T (1993) The occurrence of DBPs in Utah drinking waters. J Am Water Works Assoc, **85**(9): 98-105.

Nishikawa A, Kinae N, Furukawa F, Mitsui M, Enami T, Hasegawa T, & Takahashi M (1994) Enhancing effects of 3-chloro-4-(dichloromethyl)-5-hydroxy-2(5H)-furanone (MX) on cell proliferation and lipid peroxidation in the rat gastric mucosa. Cancer Lett, **85**: 151-157.

Noack MG & Doerr RL (1978) Reactions of chlorine, chlorine dioxide and mixtures thereof with humic acid: an interim report on water chlorination. In: Jolley RL, Gorchev H, & Hamilton DH ed. Water chlorination: Environmental impact and health effects. Ann Arbor, Michigan, Ann Arbor Science Publishers, vol 2, pp 49-65.

Nordenberg A, Delisle G, & Izukawa T (1971) Cardiac arrhythmia in a child due to chloral hydrate ingestion. Pediatrics, **47**: 134-135.

NTP (1985) Toxicology and carcinogenesis studies of chlorodibromomethane in F344/N rats and B6C3F₁ mice (Gavage studies). Research Triangle Park, North Carolina, US Department of Health and Human Services, National Toxicology Program (NTP Technical Report Series No. 282).

NTP (1987) Toxicology and carcinogenesis studies of bromodichloromethane in F344/N rats and B6C3F₁ mice. Research Triangle Park, North Carolina, US Department of Health and Human Services, National Toxicology Program (NTP Technical Report Series No. 321; NIH Publication No. 88-2537).

NTP (1989a) Toxicology and carcinogenesis studies of tribromomethane (bromoform) in F344/N rats and B6C3F₁ mice (Gavage studies). Research Triangle Park, North Carolina, US Department of Health and Human Services, National Toxicology Program (NTP Technical Report Series No. 350).

NTP (1989b) Bromoform: Reproduction and fertility assessment in Swiss CD-1 mice when administered by gavage. Research Triangle Park, North Carolina, US Department of Health and Human Services, National Toxicology Program (NTP-89-068).

NTP (1992) Technical report on the toxicology and carcinogenesis studies of chlorinated and chloraminated water in F344/N rats and B6C3F₁ mice. Research Triangle Park, North Carolina, US Department of Health and Human Services, National Toxicology Program (NTP Technical Report Series No. 392; NIH Publication No. 91-2847).

Nuckols JR, Stallones L, & Reif J (1995) Evaluation of the use of a geographic information system in drinking water epidemiology. In: Reivhard E & Zapponi G ed. Assessing and managing health risks from drinking water contamination: Approaches and applications. Wallingford, United Kingdom, International Association of Hydrological Sciences, pp 111-122 (IAHS Publication No. 233).

Nudel DB, Peterson BJ, Buckley BJ, Kaplan NA, Weinhouse E, & Gootman N (1990) Comparative effects of bicarbonate and dichloroacetate in newborn swine with hypoxic lactic acidosis. Dev Pharmacol Ther, **15**: 86-93.

Nunn JW, Davies JE, & Chipman JK (1997) Production of unscheduled DNA synthesis in rodent hepatocytes *in vitro*, but not *in vivo*, by 3-chloro-(dichloromethyl)-5-hydroxy-2[5H]-furanone (MX). Mutat Res, **373**: 67-73.

Nutley EV, Tcheong AC, Allen JW, Collins BW, Ma M, Lowe XR, Bishop JB, Moore DH, & Wyrobek AJ (1996) Micronuclei induced in round spermatids of mice after stem-cell treatment with chloral hydrate: Evaluations with centromeric DNA probes and kinetochore antibodies. Environ Mol Mutagen, **28**(2): 80-89.

Oliver BG (1983) Dihaloacetonitriles in drinking water: algae and fulvic acids as precursors. Environ Sci Technol, **15**: 1075-1080.

Omichinski JG, Soderlund EJ, Dybing E, Pearson PG, & Nelson SD (1988) Detection and mechanism of formation of the potent direct-acting mutagen 2-bromoacrolein from 1,2-dibromo-3-chloropropionic acid. Toxicol Appl Pharmacol, **92**: 286-294.

Onodera H, Tanigawa H, Matsushima Y, Maekawa A, Kurokawa Y, & Hayashi Y (1986) Eosinophilic bodies in the proximal renal tubules of rats given potassium bromate. Bull Natl Inst Hyg Sci, **103**: 15-20.

Orme J, Taylor DH, Laurie RD, & Bull RJ (1985) Effects of chlorine dioxide on thyroid function in neonatal rats. J Toxicol Environ Health, **15**: 315-322.

Osgood C & Sterling D (1991) Dichloroacetonitrile, a by-product of water chlorination induces aneuploidy in *Drosophila*. Mutat Res, **261**(2): 85-91.

Page T, Harris RH, & Epstein SS (1976) Drinking water and cancer mortality in Louisiana. Science, **193**: 55-57.

Pankow D, Damme B, Wunscher U, & Bergmann K (1997) Chlorodibromomethane metabolism to bromide and carbon monoxide in rats. Arch Toxicol, **71**(4): 203-210.

Paode RD, Amy GL, Krasner SW, Summers RS, & Rice EW (1997) Predicting the formation of aldehydes. J Am Water Works Assoc, **89**(6): 79-93.

Parnell MJ, Koller LD, Exon JH, & Arnzen JM (1986) Trichloroacetic acid effects on rat liver peroxisomes and enzyme-altered foci. Environ Health Perspect, **69**: 73-79.

Parrish JM, Austin EW, Stevens DK, Kinder DH, & Bull RJ (1996) Haloacetate-induced oxidative damage to DNA in the liver of male B6C3F$_1$ mice. Toxicology, **110**: 103-111.

Paykoc ZV & Powell JF (1945) The effect of sodium trichloroacetate. J Pharmacol Exp Ther, **85**: 289-293.

Pegram RA, Lilly PD, Thornton-Manning JR, Simmons JE, McDonald A, & Moore TC (1993) Diurnal cycle dependent renal and hepatic toxicity of bromodichloromethane. Toxicologist, **13**: 360.

Pegram RA, Andersen ME, Warren SH, Ross TM, & Claxton LD (1996) Glutathione S-transferase-mediated mutagenicity of trihalomethanes. Toxicologist, **30**: 291.

Pegram RA, Andersen ME, Warren SH, Ross TM, & Claxton LD (1997) Glutathione S-transferase-mediated mutagenicity of trihalomethanes in Salmonella typhimurium: contrasting results with bromodichloromethane and chloroform. Toxicol Appl Pharmacol, **144**: 183-188.

Penn A, Lu MX, & Parkes JL (1990) Ingestion of chlorinated water has no effect upon indicators of cardiovascular disease in pigeons. Toxicology, **63**(3): 301-313.

Pereira MA (1994) Route of administration determines whether chloroform enhances or inhibits cell proliferation in the liver of B6C3F$_1$ mice. Fundam Appl Toxicol, **23**: 87-92.

Pereira MA (1995) Effect of dichloroacetic acid and trichloroacetic acid upon cell proliferation in B6C3F$_1$ mice: Final project report. Denver, Colorado, American Water Works Association Research Foundation.

Pereira MA (1996) Carcinogenic activity of dichloroacetic acid and trichloroacetic acid in the liver of female B6C3F$_1$ mice. Fundam Appl Toxicol, **31**: 192-199.

Pereira MA & Grothaus M (1997) Chloroform in drinking water prevents hepatic cell proliferation induced by chloroform administered by gavage in corn oil to mice. Fundam Appl Toxicol, **37**(1): 82-87.

Pereira MA & Phelps BJ (1996) Promotion by dichloroacetic acid and trichloroacetic acid of N-methyl-N-nitrosourea-initiated cancer in the liver of female B6C3F$_1$ mice. Cancer Lett, **102**: 133-141.

Pereira MA, Lin LH, Lippitt JM, & Herren SL (1982) Trihalomethanes as initiators and promoters of carcinogenesis. Environ Health Perspect, **46**: 151-156.

Pereira MA, Lin LH, & Mattox JK (1984) Haloacetonitrile excretion as thiocyanate and inhibition of dimethylnitrosamine demethylase: A proposed metabolic scheme. J Toxicol Environ Health, **13**: 633-641.

Peters RJB (1991) The analysis of halogenated acetic acids in Dutch drinking water. Water Res, **25**(4): 473-477.

Peters CJ, Young RJ, & Perry R (1980) Factors influencing the formation of haloforms in the chlorination of humic materials. Environ Sci Technol, **14**: 1391-1395.

Peters RJB, De Leer EWB, & De Galan L (1990) Dihaloacetonitriles in Dutch drinking water. Water Res, **24**(6): 797-800.

Pfeiffer EH (1978) Health aspects of water chlorination with special consideration to the carcinogenicity of chlorine II. Communication: On the carcinogenicity. Zent.bl Bakteriol Hyg I. Abt Orig B, **166**: 185-211.

Piantadosi S (1994) Invited commentary: Ecologic biases. Am J Epidemiol, **139**(8): 71-64.

Piantadosi S, Byar DP, & Green SB (1988) The ecological fallacy. Am J Epidemiol, **18**: 269-274.

Pilotto LS (1995) Disinfection of drinking water, disinfection by-products and cancer: what about Australia? Aust J Public Health, **19**(1): 89-93.

Pleil JD & Lindstrom AB (1997) Exhaled human breath measurement method for assessing exposure to halogenated volatile organic compounds. Clin Chem, **43**(5): 723-730.

Pohl LR, Branchflower RV, Highet RJ, Martin JL, Nunn DS, Monks TJ, George JW, & Hinson JA (1981) The formation of diglutathionyl dithiocarbonate as a metabolite of chloroform, bromotrichloromethane, and carbon tetrachloride. Drug Metab Dispos, **9**: 334-339.

Polhuijs M, Te Koppele JM, Fockens E, & Mulder GJ (1989) Glutathione conjugation of the alpha-bromoisovaleric acid enantiomers in the rat *in vivo* and its stereoselectivity. Biochem Pharmacol, **38**: 3957-3962.

Polhuijs M, Meijer DK, & Mulder GJ (1991) The fate of diastereomeric glutathione conjugates of bromoisovalerylurea in blood in the rat *in vivo* and in the perfused rat liver. Stereoselectivity in biliary and urinary excretion. J Pharmacol Exp Ther, **256**: 458-461.

Polhuijs M, Mulder GJ, Meyer DJ, & Ketterer B (1992) Stereoselective conjugation of 2-bromocarboxylic acids and their urea derivatives by rat liver glutathione transferase 12-12 and some other isoforms. Biochem Pharmacol, **444**: 1249-1253.

Poole C (1994) Editorial: Ecologic analysis as outlook and method. Am J Public Health, **84**(5): 715-716.

Poole C (1997) Analytical meta-analysis of epidemiologic studies of chlorinated drinking water and cancer: quantitative review and re-analysis of the work published by Morris et al., Am J Public Health, 82: 955-963. Cincinnati, Ohio, US Environmental Protection Agency, National Center for Environmental Assessment.

Poon R, Levalier P, & Tryphonas H (1997) Effects of subchronic exposure of monochloramine in drinking water on male rats. Regul Toxicol Pharmacol, **25**(2): 166-175.

Potter CL, Chang LW, DeAngelo AB, & Daniel FB (1996) Effects of four trihalomethanes on DNA strand breaks, renal hyaline droplet formation and serum testosterone in male F344 rats. Cancer Lett, **106**(2): 235-242.

Prieto R & Fernandez E (1993) Toxicity and mutagenesis by chlorate are independent of nitrate reductase in *Chlamydomonas reinhardtii*. Mol Gen Genet, **237**: 429-438.

Proudlock RJ & Crouch MJ (1990) Nuclear anomaly test on MX (mouse stomach). Medmenham, United Kingdom, Water Research Centre (Report prepared by the Huntingdon Research Centre, United Kingdom).

Racey-Burns LA, Burns AH, Summer WR, & Shephard RE (1989) The effect of dichloroacetate on the isolated no flow arrested rat heart. Life Sci, **44**: 2015-2023.

Rav-Acha C & Choshen E (1987) Aqueous reactions of chlorine dioxide with hydrocarbons. Environ Sci Technol, **21**(11): 1069-1074.

Raymond P & Plaa GL (1997) Effect of dosing vehicle on the hepatotoxicity of carbon tetrachloride and nephrotoxicity of chloroform in rats. J Toxicol Environ Health, **51**(5): 463-476.

Reckhow DA & Singer PC (1985) Mechanisms of organic halide formation during fulvic acid chlorination and implications with respect to preozonation. In: Jolley RL, Bull RJ, & Davis WP ed. Water chlorination: chemistry, environmental impact and health effects. Chelsea, Michigan, Lewis Publishers, Inc., vol 5, pp 1229-1257.

Reckhow DA, Singer PC & Malcolm RL (1990) Chlorination of humic materials: by-product formation and chemical interpretation. Environ Sci Technol, **24**(11): 1655-1664.

Reddy TV, Chang LW, DeAngelo AB, Pereira MA, & Daniel FB (1992) Effect of non-genotoxic environmental contaminants on cholesterol and DNA synthesis in cultured primary rat hepato-cytes. Environ Sci, **1**: 179-189.

Reif JS, Hatch MC, Bracken M, Holmes LB, Schwetz BA, & Singer PC (1996) Reproductive and developmental effects of disinfection by-products in drinking water. Environ Health Perspect, **104**(10): 1056-1061.

Revis NW, McCauley P, Bull R, & Holdsworth G (1986a) Relationship of drinking water disinfectants to plasma cholesterol and thyroid hormone levels in experimental studies. Proc Natl Acad Sci (USA), **83**: 1485-1489.

Revis NW, McCauley P, & Holdsworth G (1986b) Relationship of dietary iodide and drinking water disinfectants to thyroid function in experimental animals. Environ Health Perspect, **69**: 243-248.

Reynolds SH, Stowers SJ, Patterson RM, Maronpot RR, Aaronson SA, & Anderson MW (1987) Activated oncogenes in B6C3F$_1$ mouse liver tumors: Implications for risk assessment. Science, **237**: 1309-1316.

Richardson AP (1937) Toxic potentialities of continued administration of chlorate for blood and tissues. J Pharmacol Exp Ther, **59**: 101-113.

Richmond RE, DeAngelo AB, Potter CL, & Daniel FB (1991) The role of hyperplastic nodules in dichloroacetic acid-induced hepatocarcinogenesis in B6C3F$_1$ mice. Carcinogenesis, **12**: 1383-1387.

Richmond RE, Carter JH, Carter HW, Daniel FB, & DeAngelo AB (1995) Immunohistochemical analysis of dichloroacetic acid (DCA)-induced hepatocarcinogenesis in male Fischer (F344) rats. Cancer Lett, **92**: 67-76.

Rijhsinghani KS, Abrahams C, Swerdlow MA, Rao KV, & Ghose T (1986) Induction of neoplastic lesions in the livers of C57BL × C3HF$_1$ mice by chloral hydrate. Cancer Detect Prev, **9**: 279-288.

Riley TJ, Cauley JA, & Murphy P (1995) Water chlorination and lipo- and apolipoproteins: the relationship in elderly white women of Pennsylvania. Am J Public Health, **85**(4): 570-573.

Ringhand HP, Kaylor WH, Miller RG, & Kopfler FC (1989) Synthesis of 3-^{14}C-3-chloro-4-(dichloro-methyl)-5-hydroxy-2(5H)-furanone and its use in a tissue distribution study in the rat. Chemosphere, **18**: 2229-2236.

Risch HA, Burch JD, Miller AB, Hill GB, Steele R, & Howe GR (1988) Dietary factors and the incidence of cancer of the urinary bladder. Am J Epidemiol, **127**(6): 1179-1191.

Risch HA, Burch JD, Miller AB, Hill GB, Steele R, & Howe GR (1992) Editorial: Chlorinated water and cancer - Is a meta-analysis a better analysis? Pediatr Alert, **17**: 91.

Robinson M, Bull RJ, Schamer M, & Long RE (1986) Epidermal hyperplasia in mouse skin following treatment with alternative drinking water disinfectants. Environ Health Perspect, **69**: 293-300.

Robinson M, Bull RJ, Olson GR, & Stober J (1989) Carcinogenic activity associated with halogenated acetones and acroleins in the mouse skin assay. Cancer Lett, **48**: 197-203.

Roby MR, Carle S, Pereira MA, & Carter DE (1986) Excretion and tissue disposition of dichloroacetonitrile in rats and mice. Environ Health Perspect, **69**: 215-220.

Rook JJ (1977) Chlorination reactions of fulvic acids in natural waters. J Environ Sci Technol, **11**: 478-482.

Rook JJ, Gras AA, van der Heijden BG, & de Wee J (1978) Bromide oxidation and organic substitution in water treatment. J Environ Sci Health, **A13**: 91-116.

Rosen JD, Segall Y, & Casida JE (1980) Mutagenic potency of haloacroleins and related compounds. Mutat Res, **78**: 113-119.

Rosenkranz HS (1973) Sodium hypochlorite and sodium perborate: preferential inhibitors of DNA polymerase-deficient bacteria. Mutat Res, **21**: 171-174.

Rosenkranz HS, Gutter B, & Speck WT (1976) Mutagenicity and DNA-modifying activity: A comparison of two microbial assays. Mutat Res, **41**: 61-70.

Rothman KJ (1986) Modern epidemiology. Boston, Massachusetts, Little Brown Co.

Ruddick JA, Villeneuve DC, Chu I, & Valli VE (1983) A teratological assessment of four trihalomethanes in the rat. J Environ Sci Health, **B18**: 333-349.

Russo A & Levis AG (1992) Detection of aneuploidy in male germ cells of mice by means of a meiotic micronucleus assay. Mutat Res, **281**(3): 187-191.

Russo A, Pacchierotti F, & Metalli P (1984) Nondisjunction induced in mouse spermatogenesis by chloral hydrate, a metabolite of trichloroethylene. Environ Mutagen, **6**: 695-703.

Russo A, Stocco A, & Majone F (1992) Identification of kinetochore-containing (CREST+) micronuclei in mouse bone marrow erythrocytes. Mutagenesis, **5**(3): 195-197.

Sai K, Takagi A, Umemura T, Hasegawa R, & Kurokawa Y (1991) Relation of 8-hydroxy-deoxyguanosine formation in rat kidney to lipid peroxidation, glutathione level and relative organ weight after a single administration of potassium bromate. Jpn J Cancer Res (Gann), **82**: 165-169.

Sai K, Hayashi M, Takagi A, Hasegawa R, Sofuni T, & Kurokawa Y (1992a) Effects of antioxidants on induction of micronuclei in rat peripheral blood reticulocytes by potassium bromate. Mutat Res, **269**: 113-118.

Sai K, Uchiyama S, Ohno Y, Hasegawa R, & Kurokawa Y (1992b) Generation of active oxygen species *in vitro* by the interaction of potassium bromate with rat kidney cell. Carcinogenesis, **13**: 333-339.

Sai K, Umemura T, Takagi A, Hasegawa R, & Kurokawa Y (1992c) The protective role of glutathione, cysteine and vitamin C against oxidative DNA damage induced in rat kidney by potassium bromate. Jpn J Cancer Res (Gann), **83**: 45-51.

Saijo T, Naito E, Ito M, Takeda E, Hashimoto T, & Kuroda Y (1991) Therapeutic effect of sodium dichloroacetate on visual and auditory hallucinations in a patient with MELAS. Neuropediatrics, **22**: 166-167.

Saillenfait AM, Langonne I, & Sabate JP (1995) Developmental toxicity of trichloroethylene, tetrachloroethylene and four of their metabolites in rat whole embryo culture. Arch Toxicol, **70**: 71-82.

Sakai M, Matsushimia-Hibiya Y, Nishizawa M, & Nishi S (1995) Suppression of rat glutathione transferase P expression by peroxisome proliferators: Interactions between Jun and peroxisome proliferator-activated receptor alpha. Cancer Res, **55**: 5370-5376.

Sanchez IM & Bull RJ (1990) Early induction of reparative hyperplasia in the liver of B6C3F$_1$ mice treated with dichloroacetate and trichloroacetate. Toxicology, **64**: 33-46.

Sanders VM, Kauffmann BM, White KL, Douglas KA, Barnes DW, Sain LE, Bradshaw TJ, Borzelleca JF, & Munson AE (1982) Toxicology of chloral hydrate in the mouse. Environ Health Perspect, **44**: 137-146.

Sans RM, Jolly WW, & Harris RA (1980) Studies on the regulation of leucine catabolism: Mechanism responsible for oxidizable substrate inhibition and dichloroacetate stimulation of leucine catabolism by the heart. Arch Biochem Biophys, **200**: 336-345.

Savin JE & Cohn PD (1996) Comparison of bladder and rectal cancer incidence with trihalomethanes in drinking water. Epidemiology, **7**(suppl 4): S63.

Savitz DA, Andrews KW, & Pastore LM (1995) Drinking water and pregnancy outcome in central North Carolina: Source, amount, and trihalomethane levels. Environ Health Perspect, **103**(6): 592-596.

Sbrana I, Di Sibio A, Lomi A, & Scarcelli V (1993) C-mitosis and numerical chromosome aberration analyses in human lymphocytes: 10 known or suspected spindle poisons. Mutat Res. **287**(1): 57-70.

Scatina J, Abdel-Rahman MS, Gerges SE, Khan MY, & Gona O (1984) Pharmacodynamics of Alcide, a new antimicrobial compound, in rat and rabbit. Fundam Appl Toxicol, **4**: 479-484.

Schechter DS & Singer F' (1995) Formation of aldehydes during ozonation. J Ozone Sci Eng, **17**(1): 53-69.

Schoonjans K, Watanabe M, Suzuki H, Mahfoudi A, Krey G, Wahli W, Grimaldi P, Staels B, Yamamoto T, & Auwerx J (1995) Induction of the acyl-coenzyme A synthetase gene by fibrates and fatty acids is mediated by a peroxisome proliferator response element of the C promoter. J Biol Chem, **270**: 19 269-19 276.

Schultz IR, Merdink JL, Gonzalez-Leon A, & Bull RJ (1999) Comparative toxicokinetics of chlorinated and brominated haloacetates in F344 rats. Toxicol Appl Pharmacol, **158**(2): 103-114.

Schwartz S (1995) The fallacy of the ecological fallacy: the potential misuse of a concept and the consequences. Am J Public Health, **84**(5): 819-823.

Schwartz DA, Smith DD, & Lakshminarayan MD (1990) The pulmonary sequelae associated with accidental inhalation of chlorine gas. Chest, **97**: 820-825.

Sclimenti MJ, Krasner SW, Glaze WH, & Weinberg HS (1990) Ozone disinfection by-products: optimization of the PFBHA derivatization method for the analysis of aldehydes. In: Proceedings of the Water Quality Conference, San Francisco, CA. Denver, Colorado, American Water Works Association.

Scully FE, Mazina KE, Ringhand HP, Chess EK, Campbell JA, & Johnson JD (1990) Identification of organic *N*-chloramines *in vitro* in stomach fluid from the rat after chlorination. Chem Res Toxicol, **3**: 301-306.

Segall Y, Kimmel EC, Dohn DR, & Casida JE (1985) 3-Substituted 2-halopropenals: mutagenicity, detoxification and formation from 3-substituted 2,3-dihalopropenal promutagens. Mutat Res, **158**: 61-68.

Sellers EM & Koch-Weser J (1970) Potentiation of warfarin-induced hypoprothrominemia by chloral hydrate. N Engl J Med, **283**: 827-831.

Sellers EM, Lang M, Koch-Weser J, LeBlanc E, & Kalant H (1972) Interaction of chloral hydrate and ethanol in man: I. Metabolism. Clin Pharmacol Ther, **13**: 37-49.

Shangraw RE, Winter R, Hromco J, Robinson T, & Gallaher EJ (1994) Amelioration of lactic acidosis with dichloroacetate during liver transplantation in humans. Anesthesiology, **81**: 1127-1138.

Sheahan BJ, Pugh DM, & Winstanley EW (1971) Experimental sodium chlorate poisoning in dogs. Res Vet Sci, **12**: 387-389.

Sherer TT, Sylvester SR, & Bull RJ (1993) Differential expression of c-erbA mRNAs in the developing cerebellum and cerevral cortex of the rat. Biol Neonate, **63**(1): 26-34.

Shih KL & Lederberg J (1976) Chloramine mutagenesis in *Bacillus subtilis*. Science, **192**: 1141-1143.

Shukairy HM & Summers RS (1992) The impact of preozonation and biodegradation on disinfection by-product formation. Water Res, **26**(9): 1217-1227.

Shy CM (1985) Chemical contamination of water supplies. Environ Health Perspect, **62**: 399-406.

Siddiqui MS (1992) Ozone-bromide interactions: Formation of DBPs. Tucson, Arizona, University of Arizona (Ph.D. Dissertation).

Siddiqui MS (1996) Chlorine-ozone interactions: Formation of chlorate. Water Res, 30(9): 2160-2170.

Siddiqui MS & Amy GL (1993) Factors affecting DBP formation during ozone-bromide reactions. J Am Water Works Assoc, 85(1): 63-72.

Siddiqui MS, Amy GL, Ozekin K, Zhai W, & Westerhoff P (1994) Alternative strategies for removing bromate. J Am Water Works Assoc, 86(10): 81-96.

Siddiqui MS, Amy GL, & Rice RG (1995) Bromate ion formation: a critical review. J Am Water Works Assoc, 87(10): 58-70.

Siddiqui MS, Zhai W, Amy GL, & Mysore C (1996a) Bromate ion removal by activated carbon. Water Res, 30(7): 1651-1660.

Siddiqui MS, Amy GL, Cooper W, Kurucz CN, Waite TD, & Nickelson GM (1996b) Bromate ion removal by high energy electron beam irradiation. J Am Water Works Assoc, 88(10): 90-101.

Siddiqui MS, Amy GL, & McCollum LJ (1996c) Bromate destruction by UV irradiation and electric arc discharge. J Ozone Sci Eng, 18(3): 271-290.

Siddiqui MS, Amy GL, & Murphy BD (1997) Ozone enhanced removal of natural organic matter. Water Res, 31(12): 3098-3106.

Silver W & Stier M (1971) Cardiac arrhythmias from chloralhydrate. Pediatrics, 48(2): 332-333.

Silver EM, Kuttab SH, Hansan T, & Hassan M (1982) Structural considerations in the metabolism of nitriles to cyanide *in vivo*. Drug Metab Dispos, 10: 495-498.

Simmon VF & Tardiff RG (1978) The mutagenic activity of halogenated compounds found in chlorinated drinking water. In: Water chlorination: Environmental impacts and health effects. Ann Arbor, Michigan, Ann Arbor Science Publishers, pp 417-431.

Singelmann E & Steffen C (1983) Increased erythrocyte rigidity in chlorate poisoning. J Clin Pathol, 36: 719.

Singelmann E, Wetzel E, Adler G, & Steffen C (1984) Erythrocyte membrane alterations as the basis of chlorate toxicity. Toxicology, 30: 135-147.

Singer PC (1993) Formation and characterization of DBPs. In: Craun GF ed. Safety of water disinfection: balancing chemical and microbial risks. Washington, DC, ILSI Press.

Singer PC (1994a) Control of disinfection by-products in drinking water. J Environ Eng, 120(4): 727-744.

Singer PC (1994b) Impacts of ozonation on the formation of chlorination and chloramination by-products. Denver, Colorado, American Water Works Association Research Foundation.

Sketchell J, Peterson HG, & Christofi N (1995) Disinfection by-product formation after biologically assisted GAC treatment of water supplies with different bromide and DOC content. Water Res, **29**(12): 2635-2642.

Slattery ML, West DW, & Robison LM (1988) Fluid intake and bladder cancer in Utah. Int J Cancer, **42**: 17-22.

Smith MK, George EL, Zenick H, Manson JM, & Stober JA (1987) Developmental toxicity of halogenated acetonitriles: Drinking water by-products of chlorine disinfection. Toxicology, **46**: 83-93.

Smith MK, Randall JL, Tocco DR, York RG, Stober JA, & Read EJ (1988) Teratogenic effects of trichloroacetonitrile in the Long-Evans rat. Teratology, **38**: 113-120.

Smith MK, Randall JL, Read EJ, & Stober JA (1989a) Teratogenic activity of trichloroacetic acid in the rat. Teratology, **40**: 445-451.

Smith MK, Randall JL, Stober JA, & Read EJ (1989b) Developmental toxicity of dichloro-acetonitrile: A by-product of drinking water disinfection. Fundam Appl Toxicol, **12**: 765-772.

Smith MK, Randall JL, Read EJ, & Stober JA (1992) Developmental toxicity of dichloroacetate in the rat. Teratology, **46**: 217-223.

Smith MK, Thrall BD, & Bull RJ (1997) Dichloroacetate (DCA) modulates insulin signaling. Toxicologist, **36**: 1133-1140.

Snyder MP & Margerum DW (1982) Kinetics of chlorine transfer from chloramine to amines, amino acids, and peptides. Inorg Chem, 21: 2545-2550.

Snyder RD, Pullman J, Carter JH, Carter HW, & DeAngelo AB (1995) *In vivo* administration of dichloroacetic acid suppresses spontaneous apoptosis in murine hepatocytes. Cancer Res, **55**: 3702-3705.

So BJ & Bull RJ (1995) Dibromoacetate (DBA) acts as a promoter of abnormal crypt foci in the colon of F344 rats. Toxicologist, **15**: 1242.

Sobti RC (1984) Sister chromatid exchange potential of the halogenated hydrocarbons produced during water chlorination. Chromosome Inf Serv, **37**: 17-19.

Sood C & O'Brien PJ (1993) Molecular mechanisms of chloroacetaldehyde-induced cytotoxicity in isolated rat hepatocytes. Biochem Pharmacol, **46**: 1621-1626.

Sora S & Carbone MJ (1987) Chloral hydrate, methylmercury hydroxide and ethidium bromide affect chromosomal segregation during meiosis of *Saccharomyces cerevisiae*. Mutat Res, **190**: 13-17.

Speitel GE, Symons JM, Diehl AC, Sorensen HW, & Cipparone LA (1993) Effect of ozone dose and subsequent biodegration on removal of disinfection by-products precursors. J Am Water Works Assoc, **85**(5): 86-95.

Spengler SJ & Singer B (1988) Formation of interstrand cross-links in chloroacetaldehyde treated DNA demonstrated by ethidium bromide fluorescence. Cancer Res, **48**: 4804-4806.

Spirtas R, Stewart PA, Lee JS, Marano DE, Forbes CD, Grauman DJ, Pettigrew HM, Blair A, Hoover RN, & Cohen JL (1991) Retrospective cohort study of workers at an aircraft maintenance facility: I. Epidemiological results. Br J Ind Med, **48**: 515-530.

Sprankle CS, Larson JL, Goldsworthy SM, & Butterworth BE (1996) Levels of myc, fos, Ha-ras, met and hepatocyte growth factor mRNA during regenerative cell proliferation in female mouse liver and male rat kidney after a cytotoxic dose of chloroform. Cancer Lett, **101**: 97-106.

Stacpoole PW (1989) The pharmacology of dichloroacetate. Metabolism, **38**: 1124-1144.

Stacpoole PW & Felts JM (1970) Diisopropylammonium dichloroacetate (DIPA) and sodium dichloroacetate (DCA): Effect on glucose and fat metabolism in normal and diabetic tissue. Metabolism, **19**: 71-78.

Stacpoole PW & Greene YJ (1992) Dichloroacetate. Diabetes Care, **15**: 785-791.

Stacpoole PW, Moore GW, & Kornhauser DM (1978) Metabolic effects of dichloroacetate in patients with diabetes mellitus and hyperlipoproteinemia. N Engl J Med, **298**: 526-530.

Stacpoole PW, Harwood HJ, & Varnado CE (1983) Regulation of rat liver hydroxymethylglutaryl coenzyme A reductase by a new class of noncompetitive inhibitors: Effects of dichloroacetate and related carboxylic acids on enzyme activity. J Clin Invest, **72**: 1575-1585.

Stacpoole PW, Harwood HJ, Cameron DF, Curry SH, Samuelson DA, Cornwell PE, & Sauberlich HE (1990) Chronic toxicity of dichloroacetate: Possible relation to thiamine deficiency in rats. Fundam Appl Toxicol, **14**: 327-337.

Stacpoole PW, Wright EC, Baumgartner TG, Bersin RM, Buchalter S, Curry SH, Duncan CA, Harman EM, Henderson GN, Jenkinson S, Lachin JM, Lorenz A, Schneider SH, Siegel JH, Summer WR, Thompson D, Wolfe CL, & Zorovich B (1992) A controlled clinical trial of dichloroacetate for treatment of lactic acidosis in adults. N Engl J Med, **327**: 1564-1569.

Stauber AJ & Bull RJ (1997) Differences in phenotype and cell replicative behavior of hepatic tumors inducted by dichloroacetate (DCA) and trichloroacetate (TCA). Toxicol Appl Pharmacol, **144**(2): 235-246.

Stauber AJ, Bull RJ, & Thrall BD (1998) Dichloroacetate and trichloroacetate promote clonal expansion of anchorage-independent hepatocytes *in vivo* and *in vitro*. Toxicol Appl Pharmacol, **150**: 287-294.

Steffen C & Seitz R (1981) Severe chlorate poisoning: Report of a case. Arch Toxicol, **48**: 281-288.

Steffen C & Wetzel E (1993) Chlorate poisoning: Mechanism of toxicity. Toxicology, **84**: 217-231.

Stenner RD, Merdink JL, Templin MV, Stevens DK, Springer DL, & Bull RJ (1996) Enterohepatic recirculation of trichloroethanol glucuronide as a significant source of trichloroacetic acid in the metabolism of trichloroethylene. Drug Metab Dispos, **25**: 529-535.

Stevens JL & Anders MW (1981) Metabolism of haloforms to cabon monoxide: IV. Studies on the reaction mechanism *in vivo*. Chem-Biol Interact, **37**: 365-374.

Stevens AA, Slocum CJ, Seeger DR, & Robeck GG (1976) Chlorination of organics in drinking water. J Am Water Works Assoc, 68(11): 615.

Stevens AA, Moore LA, & Slocum CJ (1989) By-products of chlorination at ten operating utilities. In: Disinfection by-products: Current perspectives. Denver, Colorado, American Water Works Association, pp 23-61.

Stevens DK, Eyre RJ, & Bull RJ (1992) Adduction of hemoglobin and albumin *in vivo* by metabolites of trichloroethylene, trichloroacetate and dichloroacetate in rats and mice. Fundam Appl Toxicol, 19: 336-342.

Stocker KJ, Statham J, Howard WR, & Proudlock RJ (1997) Assessment of the potential *in vivo* genotoxicity of three trihalomethanes: chlorodibromomethane, bromodichloromethane and bromoform. Mutagenesis, 12(3): 169-173.

Strauss BS (1991) The "A-rule" of mutagen specificity: a consequence of DNA polymerase bypass of noninstructional lesions. Bioessays, 13(2): 79-84.

Struba RJ (1979) Cancer and drinking water quality. Chapel Hill, North Carolina, University of North Carolina (Thesis).

Styles JA, Wyatt I, & Coutts C (1991) Trichloroacetic acid: studies on uptake and effects on hepatic DNA and liver growth in mice. Carcinogenesis, 12: 1715-1719.

Suarez-Varela MM, Gonzalez AL, Perez ML, & Caraco EF (1994) Chlorination of drinking water and cancer incidence. J Environ Pathol Toxicol Oncol, 13(1): 39-41.

Suh DH & Abdel-Rahman MS (1983) Kinetics study of chloride in rat. J Toxicol Environ Health, 12: 467-473.

Suh DH, Abdel-Rahman MS, & Bull RJ (1983) Effect of chlorine dioxide and its metabolites in drinking water on fetal developmental in rats. J Appl Toxicol, 3: 75-79.

Susser M (1994a) The logic in ecological: I. The logic of analysis. Am J Public Health, 84(5): 825-829.

Susser M (1994b) The logic in ecological: II. The logic of design. Am J Public Health, 84(5): 830-835.

Suzuki N & Nakanishi J (1995) Brominated analogues of MX (3-chloro-4-(dichloromethyl)-5-hydroxy-2(5H)-furanone) in chlorinated drinking water. Chemosphere, 30: 1557-1564.

Swan SH & Waller K (1998) Disinfection by-products and adverse pregnancy outcomes: what is the agent and how should it be measured? [Editorial; comment]. Epidemiology, 9(5): 479-481.

Swan SH, Waller K, Hopkins B, Windam G, Fenster L, Schaefer C, & Neutra RR (1998) A prospective study of spontaneous abortion: relation to amount and source of drinking water consumed in early pregnancy. Epidemiology, 9(2): 126-139.

Symons JM & Worley KL (1995) An advanced oxidation process for DBP control. J Am Water Works Assoc, 87(11): 66-75.

Symons JM, Stevens AA, Clark RM, Geldreich EE, Love OT, & De Marco J (1981) Treatment techniques for controlling trihalomethanes in drinking water. Washington, DC, US Environmental Protection Agency (EPA 600/2-81-156).

Takamura N, Kurokawa Y, Matsushima Y, Imazawa T, Onodera H, & Hayashi Y (1985) Long-term oral administration of potassium bromate in male Syrian golden hamsters. Sci Rep Res Inst Tohoku Univ, 32(1-4): 43-46.

Tao L, Kramer PM, Latendresse JR, & Pereira MA (1996) Expression of the protooncogenes, TGF-α and β in the liver of B6C3F$_1$ mice treated with trichloroethylene, dichloroacetic and trichloroacetic acid. Toxicologist, 15: 1495.

Taylor DH & Pfohl RJ (1985) Effects of chlorine dioxide on neurobehavioral development of rats. In: Jolley RL, Bull RJ, & Davis WP ed. Water chlorination: Chemistry, environmental impact and health effects. Chelsea, Michigan, Lewis Publishers, Inc., vol 5, pp 355-364.

Temperman J & Maes R (1966) Suicidal poisoning by sodium chlorate: A report of three cases. J Forensic Med, 13: 123-129.

Templin MV, Parker JC, & Bull RJ (1993) Relative formation of dichloroacetate and trichloroacetate from trichloroethylene in male B6C3F$_1$ mice. Toxicol Appl Pharmacol, 123: 1-8.

Templin MV, Stevens DK, Stenner RD, Bonate PL, Tuman D, & Bull RJ (1995) Factors affecting species differences in the kinetics of metabolites of trichloroethylene. J Toxicol Environ Health, 44: 435-447.

Templin MV, Jamison KC, Wolf DC, Morgan KT, & Butterworth BE (1996a) Comparison of chloroform-induced toxicity in the kidneys, liver, and nasal passages of male Osborne-Mendel and F-344 rats. Cancer Lett, 104: 71-78.

Templin MV, Jamison KC, Sprankle CS, Wolf DC, Wong BA, & Butterworth BE (1996b) Chloroform-induced cytotoxicity and regenerative cell proliferation in the kidneys and liver of BDF$_1$ mice. Cancer Lett, 108: 225-231.

Templin MV, Larson JL, Butterworth BE, Jamison KC, Leininger JR, Mery S, Morgan KT, Wong BA, & Wolf DC (1996c) A 90-day chloroform inhalation study in F-344 rats: profile of toxicity and relevance to cancer studies. Fundam Appl Toxicol, 32: 109-125.

Templin MV, Constan AA, Wolf DC, Wong BA, & Butterworth BE (1998) Patterns of chloroform-induced regenerative cell proliferation in BDF$_1$ mice correlate with organ specificity and dose-response of tumor formation. Carcinogenesis, 19(1): 187-193.

Teng H & Veenstra J (1995) Disinfection by-products formed using four alternative disinfectants as a function of precursor characteristics. In: Minear R & Amy G ed. Disinfection by-products in water treatment. Chelsea, Michigan, Lewis Publishers, Inc.

TERA (1998) Toxicology excellence for risk assessment - Health risk assessment/ characterization of the drinking water disinfection byproducts chlorine dioxide and chlorite (8W-0766-NTLX). Cincinnati, Ohio.

Testai E, Di Marzio S, di Domenico A, Piccardi A, & Vittozzi L (1995) An in vitro investigation of the reductive metabolism of chloroform. Arch Toxicol, 70: 83-88.

Testai E, De Curtis V, Gemma S, Fabrizi L, Gervasi P, & Vittozzi L (1996) The role of different cytochrome P450 isoforms in *in vitro* chloroform metabolism. J Biochem Toxicol, **11**: 305-312.

Thier R, Taylor JB, Pemble SE, Humphreys WG, Persmark M, Ketterer B, & Guengerich FP (1993) Expression of mammalian glutathione *S*-transferase 5-5 in *Salmonella typhimurium* TA1535 leads to base-pair mutations upon exposure to dihalomethanes. Proc Natl Acad Sci (USA), **90**: 8576-8580.

Thier R, Pemble SE, Kramer H, Taylor JB, Guengerich FP, & Ketterer B (1996) Human glutathione *S*-transferase T1-1 enhances mutagenicity of 1,2-dibromoethane, dibromomethane, and 1,2,3,4-diepoxybutane in *Salmonella typhimurium*. Carcinogenesis, **17**: 163-166.

Thomas EL, Jefferson MM, Bennett JJ, & Learn DB (1987) Mutagenic activity of chloramines. Mutat Res, **188**: 35-41.

Thornton-Manning JR, Gao P, Lilly PD, & Pegram RA (1993) Acute bromodichloromethane toxicity in rats pretreated with cytochrome P450 inducers and inhibitors. Toxicologist, **13**: 361 (abstract).

Thornton-Manning JR, Seely JR, & Pegram RA (1994) Toxicity of bromodichloromethane in female rats and mice after repeated oral dosing. Toxicology, **94**: 3-18.

Thurman EM (1985) Developments in biochemistry: Organic geochemistry of natural waters. Dordrecht, The Netherlands, Nijhoff M & Junk W Publishers.

Tomasi A, Albano E, Biasi F, Slater TF, Vannini V, & Dianzani M (1985) Activation of chloroform and related trihalomethanes to free radical intermediates in isolated hepatocytes and in the rat *in vivo* as detected by the ESR-spin trapping technique. Chem-Biol Interact, **55**: 303-316.

Tong Z, Board PG, & Anders MW (1998) Glutathione transferase zeta catalyzes the oxygenation of the carcinogen dichloroacetic acid to glyoxylic acid. Biochem J, **331**: 371-374.

Toth GP, Long RE, Mills TS, & Smith MK (1990) Effects of chlorine dioxide on the developing rat brain. J Toxicol Environ Health, **31**: 29-44.

Toth GP, Kelty KC, George EL, Read EJ, & Smith MK (1992) Adverse male reproductive effects following subchronic exposure of rats to sodium dichloroacetate. Fundam Appl Toxicol, **19**: 57-63.

Toth PP, El-Shanti H, Elvins S, Rhead WJ, & Klein JM (1993) Transient improvement of congenital lactic acidosis in a male infant with pyruvate decarboxylase deficiency treated with dichloro-acetate. J Pediatr, **123**: 427-430.

Tratnyek PG & Hoigne J (1994) Kinetics of reactions of chlorine dioxide in water - II: quantitative structure-activity relationships for phenolic compounds. Water Res, **28**(1): 57-66.

Trehy ML & Bieber TI (1981) Detection, identification and quantitative analysis of dihalo-acetonitriles in chlorinated natural waters. In: Keith LH ed. Advances in the identification and analysis of organic pollutants in water. Ann Arbor, Michigan, Ann Arbor Science Publishers, vol 2, pp 941-975.

Trehy ML, Yost RA, & Miles CJ (1986) Chlorination by-products of amino acids in natural waters. Environ Sci Technol, **20**: 1117-1122.

Trussell RR & Umphres MD (1978) The formation of trihalomethanes. J Am Water Works Assoc, 70(11): 604.

Tuomisto J, Hythinen J, Jansson K, Komulainen H, Kosma VM, Maki-Paakkanen J, Vaittinen SL, & Vartiainen T (1995) Genotoxicity and carcinogenicity of MX and other chlorinated furanones. In: Disinfection by-products in drinking water: Critical issues in health effects research. Washington, DC, International Life Sciences Institute, pp 30-31.

Tuppurainen K, Lotjonen S, Laatikainen R, Vartiainen T, Maran U, Strandberg M, & Tamm T (1991) About the mutagenicity of chlorine substituted furanones and halopropenals. A QSAR study using molecular orbital indices. Mutat Res, 247: 97-102.

Tuthill RW & Moore GS (1980) Drinking water chlorination: A practice related to cancer mortality. J Am Water Works Assoc, 72: 570-573.

Umemura T, Sai K, Takagi A, Hasegawa R, & Kurokawa Y (1993) A possible role for cell proliferation in potassium bromate ($KBrO_3$). J Cancer Res Clin Oncol, 119: 463-469.

Urano K, Wada H, & Takemasa T (1983) Empirical rate equation for trihalomethane formation with chlorination of humic substances in water. Water Res, 17(12): 1797-1802.

US EPA (1994a) Workshop report and recommendations for conducting epidemiologic research on cancer and exposure to chlorinated drinking water. Cincinnati, Ohio, US Environmental Protection Agency, pp 2/13-2/19.

US EPA (1994b) Drinking water criteria for trihalomethanes. Washington, DC, US Environmental Protection Agency, Office of Water.

US EPA (1997) Workshop report and recommendations for conducting epidemiologic research on reproductive and developmental effects and exposure to disinfected drinking water. Research Triangle Park, North Carolina, US Environmental Protection Agency.

US EPA (1998) Dichloroacetic acid - Carcinogenicity identification characterization summary. Washington, DC, US Environmental Protection Agency, Office of Research and Development.

Vagnarelli P, De Sario A, & De Carli L (1990) Aneuploidy induced by chloral hydrate detected in b human lymphocytes with Y97 probe. Mutagenesis, 5: 591-592.

Vaittinen SL, Komulainen H, Kosma VM, Julkunen A, Maki-Paakkanen J, Jansson K, Vartiainen T, & Tuomisto J (1995) Subchronic toxicity of 3-chloro-4-(dichloromethyl)-5-hydroxy-2(5H)-furanone (MX) in Wistar rats. Food Chem Toxicol, 33(12): 1027-1037.

Valentine RL & Solomon WL (1987) Effect of inorganic composition on the kinetics of chloramine decomposition In the presence of excess ammonia. Water Res, 21: 1475-1483.

Van Duuren BL, Goldschmidt BM, Loewengart G, Smith AC, Melchionne S, Seidman I, & Roth D (1979) Carcinogenicity of halogenated olefinic and aliphatic hydrocarbons in mice. J Natl Cancer Inst, 63: 1433-1439.

van Heijst AN, Zimmerman AN, & Pikaar SA (1977) [Chloral hydrate - the forgotten poison.] Ned Tijdschr Geneesk, 121(40): 1537-1539 (in Dutch).

Van Hoof F, Janssens JG, & van Dijck H (1986) Formation of mutagenic activity during surface water pre-ozonation and its removal in drinking water treatment. Chemosphere, 14(5): 501-509.

Varanasi U, Chu RY, Huang Q, Castellon R, Yeldandi AV, & Reddy JK (1996) Identification of a peroxisome proliferator-responsive element upstream of the human peroxisomal fatty acyl coenzyme A oxidase gene. J Biol Chem, 271: 2147-2155.

Varma MM, Ampy FR, Verma K, & Talbot WW (1988) In vitro mutagenicity of water contaminants in complex mixtures. J Appl Toxicol, 8: 243-248.

Vartiainen T, Liimatainen A, Kauranen P, & Hiisvirta L (1988) Relations between drinking water mutagenicity and water quality parameters. Chemosphere, 17: 189-202.

Velazquez SF, McGinnis PM, Vater ST, Stiteler WS, Knauf LA, & Schoeny RS (1994) Combination of cancer data in quantitative risk assessments: case study using bromodichloromethane. Risk Anal, 14: 285-291.

Vena JE, Graham S, Freudenheim J, Marshall J, Zielezny M, Swanson M, & Sufrin G (1993) Drinking water, fluid intake, and bladder cancer in Western New York. Arch Environ Med, 48(3): 191-198.

Vesselinovitch SD, Rao KV, Mihailovich N, Rice JM, & Lombard LS (1974) Development of broad spectrum of tumors by ethylnitrosourea in mice and the modifying role of age, sex and strain. Cancer Res, 34: 2530-2538.

Vogt CR, Liao JC, Sun GY, & Sun AY (1979) In vivo and in vitro formation of chloroform in rats with acute dosage of chlorinated water and the effect of membrane function. In: Trace substances in environmental health: XIII. Proceedings of the University of Missouri 13th Annual Conference on Trace Substances in Environmental Health. Columbia, Missouri, University of Missouri, pp 453-459.

Von der Hude W, Scheutwinkel M, Gramlich U, Fisler B, & Basler A (1987) Genotoxicity of three-carbon compounds evaluated in the SCE test in vitro. Environ Mutagen, 9: 401-410.

von Gunten U & Hoigne J (1994) Bromate formation during ozonation of bromide-containing waters: Interactions of ozone and hydroxyl radical reactions. Environ Sci Technol, 28(7): 1234.

Voudrias EA, Dielmann LM, Snoeyink VL, Larson RA, McCreary JJ, & Chen AS (1983) Reactions of chlorite ion with activated carbon and with vanillic acid and indan adsorbed on activated carbon. Water Research, 17: 1107-1112.

Wahli W, Braissant O, & Desvergne B (1995) Peroxisome proliferator activated receptors: transcriptional regulators of adipogenesis, lipid metabolism and more... Chem Biol, 2: 261-266.

Waller CL & McKinney JD (1993) Theoretical investigation into the potential of halogenated methanes to undergo reproductive metabolism. J Comput Chem, 14(12): 1575-1579.

Waller K, Swan SH, DeLorenze G, & Hopkins B (1998) Trihalomethanes in drinking water and spontaneous abortion. Epidemiology, 9: 134-140.

Warr TJ, Parry EM, & Parry JM (1993) A comparison of two *in vivo* mammalian cell cytogenetic assays for the detection of mitotic aneuploidy using 10 known or suspected aneugens. Mutat Res, **287**(1): 29-46.

Warshaw BL, Carter MC, Hymes LC, Bruner BS, & Rauber AP (1985) Bromate poisoning from hair permanent preparations. Pediatrics, **76**: 975-978.

Waskell L (1978) A study of the mutagenicity of anesthetics and their metabolites. Mutat Res, **57**: 141-153.

Watanabe M, Kobayashi H, & Ohta T (1994) Rapid inactivation of 3-chloro-4-(dichloromethyl)-5-hydroxy-2(5H)-furanone (MX), a potent mutagen in chlorinated drinking water, by sulfhydryl compounds. Mutat Res, **312**: 131-138.

Water Research Centre (1980) Trihalomethanes in water: Seminar held at the Lorch Foundation, Lane End, Buckinghamshire, UK, 16-17 January 1980. Medmenham, United Kingdom, Water Research Centre.

Weil I & Morris JC (1949) Kinetic studies of chloramine: The rates of formation of monochloramine, *N*-chloromethylamine and *N*-chlorodimethylamine. J Am Chem Soc, **71**: 1664-1671.

Weinberg HS, Glaze WH, Krasner SW, & Sclimenti MJ (1993) Formation and removal of aldehydes in plants that use ozone. J Am Water Works Assoc, **85**(5): 72-85.

Weinberg HS, Yamada H, & Joyce RJ (1998) New, sensitive and selective method for determining submicrogram/l levels of bromate in drinking water. J Chromatogr, **A804**(1/2): 137-142.

Weiss NS (1996) Cancer in relation to occupational exposure to trichloroethylene. Occup Environ Med, **53**: 1-5.

Wells PG, Moore GW, Rabin D, Wilkinson GR, Oates JA, & Stacpoole PW (1980) Metabolic effects and pharmacokinetics of intravenously administered dichloroacetate in humans. Diabetologia, **19**: 109-113.

Whitehouse S & Randle PJ (1973) Activation of pyruvate dehydrogenase in perfused rat heart by dichloroacetate. Biochem J, **134**: 651-653.

Whitehouse S, Cooper RH, & Randle PJ (1974) Mechanism of activation of pyruvate dehydrogenase by dichloroacetate and other halogenated carboxylic acids. Biochem J, **141**: 761-774.

WHO (1993) Guidelines for drinking-water quality - Volume 1: Recommendations. Geneva, World Health Organization.

WHO (1996) Guidelines for drinking-water quality - Volume 2: Health criteria and other supporting information. Geneva, World Health Organization.

WHO (1998) Guidelines for drinking-water quality - Addendum to Volume 2: Health criteria and other supporting information. Geneva, World Health Organization.

Wigle DT, Mao Y, Semenci WR, Smith MH, & Toft P (1986) Contaminants in drinking water and cancer risks in Canadian cities. Can J Public Health, **77**: 335-342.

Wilkins JR & Comstock GW (1981) Source of drinking water at home and site-specific cancer incidence in Washington County, Maryland. Am J Epidemiol, **114**: 178-190.

Wilson JR, Mancini DM, Ferraro N, & Egler J (1988) Effect of dichloroacetate on the exercise performance of patients with heart failure. J Am Coll Cardiol, **12**: 1464-1469.

Wlodkowski TJ & Rosenkranz HS (1975) Mutagenicity of sodium hypochlorite for *Salmonella typhimurium*. Mutat Res, **31**: 39-42.

Wolf CR, Mansuy D, Nastainczyk W, Deutschmann G, & Ullrich V (1977) The reduction of polyhalogenated methanes by liver microsomal cytochrome P-450. Mol Pharmacol, **13**: 698-705.

Wones RG & Glueck CJ (1986) Effect of chlorinated drinking water on human lipid metabolism. Environ Health Perspect, **69**: 255-258.

Wones RG, Mieczkowski L, & Frohman LA (1990) Chlorinated drinking water and human lipid and thyroid metabolism. In: Jolley RL, Condie LW, & Johnson JD ed. Water chlorination: Chemistry, environmental impact and health effects. Chelsea, Michigan, Lewis Publishers, Inc., vol 6, p 301.

Wones RG, Deck CC, & Stadler B (1993a) Lack of effect of drinking water chlorine on lipid and thyroid metabolism in healthy humans. Environ Health Perspect, **99**: 375-381.

Wones RG, Deck CC, & Stadler B (1993b) Effects of drinking water monochloramine on lipid and thyroid metabolism in healthy men. Environ Health Perspect, **99**: 369-374.

Wones RG, Deck CC, Stadler B, Roark S, Hogg E, & Frohman LA (1993c) Lack of effect of drinking water chlorine on lipid and thyroid metabolism in healthy humans. Environ Health Perspect, **99**: 375-381.

Woodard G, Lange SW, Nelson KW, & Calvery HO (1941) The acute oral toxicity of acetic, chloroacetic, dichloroacetic and trichloroacetic acids. J Ind Hyg Toxicol, **23**: 78-82.

Woodruff RC, Mason JM, Valencia R, & Zimmering S (1985) Chemical mutagenesis testing in *Drosophila*: V. Results of 53 coded compounds tested for the National Toxicology Program. Environ Mutagen, **7**(5): 677-702.

Worley KL (1994) Oxidation of NOM using peroxide and visible-UV irradiation. Houston, Texas, University of Houston, Civil and Environmental Engineering Department (M.S. Thesis).

Wyatt I, Gyte A, Mainwaring G, Widdowson PS, & Lock EA (1996) Glutathione depletion in the liver and brain produced by 2-chloropropionic acid: Relevance to cerebellar granule cell necrosis. Arch Toxicol, **70**: 380-389.

Xie Y & Reckhow DA (1993) Identification of trihaloacetaldehydes in ozonated and chlorinated fulvic acid solutions. Analyst, **118**: 71-72.

Xu W & Adler ID (1990) Clastogenic effects of known and suspect spindle poisons studied by chromosome analysis in mouse bone marrow cells. Mutagenesis, **5**(4): 371-374.

Xu G, Stevens DK, & Bull RJ (1995) Metabolism of bromodichloroacetate in B6C3F$_1$ mice. Drug Metab Dispos, **23**: 1412-1416.

Yamada H (1993) By-products of ozonation of low bromide waters and reduction of the by-products by activated carbon. In: Ozone in water and wastewater treatment - Proceedings of the Eleventh Ozone World Congress, San Francisco, California, 29 August - 3 September 1993. Lille, France, International Ozone Association, pp 9-58.

Yamamoto K, Fukushima M, & Oda K (1988) Disappearance rates of chloramines in river water. Water Res, 22(1): 79-84.

Yang CY, Chiu HF, Cheng MF, & Tsai SS (1998) Chlorination of drinking water and cancer mortality in Taiwan. Environ Res, 78(1): 1-6.

Yang TC & Neely WC (1986) Relative stoichiometry of the oxidation of ferrous ion by ozone in aqueous solution. Anal Chem, 58: 1551-1555.

Yarington CT (1970) The experimental causticity of sodium hypochlorite in the esophagus. Ann Otol Rhinol Laryngol, 79(5): 895-988.

Yllner S (1971) Metabolism of chloroacetate-^{14}C in the mouse. Acta Pharmacol Toxicol, 30: 69-80.

Yokose Y, Uchhida K, Nakae D, Shiraiwa K, Yamamoto K, & Konishi Y (1987) Studies of carcinogenicity of sodium chlorite in B6C3F$_1$ mice. Environ Health Perspect, 76: 205-210.

Yoshida Y, Hirose Y, Konda S, Kitada H, & Shinoda A (1977) A cytological study of Heinz body-hemolytic anemia. Report of a case of sodium chlorate poisoning complicated by methemoglobinemia and acute renal failure. Acta Haematol Jpn, 40: 147-151.

Young TB, Kanarek MS, & Tsiatis AA (1981) Epidemiologic study of drinking water chlorination and Wisconsin female cancer mortality. J Natl Cancer Inst, 67: 1191-1198.

Young TB, Wolf DA, & Kanarek MS (1987) Case-control study of colon cancer and drinking water trihalomethanes in Wisconsin. Int J Epidemiol, 16: 190-197.

Young TB, Kanarek MS, Wolf DA, & Wilson DA (1990) Case-control study of colon cancer and volatile organics in Wisconsin municipal groundwater supplies. In: Jolley RL, Condie LW, & Johnson JD ed. Water chlorination: Chemistry, environmental impact and health effects. Chelsea, Michigan, Lewis Publishers, Inc., vol 6, p 373.

Yount EA & Harris RA (1980) Studies on the inhibition of gluconeogenesis by oxalate. Biochim Biophys Acta, 633: 122-133.

Yount EA, Felten SY, O'Connor BL, Peterson RG, Powell RS, Yum MN, & Harris RA (1982) Comparison of the metabolic and toxic effects of 2-chloropropionate and dichloroacetate. J Pharmacol Exp Ther, 222: 501-508.

Zajdela F, Croisy A, Barbin A, Malaveille C, Tomatis L, & Bartsch H (1980) Carcinogenicity of chloroethylene oxide, an ultimate reactive metabolite of vinyl chloride, and bis(chloromethyl)ether after subcutaneous administration and in initiation-promotion experiments in mice. Cancer Res, 40: 352-356.

Zeiger E (1990) Mutagenicity of 42 chemicals in *Salmonella*. Environ Mol Mutagen, 16(suppl 18): 32-54.

Zeighami EA, Watson AP, & Craun GF (1990a) Chlorination, water hardness and serum cholesterol in forty-six Wisconsin communities. Int J Epidemiol, **19**: 49-58.

Zeighami EA, Watson AP & Craun GF (1990b) Serum lipid levels in neighboring communities with chlorinated and nonchlorinated drinking water. In: Jolley RL, Condie LW, & Johnson JD ed. Water chlorination: Chemistry, environmental impact and health effects. Chelsea, Michigan, Lewis Publishers, Inc., vol 6, p 421.

Zierler S, Danley RA, & Feingold L (1986) Type of disinfectant in drinking water and patterns of mortality in Massachusetts. Environ Health Perspect, **69**: 275-279.

Zierler S, Feingold L, Danley RA, & Craun G (1988) Bladder cancer in Massachusetts related to chlorinated and chloraminated drinking water: A case-control study. Arch Environ Health, **43**: 195-200.

Zierler S, Feingold L, Danley RA, & Craun GF (1990) A case-control study of bladder cancer in Massachusetts among populations receiving chlorinated and chloraminated drinking water. In: Jolley RL, Condie LW, & Johnson JD ed. Water chlorination: Chemistry, environmental impact and health effects. Chelsea, Michigan, Lewis Publishers, Inc., vol 6, p 399.

RESUME ET EVALUATION

Le chlore (Cl$_2$) est largement utilisé partout dans le monde comme désinfectant chimique et c'est lui qui constitue la principale barrière à la contamination microbienne de l'eau de boisson. Les qualités biocides remarquables du chlore sont toutefois quelque peu atténuées par la formation, lors du processus de chloration, de sous-produits de ce désinfectant (SPC) qui posent un problème de santé publique. C'est d'ailleurs la raison pour laquelle on utilise de plus en plus d'autres désinfectants chimiques comme l'ozone (O$_3$), le dioxyde de chlore (ClO$_2$) et les chloramines (NH$_2$Cl). Toutefois chacun d'entre eux donne aussi naissance à des SPC. Il est certain qu'aucun compromis n'est tolérable en ce qui concerne la qualité de l'eau, mais il faut cependant mieux connaître la chimie, la toxicologie et l'épidémiologie des désinfectants chimiques et de leurs sous-produits afin d'établir avec plus de sûreté les risques (d'ordre chimique ou microbien) que comporte la consommation d'eau et de trouver un compromis entre le risque chimique et le risque microbiologique. Il est possible de réduire le risque chimique dû aux SPC sans nuire à la qualité microbiologique de l'eau.

1. Chimie des désinfectants et de leurs sous-produits

Les désinfectants les plus utilisés sont le chlore, l'ozone, le dioxyde de chlore et la chloramine. Les propriétés physiques et chimiques des désinfectants et de leurs SPC conditionnent leur comportement dans l'eau ainsi que leur toxicologie et leur épidémiologie. Tous les désinfectants envisagés ici sont des oxydants solubles dans l'eau que l'on produit soit sur place (comme l'ozone) soit ailleurs (comme le chlore). Ils sont introduits dans l'eau sous forme de gaz (ozone) ou de liquide (hypochlorite par ex.) à des doses de l'ordre de quelques mg par litre, soit seuls, soit en association. Les SPC étudiés dans ce qui suit sont dosables par chromatographie en phase gazeuse ou liquide et peuvent être classés en dérivés organiques ou minéraux halogénés (chlorés ou bromés) ou non halogénés, volatils ou non volatils. Une fois formés, les SPC peuvent être stables ou instables (par exemple, être décomposés par hydrolyse).

Les SPC se forment par réaction des désinfectants sur un certain nombre de précurseurs. Les matières organiques naturelles (NOM) que l'on dose habituellement sous la forme de carbone organique total (TOC) constituent le précurseur organique, tandis que les ions bromure (Br⁻) sont les précurseurs minéraux. La formation des SPC dépend de la nature de l'eau (teneur en carbone organique total, bromures, pH, température, ammoniaque, alcalinité due à la présence de carbonates) et des conditions de traitement (par exemple, dose de désinfectant, durée de contact, élimination des matières organiques naturelles en amont du point d'introduction du désinfectant, adjonction préalable de désinfectant).

Sous la forme d'acide hypochloreux ou d'ion hypochlorite (HOCl/OCl⁻), le chlore réagit sur l'ion bromure en l'oxydant en acide hypobromeux ou ion hypobromite (HOBr/OBr⁻). L'acide hypo-chloreux (un oxydant plus énergique) et l'acide hypobromeux (un agent d'halogénation plus efficace) réagissent collectivement sur les NOM pour former des SPC halogénés tels que trihalogénométhanes (THM), acides halogénoacétiques (HAA), halogénoacétonitriles (HAN), halogénocétones, hydrate de chloral et chloropicrine. En général, ces SPC se classent par ordre d'importance selon la séquence THM > HAA > HAN. La teneur relative en TOC, bromures et chlore influe sur la distribution des différents THM (on en compte quatre espèces : le chloroforme, le bromoforme, le bromodichlorométhane - BDCM - et le dibromochlorométhane - DBCM), des HAA (jusqu'à neuf espèces chlorées ou bromées) et des HAN (plusieurs espèces chlorées ou bromées). Généralement les THM, HAA et HAN chlorés sont plus abondants que leurs homologues bromés, mais c'est l'inverse dans les eaux à forte teneur en bromures. On a identifié de nombreux SPC dérivant du chlore mais une proportion importante des halo-génures organiques totaux reste à caractériser. Dans les solutions concentrées d'hypochlorite, le chlore donne également naissance à des chlorates (ClO₃⁻).

L'ozone peut réagir directement ou indirectement sur les bromures pour donner des sous-produits bromés et notamment des bromates (BrO₃⁻). En présence de NOM, il se forme des sous-produits organiques non halogénés au cours de l'ozonisation, par exemple des aldéhydes, des cétoacides et des acides carboxyliques, les aldéhydes (comme le formaldéhyde) étant prédominants. En présence de NOM et de bromures, l'ozonisation conduit à la formation d'acide hypo-bromeux qui conduit à son tour à la formation d'halogénures organiques comme le bromoforme.

Les principaux SPC qui se forment en présence de dioxyde de chlore sont les ions chlorite (ClO_3^-) et chlorate, sans formation directe de SPC organohalogénés. A l'inverse des SPC des autres désinfectants, les principaux sous-produits du dioxyde de chlore proviennent de la décomposition du désinfectant lui-même et non pas d'une réaction sur des précurseurs.

Lorsqu'on utilise de la chloramine comme désinfectant secon-daire, il se forme en général un dérivé azoté, le chlorure de cyanogène (CNCl) et des SPC en quantité sensiblement moindre. Il se pose égale-ment la question de la présence de nitrites (NO_2^-) dans les réseaux de distribution traités par la chloramine.

Autant qu'on sache, ce sont les THM, les HAA, les bromates et les chlorites qui sont les SPC les plus fréquents et les plus intéressants du point de vue de leurs effets sur la santé.

Le groupe de SPC prédominant, lorsqu'on traite par le chlore, est celui des THM, dont les représentants principaux sont, dans l'ordre, le chloroforme et le BDCM. Viennent ensuite les HAA dont les espèces les plus abondantes sont, dans l'ordre, l'acide dichloracétique (DCA) et l'acide trichloracétique (TCA).

La transformation des bromures en bromates au cours de l'ozonisation dépend, entre autres, de la teneur en NOM, du pH et de la température. La concentration peut aller de teneurs indétectables (2 µg/litre) à plusieurs dizaines de milligrammes par litre. Il est en général tout à fait possible de prévoir la concentration en chlorites, qui va d'environ 50 à 70 % de la dose de dioxyde de chlore utilisée.

Les SPC se présentent sous la forme de mélanges complexes qui sont fonction du désinfectant utilisé, de la qualité de l'eau et des traitements qu'elle subit. Les autres facteurs qui entrent en ligne de compte sont l'utilisation simultanée ou successive de plusieurs désinfectants ou oxydants. En outre, la composition de ces mélanges peut changer selon la saison. Il est clair que les effets sur la santé qui pourraient résulter de la présence de ces composés chimiques dans l'eau dépendent du degré d'exposition aux mélanges de SPC.

Indépendamment de ces SPC (et des THM en particulier), on ne possède que très peu de données sur la présence de SPC dans l'eau qui sort des installations de traitement pour pénétrer dans le réseau d'adduction. A partir des bases de données des laboratoires, on a mis au point des modèles empiriques qui permettent de prévoir la concentration en THM (THM totaux et différentes espèces de THM), HAA (HAA totaux et différentes espèces de HAA) et en bromates. Ces modèles peuvent être utilisés pour évaluer l'efficacité des traitements et calculer à l'avance les conséquences d'une modification de ces traitements. On peut aussi les utiliser lors d'une évaluation de l'exposition, pour simuler des données manquantes ou anciennes (par exemple, pour calculer la concentration en HAA d'après celle des THM).

On peut agir sur les SPC en agissant en amont, c'est-à-dire sur le précurseur - notamment en l'éliminant - ou en choisissant une autre méthode de désinfection. Par exemple, on peut éliminer les matières organiques naturelles (NOM) par coagulation, passage sur granulés de charbon actif, filtration sur membrane et biofiltration en présence d'ozone. A part l'utilisation de membranes, il n'y a guère d'autres possibilités pour se débarrasser efficacement des bromures. Si on veut éviter d'avoir à traiter l'eau, il faut protéger et contrôler les sources. L'élimination des SPC une fois formés n'est pas une solution valable dans le cas des SPC organiques; par contre on peut éliminer les bromates et les chlorites par passage sur charbon actif ou par réduction. Il y a encore la possibilité de réduire la teneur en SPC en associant les désinfectants de façon optimale, qu'on utilise comme désinfectants primaires,ou comme désinfectants secondaires. La tendance actuelle est à l'utilisation simultanée ou successive de divers désinfectants; l'ozone est utilisée exclusivement comme désinfectant primaire, les chloramines comme désinfectants secondaires, tandis que le chlore et le dioxyde de chlore peuvent l'être dans les deux cas.

2. Cinétique et métabolisme chez les animaux de laboratoire et l'Homme

2.1 Désinfectants

Les désinfectants résiduels sont des substances chimiques susceptibles de réagir sur les composés organiques présents dans la salive et dans le contenu stomacal, entraînant la formation de produits secondaires. Il existe d'importantes différences dans la pharmaco-cinétique du ^{36}Cl selon qu'il provient du chlore lui-même, de la chloramine ou du dioxyde de chlore.

2.2 Trihalogénométhanes

Les THM sont absorbés, métabolisés et éliminés rapidement par les mammifères après ingestion ou inhalation. Après absorption, c'est au niveau des graisses, du foie et des reins que la concentration tissulaire est la plus élevée. La demi-vie varie généralement de 0,5 à 3 h et la voie d'élimination principale est une métabolisation en dioxyde de carbone. Pour que la toxicité se manifeste, il faut que les THM subissent une activation métabolique en intermédiaires réactifs et les trois espèces bromées sont métabolisées plus rapidement et en proportion plus importante que le chloroforme. La principale voie métabolique est dans tous les cas une oxydation par l'intermédiaire du cytochrome P450 (CYP) 2E1, qui conduit à la formation de dérivés carbonylés halogénés (par exemple le phosgène et ses homologues bromés), après quoi ceux-ci peuvent être hydrolysés en dioxyde de carbone ou se fixer à des macromolécules tissulaires. Il existe des voies métaboliques secondaires, comme la déshalogénation réductrice par l'intermédiaire de la CYP2B1/2/2E1 (qui conduit à la formation de radicaux libres) ou la conjugaison avec le glutathion (GSH) par l'intermédiaire de la glutathion-S-transférase (GST) T1-1, qui entraîne la formation d'intermédiaires mutagènes. Les THM bromés ont beaucoup plus de chances d'emprunter les voies métaboliques secondaires que le chloroforme et la conjugaison de ce dernier composé avec le GSH sous l'action de la GST peut s'effectuer à des concentrations ou à des doses de chloroforme extrêmement élevées.

2.3   Acides halogénoacétiques

Le métabolisme et la cinétique des acides trihalogénoacétiques et dihalogénoacétiques diffèrent sensiblement. Dans la mesure où ils sont métabolisés, les principales réactions des acides trihalogénoacétiques se produisent dans la fraction microsomique, alors que le métabolisme des acides dihalogénoacétiques, qui s'effectue essentiellement sous l'action des glutathion-transférases, se déroule à plus de 90 % dans le cytosol. Le TCA a une demi-vie biologique de 50 h chez l'Homme. La demi-vie des autres acides trihalogénoacétiques diminue sensiblement avec la substitution par le brome et on peut déceler des quantités mesurables d'acides dihalogénoacétiques comme produits à côté d'acides trihalogénoacétiques bromés. La demi-vie des acides dihalogénoacétiques est très courte à faible dose, mais elle augmente très fortement avec la dose.

2.4   Halogénoaldéhydes et halogénocétones

On ne possède que des données limitées sur la cinétique de l'hydrate de chloral. Ses deux principaux métabolites sont le trichloréthanol et le TCA. Le trichloréthanol subit une glucuronidation rapide puis il passe dans le circuit entérohépatique, il est hydrolysé et enfin oxydé en TCA. La déchloration du trichloréthanol ou de l'hydrate de chloral conduirait à la formation de DCA. Le DCA pourrait être ensuite transformé en monochloracétate (MCA), en glyoxalate, en glycolate et en oxalate, probablement par le canal d'un intermédiaire réactif. On n'a trouvé aucune donnée concernant les autres aldéhydes ou cétones halogénés.

2.5   Halogénoacétonitriles

Ni le métabolisme ni la cinétique des HAN n'ont été étudiés. Les données quantitatives indiquent que parmi les produits du métabolisme on trouve du cyanure, du formaldéhyde, ainsi que du cyanure et des halogénures de formyle.

2.6   Dérivés halogénés de l'hydroxyfuranone

La 3-chloro-4-(dichlorométhyl)-5-hydroxy-2(5H)-furanone (MX) est, parmi les hydroxyfuranones, celle qui a été le plus largement étudiée. Il ressort des études sur l'animal que le radiomarqueur (^{14}C) est rapidement résorbé au niveau des voies digestives et qu'il passe dans la circulation générale. On n'a pas procédé au dosage de la MX elle-même dans le sang. Le radiomarqueur est en grande partie excrété dans les urines et les matières fécales, mais c'est la voie urinaire qui est la principale voie d'excrétion. Au bout de cinq jours, il ne reste dans l'organisme qu'une proportion minime du radiomarqueur initial.

2.7 Chlorites

Le ^{36}Cl provenant de l'ion chlorite est rapidement absorbé. La dose initiale de chlorite se retrouve à moins de 50 % sous forme de chlorure dans les urines et en faible proportion sous sa forme initiale. Il est probable qu'une proportion s'intègre à la réserve de chlorures de l'organisme, mais comme on ne dispose pas de méthode d'analyse permettant de caractériser les chlorites présents dans les échantillons biologiques, on ne possède pas de données détaillées à ce sujet.

2.8 Chlorates

Les chlorates ont un comportement analogue à celui des chlorites. Les problèmes analytiques sont les mêmes.

2.9 Bromates

Les bromates sont rapidement absorbés et excrétés, principalement dans les urines, sous forme de bromures. On peut les mettre en évidence dans les urines à des doses supérieures ou égales à 5 mg/kg de poids corporel. La concentration urinaire des bromates culmine au bout d'environ 1 h et au bout de 2 h ils ne sont plus décelables dans le plasma.

3. Toxicologie des désinfectants et de leurs sous-produits

3.1 Désinfectants

Le chlore, la chloramine et le dioxyde de chlore sont très irritants pour les voies respiratoires. L'hypochlorite de sodium, qui entre dans la composition de l'eau de Javel, est souvent la cause d'intoxications chez l'Homme. Il s'agit toutefois de cas qui n'ont rien à voir avec une exposition par consommation d'eau de boisson. On a relativement peu étudié les effets toxiques que ces désinfectants peuvent avoir sur l'Homme ou l'animal d'expérience lorsqu'ils sont présents dans l'eau de boisson. Les quelques études dont on dispose indiquent que le chlore, les solutions d'hypochlorite ainsi que la chloramine et le dioxyde de chlore eux-mêmes ne sont probablement pas à l'origine de cancers ou d'un quelconque effet toxique. On s'intéresse surtout aux produits secondaires très divers qui résultent de l'action du chlore et d'autres désinfectants sur les matières organiques naturelles présentes dans presque toutes les eaux quelle que soit leur origine.

3.2   Trihalogénométhanes

A la dose d'environ 0,5 mmol/kg de poids corporel, les THM se révèlent hépatotoxiques et néphrotoxiques chez les rongeurs. Le véhicule utilisée pour l'administration influe sensiblement sur la toxicité. Les THM ont peu d'effets toxiques sur la reproduction ou le développement, mais le BDCM s'est révélé capable de réduire la mobilité des spermatozoïdes chez des rats à qui on en avait fait consommer une dose quotidienne de 39 mg/kg p.c. dans leur eau de boisson. Comme le chloroforme, le BDCM, lorsqu'il est administré dans de l'huile de maïs, provoque des cancers du foie et du rein après une exposition à forte dose pendant toute la vie. Au rebours du chloroforme et du DBCM, le BDCM et le bromoforme provoquent des tumeurs du côlon chez des rats a qui on les administre par gavage dans de l'huile de maïs. Le BDCM provoque des cancers ayant ces trois localisations et à des doses inférieures à celles des autres THM. Depuis la publication en 1994 des Critères d'hygiène de l'environnement relatifs au chloroforme, des études supplémentaires sont venues compléter la somme de données selon lesquelles le chloroforme n'est pas un cancérogène exerçant une action mutagène directe par réaction sur l'ADN. En revanche, les THM bromés se révèlent être faiblement mutagènes, probablement par suite de leur conjugaison au GSH.

3.3   Acides halogénoacétiques

Les HAA exercent différents effets toxiques sur les animaux de laboratoire. Dans les cas les plus inquiétants, il s'agit d'effets cancéro-gènes ou encore d'effets sur la reproduction et le développement.

L'acide dichloracétique a des effets neurotoxiques sensibles aux fortes doses utilisées dans un but thérapeutique. Les effets cancérogènes sont limités au foie et aux fortes doses. Il existe une somme de données qui tendent à prouver que les effets tumorigènes de l'acide dichloracétique et de l'acide trichloracétique tiennent au fait que ces composés agissent sur la division et la mort cellulaire plutôt qu'à leur faible activité mutagène. Le stress oxydatif est également une caractéristique de la toxicité des dérivés bromés appartenant à ce groupe. A forte dose, les acides dichloracétique et trichloracétique provoquent des malformations cardiaques chez le rat.

3.4   Halogénoaldéhydes et halogénocétones

Chez le rat, l'hydrate de chloral provoque une nécrose hépatique à des doses quotidiennes égales ou supérieures à 120 mg/kg de poids corporel. Chez l'Homme, son effet dépresseur sur le système nerveux central est probablement en rapport avec un métabolite, le trichloréthanol. On ne possède que des données toxicologiques limitées sur les autres cétones et aldéhydes halogénés. Une exposition au chloracétaldéhyde entraîne des anomalies hématologiques chez le rat. Chez la souris, on constate que l'exposition à la 1,1-dichloropropanone (1,1-DCPN) a des effets hépatotoxiques, effets qui ne s'observent pas avec l'isomère 1,3 (1,3-DCPN).

La plupart des tests sur bactéries à la recherche de mutations ponctuelles se sont révélés négatifs dans le cas de l'hydrate de chloral et il en a été de même pour la recherche de lésions chromosomiques *in vivo*. On a toutefois montré que l'hydrate de chloral peut provoquer des aberrations chromosomiques structurales *in vivo* et *in vitro*. L'hydrate de chloral provoquerait également la formation de tumeurs hépatiques chez la souris. On ne sait pas très bien si c'est l'hydrate de chloral lui-même ou ses métabolites qui sont à l'origine des effets cancérogènes. Les deux métabolites de l'hydrate de chloral, à savoir l'acide trichloracétique et l'acide dichloracétique, se sont révélés capables de provoquer des tumeurs hépatiques chez la souris.

Un certain nombre d'aldéhydes et de cétones se révèlent être puissamment mutagènes pour les bactéries. On observés des effets clastogènes dus aux chloropropanones. Dans une étude au cours de laquelle les animaux ont été exposés leur vie durant à du chloracétaldéhyde contenu dans leur eau de boisson, on a observé la formation de tumeurs hépatiques. D'autres aldéhydes halogénés comme le 2-chloropropénal, se sont révélés avoir un effet tumoro-initiateur sur la peau de souris. On n'a pas étudié les propriétés cancérogènes des halogénocétones présentes dans l'eau de boisson, mais la 1,3-DCPN se comporte comme un initiateur tumoral cutané chez la souris.

3.5   Halogénoacétonitriles

Jusqu'ici on n'a procédé qu'à des études toxicologiques limitées sur ces composés. Certains d'entre eux sont mutagènes, mais ces effets sont difficiles à mettre en rapport avec le fait que ces composés se comportent comme des initiateurs tumoraux cutanés. On ne dispose que d'études très limitées sur la cancérogénicité de ce groupe de composés. Les premiers indices d'effets toxiques sur le développement relevés dans le cas de certains de ces composés, sont semble-t-il en grande partie attribuables au véhicule utilisé pour les administrer.

3.6   Dérivés halogénés de l'hydroxyfuranone

D'après les études expérimentales, les effets toxiques de la MX sont essentiellement des effets cancérogènes et mutagènes. Plusieurs études *in vitro* ont mis en évidence une activité mutagène de ce composé sur cellules bactériennes et mammaliennes. Il provoque également des aberrations chromosomiques et des lésions de l'ADN sur des cellules hépatiques et testiculaires isolées et on observe *in vivo* des échanges entre chromatides soeurs dans les lymphocytes périphériques de rats. Une évaluation globale des données relatives à la mutagénicité montre que la MX est mutagène *in vitro* et *in vivo*. Une étude de cancérogénicité sur des rats a montré qu'il y avait augmentation de la fréquence des tumeurs au niveau de plusieurs organes.

3.7   Chlorites

L'action toxique des chlorites est due principalement aux lésions qu'ils causent par oxydation aux érythrocytes (stress oxydatif) à des doses ne dépassant pas 10 mg/kg de poids corporel. On a également relevé des indices d'effets neurocomportementaux légers chez des ratons à des doses quotidiennes de 5,6 mg/kg de poids corporel. En ce qui concerne la génotoxicité, les données sont contradictoires. Chez des animaux exposés de manière chronique à cet ion, on ne relève pas d'augmentation dans la fréquence des tumeurs.

3.8   Chlorates

Sur le plan toxicologique, les chlorates sont analogues aux chlorites, mais en tant qu'oxydants, leur pouvoir lésionnel est moindre. Il ne semblent pas être tératogènes ni génotoxiques *in vivo*. On ne possède pas de données provenant d'études de cancérogénicité à long terme.

3.9   Bromates

A haute dose, les bromates provoquent des lésions au niveau des tubules rénaux chez le rat. Administrés de manière chronique ils provoquent des tumeurs rénales, péritonéales et thyroïdiennes chez le rat aux doses supérieures ou égales à 6 mg/kg p.c. Le hamster est moins sensible et les souris beaucoup moins. Les bromates sont également génotoxiques *in vivo* à forte dose chez le rat. Le pouvoir cancérogène se révèle être la conséquence du stress oxydatif subi par la cellule.

4.   Etudes épidémiologiques

4.1   Cardiopathies

Les études épidémiologiques ont mis en évidence une augmentation du risque de cardiopathies qui serait liée à la consommation d'eau traitée par le chlore ou la chloramine. On n'a pas effectué d'études de ce genre sur les autres désinfectants.

4.2   Cancer

Les données épidémiologiques ne sont pas suffisantes pour qu'on puisse parler d'une relation causale entre le cancer de la vessie et la consommation prolongée d'eau traitée par le chlore ou une exposition à des THM comme le chloroforme. Il en va de même pour le cancer du côlon, les données épidémiologiques étant dans ce cas équivoques et non concluantes. On ne dispose pas de renseignements suffisants pour évaluer le risque de cancer du rectum ni le risque d'autres cancers observés lors d'une seule et unique étude analytique.

Des études épidémiologiques diverses se sont efforcées d'évaluer le risque de cancer résultant de la consommation d'eau chlorée. Deux de ces études ont porté sur de l'eau traitée à la chloramine. Plusieurs autres sont consacrées à l'évaluation de l'exposition aux THM totaux ou à certains d'entre eux comme le chloroforme, mais elles ne prennent pas en considération les autres SPC ou contaminants de l'eau, lesquels ne sont pas forcément les mêmes selon qu'il s'agit de nappes souterraines ou d'eaux superficielles. Dans un cas, on a évalué le pouvoir mutagène de l'eau de boisson par un test sur *Salmonella typhimurium*. On n'a pas essayé de déterminer le risque de cancer que pourrait comporter la consommation d'eau désinfectée par l'ozone ou le dioxyde de chlore.

Des études cas-témoins écologiques ou basées sur l'examen des certificats de décès ont permis d'échafauder un certain nombre d'hypothèses qui devront être approfondies par des études analytiques prenant en considération la consommation individuelle d'eau de boisson, compte tenu d'éventuels facteurs de confusion.

Selon les études analytiques auxquelles il a été procédé, il y aurait une augmentation faible à modérée du risque de cancer de la vessie, du côlon, du rectum, du pancréas, du sein, du cerveau ou du poumon en cas de consommation prolongée d'eau traitée par le chlore. Un certain nombre d'études ont relevé, individuellement, une association entre l'exposition à l'eau chlorée et le cancer du pancréas, du sein et du cerveau. Toutefois, pour déterminer si ces associations épidémiologiques correspondent effectivement à un lien causal, une seule et unique étude ne suffit pas. Par exemple, une étude relevé une légère augmentation du risque relatif de cancer du poumon lié à la consommation d'eau de surface, mais ce risque est trop faible pour qu'on puisse exclure la présence d'un facteur de confusion résiduel.

Selon une étude cas-témoins, il y a aurait une corrélation modérément forte entre le cancer du rectum et la consommation prolongée d'eau chlorée ou une exposition cumulée à des THM, mais les études de cohortes portant sur ce problème n'ont relevé aucune augmentation du risque ou tout du moins un risque trop faible pour qu'on puisse exclure la présence de facteurs de confusion résiduels.

On a aussi trouvé que l'augmentation de la durée de consommation d'eau chlorée à la chloramine était associée à une diminution du risque de cancer de la vessie, mais rien sur le plan biologique ne permet de considérer que l'eau traitée à la chloramine puisse avoir un tel effet protecteur.

A en juger par plusieurs études, il y aurait une association entre l'augmentation du risque de cancer de la vessie et la consommation prolongée d'eau chlorée ou une exposition de longue durée à des THM, mais pour le même type de cancer les comparaisons entre fumeurs et non fumeurs ou entre hommes et femmes donnent des résultats incohérents. Dans trois de ces études, on a étudié le risque découlant d'une exposition aux THM. L'une d'entre elles n'a mis aucune corrélation en évidence, une autre a trouvé que le risque relatif était modérément accru pour les hommes, mais pas pour les femmes. Selon la troisième étude, une légère augmentation du risque relatif serait associée à une exposition cumulée à des THM évaluée à 1957-6425 µg de THM par année-litre. On a également fait état d'une association modérée entre le risque de cancer et une exposition à des concentrations de THM supérieures à 24, 49 ou 74 µg/litre, selon le cas. Il n'a pas été constaté d'association entre l'augmentation du risque de cancer de la vessie dans une cohorte de femmes et la consommation d'eau de surface chlorée délivrée par les services municipaux ou l'exposition à du chloroforme ou d'autres THM, mais la durée de suivi a été très courte (8 ans), d'où la rareté des cas à étudier.

Comme on s'est insuffisamment intéressé, d'un point de vue épidémiologique, à la détermination de l'exposition aux contaminants présents dans l'eau, il n'est pas possible d'évaluer correctement l'accroissement du risque de cancer qui ressort de ces différentes études. Il peut y avoir des risques particuliers dus à d'autres SPC, à des mélanges de produits secondaires ou à d'autres contaminants, mais il est également possible que cet accroissement du risque soit dû à d'autres facteurs dont on attribuerait les effets à l'eau chlorée et aux THM.

4.3   Grossesses à issue défavorable

Des études ont été consacrées au lien qu'il pourrait y avoir entre des grossesses à issue défavorable et la consommation d'eau chlorée ou l'exposition à des THM. Un groupe de scientifiques qui s'est récemment réuni sous l'égide de l'Environmental Protection Agency des Etats-Unis a passé en revue les études épidémiologiques consacrées à cette question et conclu que les résultats publiés ne prouvent pas de manière convaincante que l'eau chlorée ou les THM sont responsables d'accidents au cours de la grossesse.

Les résultats des premières études sont difficiles à interpréter à cause d'insuffisances d'ordre méthodologique et de biais probables.

Une étude cas-témoins récemment achevée mais non encore publiée fait état d'une augmentation modérée du risque relatif de malformation du tube neural chez les enfants dont la mère a résidé au début de sa grossesse dans une zone où la concentration des THM était supérieure à 40 µg/litre. Il faudra confirmer ces résultats dans une autre zone pour pouvoir procéder à une évaluation en bonne et due forme. Une étude menée antérieurement dans la même région avait fait état d'une association similaire, mais elle présentait des insuffisances sur le plan méthodologique.

Un récente étude de cohorte a révélé l'existence d'un risque accru d'avortement prématuré chez les femmes enceintes ayant consommé de grandes quantités (au moins 5 verres par jour) d'eau du robinet froide contenant ≳75 µg de THM par litre. En considérant le cas de chaque espèce chimique en particulier, on a constaté que seule une forte consommation de BDCM (≥ 18 µg/litre) était associée à un risque d'avortement. Comme il s'agit de la première étude qui fasse état d'un effet génésique indésirable imputable à un produit secondaire bromé, un groupe scientifique a recommandé de procéder à une autre étude dans une région différente afin de voir s'il est possible de reproduire ces résultats et il a également indiqué qu'il serait souhaitable d'essayer d'évaluer l'exposition des membres de la cohorte à d'autres contaminants.

5. Caractérisation du risque

Il est à noter que le traitement de l'eau par des désinfectants conduit habituellement à la formation de sous-produits dont certains peuvent être dangereux. Toutefois, aux concentrations auxquelles ils sont présents dans l'eau de boisson, le risque que ces composés représentent pour la santé est extrêmement faible par rapport à celui d'une désinfection insuffisante. Il ne faut pas que les tentatives en vue de réduire ces produits secondaires conduisent à une désinfection insuffisante.

5.1 *Caractérisation du risque et relation dose-réponse*

5.1.1 *Toxicologie*

1) Chlore

Le Groupe de travail de l'OMS qui s'est réuni en 1993 pour préparer les *Directives pour l'eau de boisson* s'est penché sur le problème du chlore. Il a fixé une dose journalière tolérable (TDI) pour cet élément égale à 150 µg/kg de poids corporel de chlore libre, en se basant sur la dose sans effet observable (NOAEL) qui est d'environ 15 mg/kg p.c. par jour selon des études de 2 ans sur le rat et la souris, avec une marge d'incertitude correspondant à un facteur 100 (10 pour à chaque fois pour tenir compte des variation intra- et interspécifiques). On ne possède pas de nouvelles données selon lesquelles il y aurait lieu de modifier cette dose journalière tolérable.

2) Monochloramine

Le Groupe de travail précité a également étudié le cas de la monochloramine. Il a fixé à 94 µg/kg p.c. la dose journalière tolérable de ce composé en s'appuyant sur la NOAEL d'environ 9,4 mg/kg p.c. obtenue à l'issue d'une étude toxicologique de 2 ans sur le rat (dose maximale utilisée), avec une marge d'incertitude correspondant à un facteur 100 (10 à chaque fois pour tenir compte des variations intra- et interspécifiques). On ne possède pas de nouvelles données selon lesquelles il y aurait lieu de modifier cette dose journalière tolérable.

3)   Dioxyde de chlore

Dans l'eau, la chimie du dioxyde de chlore se révèle complexe, mais le principal produit de décomposition est l'ion chlorite. Pour fixer une dose journalière tolérable, on peut prendre en considération les données relatives au dioxyde de chlore et aux chlorites. Dans ces conditions, la dose journalière tolérable de dioxyde de chlore est égale à 30 µg/kg p.c.; elle a été obtenue sur la base d'une NOAEL de 2,9 mg/kg p.c. par jour, le critère pris en compte étant les anomalies du développement neural chez le rat provoquées par l'ion chlorite.

4)   Trihalogénométhanes

C'est le cancer qui constitue le principal risque d'une exposition prolongée à ce groupe de SPC. Vu que les données relatives au chloroforme n'indiquent la possibilité d'apparition de cancers du foie chez l'animal qu'après exposition de longue durée à des doses cytotoxiques, il est clair qu'une exposition à de faibles concentrations de ce composé dans l'eau de boisson ne fait guère courir de risque de cancer. On a obtenu une NOAEL de 10 mg/kg p.c. par jour avec comme critères la cytolétalité et l'hyperplasie régénérative, après administration du composé à des souris dans de l'huile de maïs sur une période de 3 semaines. Compte tenu des données relatives au mode d'action du chloroforme en tant que cancérogène, on a fixé à 10 µg/kg p.c. la dose journalière tolérable de ce composé en se basant sur la NOAEL relative à la cytotoxicité obtenue sur la souris, avec une marge d'incertitude correspondant à un facteur 1000 (un facteur 10 à chaque fois pour les variations intra- et interspécifiques plus 10 pour tenir compte de la brève durée de l'étude). Cette façon de faire est justifiée par un certain nombre d'autres études. Cette dose journalière tolérable a une valeur du même ordre que celle que figure dans la dernière édition des *Directives pour l'eau de boisson*, valeur qui est tirée d'une étude de 1979 au cours de laquelle des chiens ont été exposés pendant 7,5 années à du chloroforme.

Parmi les THM bromés, le BDCM est particulièrement intéressant car il provoque des tumeurs de diverses localisations chez le rat et la souris (foie, rein, côlon) après administration par gavage dans de l'huile de maïs. La formation de tumeurs coliques chez le rat sous l'action du BDCM (et du bromoforme) est également intéressante en raison de l'existence d'associations épidémiologiques avec le cancer colo-rectal. On estime également que BDCM et les autres THM bromés sont faiblement mutagènes. Il est généralement admis que les cancérogènes dotés de propriétés mutagènes donnent lieu à une relation dose-réponse linéaire à faible dose, la mutagenèse étant généralement considérée comme un effet irréversible et cumulatif.

Lors d'une étude toxicologique de 2 ans, du BDCM a été administré par gavage dans de l'huile de maïs à des souris et des rats. On a observé la formation de tumeurs (ainsi qu'une cytotoxicité et une augmentation de la prolifération cellulaire) au niveau du rein aux doses quotidienne de 50 mg/kg p.c. chez les souris et de 100 mg/kg p.c. chez le rat. Des tumeurs du côlon ont été observées chez le rat après exposition à des doses quotidiennes de 50 et 100 mg/kg p.c. En s'appuyant sur la valeur de l'incidence des tumeurs rénales obtenue lors de cette étude, on a pu procéder à une estimation quantitative du risque. On a ainsi obtenu un CSF (*cancer slope factor*) de $4,8 \times 10^{-3}$ [mg/kg p.c. par jour]$^{-1}$ et pour un niveau de risque de 10^{-5}, la dose est de 2,1 µg/kg p.c. par jour. En se fondant sur la valeur de l'incidence des cancers du côlon chez le rat, on a obtenu un CSF égal à $4,2 \times 10^{-3}$ [mg/kg p.c. par jour]$^{-1}$ (2,4 µg/kg p.c. par jour pour un risque de 10^{-5}). Le Centre international de recherche sur le cancer (CIRC) a classé le BDCM dans le groupe 2B (peut-être cancérogène pour l'Homme).

Le DBCM et le bromoforme ont fait l'objet d'études toxicologiques à long terme. Lors d'une étude au cours de laquelle on a gavé des rats et des souris pendant deux ans avec ces produits incorporés à de l'huile de maïs, on a constaté que le DBCM provoquait des tumeurs hépatiques chez les souris femelles - mais pas chez les rats - à la dose quotidienne de 100 mg/kg p.c. Il avait été avancé, lors d'évaluations antérieures, que l'huile de maïs aurait pu jouer un rôle dans l'apparition de ces tumeurs chez les souris femelles. Dans le cas du bromoforme, on a observé des tumeurs du côlon en légère augmentation chez le rat à la dose quotidienne de 200 mg/kg p.c. La valeur du CSF obtenue dans le cas de ces tumeurs est égale à $6,5 \times 10^{-3}$ [mg/kg p.c. par jour]$^{-1}$ dans le cas du DBCM pour un risque de 10^{-5} et à $1,3 \times 10^{-3}$ [mg/kg p.c. par jour]$^{-1}$ ou 7,7 µg/kg p.c. par jour dans le cas du bromoforme pour un risque de 10^{-5}.

Ces deux THM bromés sont faiblement mutagènes dans un certain nombre de tests et ce sont en tous cas de loin les SPC qui se révèlent les plus mutagènes du groupe dans le système d'épreuve utilisant les GST. Comme ce sont en outre les plus lipophiles, il faut se demander si l'huile de maïs n'a pas réduit la biodisponibilité dans le cas des études à long terme. En ce qui concerne le DBCM, on a obtenu une NOAEL de 30 mg/kg p.c. par jour en se basant sur l'absence d'effets histopathologiques sur le foie chez des rats qui avaient reçu par gavage pendant 13 semaines ce composé incorporé à de l'huile de maïs. Le CIRC a placé ce composé dans le groupe 3 (composés ne pouvant être classés par rapport à leur cancérogénicité pour l'Homme). On a fixé une dose journalière tolérable de 30 µg/kg p.c. en se basant sur la NOAEL de 30 mg/kg p.c. j^{-1} (critère : hépatotoxicité) avec une marge d'incertitude correspondant à un facteur 1000 (un facteur de 10 à chaque fois pour tenir compte des variations intra- et interspécifiques, plus un autre facteur de 10 pour prendre en compte la faible durée de l'étude et un pouvoir cancérogène éventuel).

De même, il est possible d'obtenir pour le bromoforme une NOAEL de 25 mg/kg p.c. j^{-1} en se basant sur l'absence de lésions hépatiques chez le rat après 13 semaines d'administration par gavage dans de l'huile de maïs. A partir de cette valeur, on a fixé à 25 µg/kg p.c., la dose journalière tolérable, avec une marge d'incertitude correspondant à un facteur 1000 (un facteur de 10 à chaque fois pour tenir compte des variations intra- et interspécifiques, plus un autre facteur 10 pour prendre en compte de la courte durée de l'étude et de la cancérogénicité éventuelle du produit). Le CIRC a placé le bromoforme dans le groupe 3 (composés ne pouvant être classés par rapport à leur cancérogénicité pour l'Homme).

5) Acides halogénoacétiques

Il est très improbable que le DCA provoque des mutations aux faibles doses correspondant à sa concentration habituelle dans l'eau de boisson chlorée. D'après les données disponibles, il affecte différemment la vitesse de réplication des hépatocytes selon qu'il y a eu ou non action d'un initiateur. Les relations dose-réponse sont complexes, la DCA commençant par stimuler la division des hépatocytes normaux. Toutefois, aux doses plus faibles utilisées dans les études à long terme sur l'animal (ces doses sont tout de même beaucoup plus élevées que les concentrations présentes habituellement dans l'eau de boisson), la vitesse de réplication des hépatocytes normaux finit par diminuer fortement. On peut en déduire que les hépatocytes normaux finissent par provoquer une régulation négative des voies de stimulation par la DCA. Cependant, les cellules modifiées, notamment celles qui expriment de grandes quantités de protéines réagissant sur les anticorps c-Jun, ne semblent pas capables de réguler négativement cette réponse. C'est pourquoi les cellules porteuses de ce phénotype se divisent très rapidement dans les lésions précancéreuses aux doses de DCA provoquant l'apparition de tumeurs à très faible temps de latence. D'après les données les premières données, il semblerait que cette modification permanente de la naissance et de la mort cellulaires soit également nécessaire pour qu'il y ait cancérisation des lésions. Les études dans lesquelles on fait également intervenir un initiateur ou un promoteur tumoral appuient cette interprétation.

En se fondant sur les considérations précédentes, on peut penser que les estimations actuelles du risque de cancer imputable à l'acide dichloracétique devront être modifiées pour tenir compte des nouveaux résultats concernant le métabolisme et le mode d'action comparés de ce composé, afin que l'on puisse élaborer un modèle dose-réponse qui s'appuie sur les données biologiques. Ces résultats ne sont pas encore disponibles, mais ils devraient l'être d'ici 2 à 3 ans.

Les effets de l'acide dichloracétique se révèlent être en rapport très étroit avec les doses qui provoque une hépatomégalie et une accumulation de glycogène chez la souris. La dose la plus faible produisant un effet nocif observable (LOAEL) dans ce cas a été évaluée à 0,5 g/litre lors d'une étude de 8 semaines sur la souris. Cette dose correspond à environ 100 mg/kg p.c. par jour. La même étude a fourni une NOAEL de 0,2 g/litre, soit environ 40 mg/kg j^{-1}. On a fixé la dose journalière tolérable à 40 µg par kg de poids corporel en appliquant un coefficient d'incertitude de 1000 à cette NOAEL (un facteur de 10 à chaque fois pour tenir compte des variations intra- et interspécifiques plus un autre facteur de 10 pour prendre en compte la courte durée d'étude et une cancérogénicité éventuelle). Le CIRC a placé l'acide dichloracétique dans le groupe 3 (composés ne pouvant être classés par rapport à leur cancérogénicité pour l'Homme).

L'acide trichloracétique est l'un des plus faibles activateurs des récepteurs PPAR (*peroxisome proliferator-activated receptors*) que l'on connaisse. En tant que proliférateur des peroxysomes, il n'a qu'une activité marginale, même chez le rat. Par ailleurs, lorsqu'on donne à des rats une eau de boisson à forte teneur en acide trichloracétique, il ne se forme pas de tumeurs du foie. Tous ces résultats incitent fortement à penser que l'acide trichloracétique ne présente qu'un faible risque cancérogène pour l'Homme étant donné sa faible concentration dans l'eau de boisson.

Si on considère le problème toxicologique dans sa généralité, ce sont les effets de ce composé sur le développement qui constituent le point d'aboutissement le plus préoccupant de son action toxique. Les animaux de laboratoire présentent une bonne tolérance à ce composé à la dose de 0,5 g/litre (soit une dose quotidienne d'environ 50 mg/kg de poids corporel) et ne présentent guère d'effets indésirables à cette concentration. A la dose de 2 g/litre, le seul effet indésirable consiste en une hépatomégalie. Chez la souris, on n'observe pas d'hépatomégalie à la dose de 0,35 g/litre, c'est à dire pour une dose quotidienne de 40 mg/kg p.c.

Dans une autre étude, on a observé environ trois fois plus d'anomalies au niveau des tissus mous que chez les témoins à la dose la plus faible administrée, soit 330 mg/kg j^{-1}. A cette dose, il s'agissait d'anomalies légères et la dose est bien du même ordre que celle qui provoque une hépatomégalie (et certains effets cancérogènes). Etant donné qu'il y a interaction entre les récepteurs PPAR et les mécanismes de signalisation cellulaire susceptibles d'intervenir dans les processus normaux de développement, il faut envisager l'existence d'un mécanisme commun à l'hépatomégalie, aux effets cancérogènes et aux effets sur le développement.

La dose journalière tolérable d'acide trichloracétique est basée sur une NOAEL de 40 mg par kg de poids corporel par jour, obtenue à la suite d'une étude à long terme sur la souris, le critère retenu étant l'hépatotoxicité. En se donnant une marge d'incertitude correspondant à un facteur 1000 (un facteur de 10 à chaque fois pour tenir compte des variations intra- et interspécifiques plus un autre facteur de 10 pour prendre en compte la cancérogénicité éventuelle du produit), on arrive à une dose journalière tolérable de 40 µg/kg p.c. Le CIRC a placé l'acide trichloracétique dans le groupe 3 (composés ne pouvant être classés par rapport à leur cancérogénicité pour l'Homme).

Les données relatives à la cancérogénicité des acides brom-acétiques ont un caractère trop préliminaire pour permettre la caractérisation du risque. Les données que l'on peut tirer des résumés analytiques incitent cependant à penser que ces composés sont susceptibles d'avoir des effets hépatocancérogènes chez la souris à des doses qui ne sont pas tellement différentes ce celles des acides chloracétiques. Outre des mécanismes analogues à ceux qui sont à la base des processus malins dont sont responsables les acides dichlor-acétique et trichloracétique, il est possible que le stress oxydatif découlant de leur métabolisation joue un rôle dans leurs effets.

On possède un nombre non négligeable de données concernant les effets que l'acide dibromacétique exerce sur la fonction reproductrice chez le mâle. On n'a pas observé d'effets chez des rats à la dose quotidienne de 2 mg/kg de poids corporel sur une durée de 79 jours, mais à la dose de 10 mg/kg, il y avait augmentation de la rétention des spermatides au stade 19. A mesure que les doses ont été augmentées, on a noté une aggravation des effets, notamment une atrophie importante des tubes séminifères à 250 mg/kg j^{-1}. Il n'y a pas eu retour à la normale dans les six mois suivant la cessation de l'exposition. Pour déterminer la dose journalière tolérable, on est parti d'une NOAEL journalière de 2 mg/kg p.c. en se donnant une marge d'incertitude correspondant à un facteur 100 (un facteur de 10 à chaque fois pour tenir compte des variations intra- et interspécifiques).

6)   Hydrate de chloral

A la concentration de 1 g par litre d'eau de boisson (166 mg/kg j^{-1}), il y a eu formation de tumeurs hépatiques chez des souris exposée à ce produit pendant 104 semaines. On n'a pas étudié les effets des doses inférieures à cette valeur. Il a été montré que l'hydrate de chloral provoquait l'apparition d'anomalies chromosomiques dans un certain nombre de systèmes d'épreuve *in vitro*, mais *in vivo* les résultats se sont révélés largement négatifs. Il est probable que si l'hydrate de chloral provoque des tumeurs du foie, c'est parce qu'il est métabolisé en acide dichloracétique ou trichloracétique. Comme on l'a vu plus haut, ces composés sont considérés comme des promoteurs tumoraux.

Le CIRC a placé l'hydrate de chloral dans le groupe 3 (composés qui ne peuvent être classés par rapport à leur cancérogénicité pour l'Homme).

Administré à des rats pendant 90 jours dans leur eau de boisson, l'hydrate de chloral a provoqué une nécrose des hépatocytes aux concentrations supérieures ou égales à 1200 mg/litre. En revanche, aucun effet n'a été observé à 600 mg/litre (soit environ 60 mg/kg j^{-1}) On a observé une hépatomégalie chez des souris à la dose quotidienne de 144 mg/kg p.c., lorsque le produit était administré par gavage sur une période de 14 jours. Lors de cette même étude, aucun effet n'a été observé à la dose quotidienne de 14,4 mg/kg, mais une étude de 90 jours effectuée dans le prolongement de la précédente a montré qu'à la dose de 70 mg/litre dans l'eau de boisson (c'est-à-dire 16 mg/kg j^{-1}), il y avait une légère hépatomégalie. En se donnant une marge d'incertitude correspondant à un facteur 1000 (un facteur de 10 à chaque fois pour tenir compte des variation inter- et intraspécifiques plus un autre facteur 10 pour prendre en considération le fait qu'on est parti de la LOAEL au lieu de la NOAEL), on aboutit à une dose journalière tolérable de 16 µg/kg de poids corporel.

7) Halogénoacétonitriles

Faute de données humaines suffisantes ou d'une étude sur l'animal qui porte sur une fraction substantielle de la vie des animaux de laboratoire, on ne dispose d'aucun élément d'appréciation du risque cancérogène qui fasse l'unanimité.

Les données tirées des études subchroniques permettent d'avoir un certain nombre d'indications sur les NOAEL relatives à la toxicité générale du dichloracétonitrile (DCAN) et du dibromacétonitrile (DBAN). C'est ainsi que l'on a obtenu une NOAEL respectivement égale à 8 et 23 mg/kg p.c. j^{-1} pour le DCAN et le DBAN à l'occasion d'études de 90 jours sur des rats et des souris, le critère pris en considération étant une diminution du poids corporel notée aux doses respectives de 33 et 45 mg/kg p.c. j^{-1}.

Le groupe de travail de l'OMS qui s'est réuni en 1993 pour la préparation des *Directives de qualité pour l'eau de boisson* a étudié le cas du DCAN et du DBAN. Il a fixé à 15 µg/kg j^{-1} la dose journalière tolérable de DCAN en se basant sur une NOAEL de 15 mg/kg j^{-1} obtenue à la suite d'une étude sur la toxicité génésique du DCAN chez le rat. Le groupe a considéré qu'il y avait une marge d'incertitude correspondant à un facteur 1000 (un facteur de 10 à chaque fois pour tenir compte des variation intra- et interspécifiques plus un autre facteur 10 afin de prendre également en considération la gravité des effets). En ce qui concerne le DBAN, on n'a observé d'effets sur la reproduction et le développement qu'aux doses dépassant celles entraînant une intoxication générale (soit environ 45 mg/kg p.c. j^{-1}). En se basant sur la NOAEL de 23 mg/kg p.c. j^{-1} tirée de l'étude de 90 jours sur le rat et en se donnant une marge d'incertitude correspondant à un facteur 1000 (un facteur de 10 à chaque fois pour tenir compte des variations intra- et interspécifiques plus un autre facteur 10 en considération de la brièveté de l'étude), on a abouti à une valeur de la dose journalière tolérable égale à 23 µg/kg p.c. j^{-1}). On ne dispose d'aucune donnée nouvelle qui justifierait de modifier cette dose.

En ce qui concerne le trichloracétonitrile (TCA), on a obtenu une LOAEL de 7,5 mg/kg j^{-1} en prenant l'embryotoxicité comme critère et une LOAEL de 15 mg/kg j^{-1} en prenant en considération les effets sur le développement. Des résultats ultérieurs incitent toutefois à penser que les effets constatés étaient liés au véhicule utilisé.

On ne possède aucune donnée qui permettrait de caractériser le risque imputable à d'autres halogénoacétonitriles.

8)   MX

Le MX, qui possède des propriétés mutagènes, a récemment fait l'objet d'une étude à long terme sur le rat au cours de laquelle on a observé des effets cancérogènes. Selon cette étude, le MX provoque des tumeurs de la thyroïde et des voies biliaires. A la dose la plus faible administrée (0,4 mg/kg p.c. j^{-1}), on a constaté que l'incidence des tumeurs thyroïdiennes était en augmentation. On estime depuis longtemps que la formation de tumeurs de la thyroïde après exposition à de fortes doses de produits chimiques est une caractéristique des composés halogénés. Il se pourrait que les tumeurs folliculaires de la thyroïde soient la conséquence d'un dérèglement de la fonction thyroïdienne ou d'une mutagenèse. On a également observé un accroissement de l'incidence des cholangiomes et des cholangiocarcinomes qui était lié à la dose; cet effet à commencé à se manifester à faible dose chez les femelles; il était moins marqué chez les mâles. C'est précisément cette augmentation de l'incidence des cholangiomes et des cholangiocarcinomes chez les rattes que l'on a utilisé pour déterminer la valeur du CSF (*cancer slope factor*). La limite supérieure de confiance à 95 % pour un risque de 10^{-5} sur toute la durée de l'existence a été trouvée égale à 0,06 µg/kg p.c. j^{-1} sur la base d'un modèle linéaire multistade.

9) Chlorites

L'exposition aux chlorites conduit systématiquement à un stress oxydatif qui en constitue le principal effet avec pour conséquence des modifications au niveau des érythrocytes. Ce point d'aboutissement de l'action toxique de l'ion chlorite s'observe chez les animaux de laboratoire et, comme dans le cas des chlorates, chez les sujets humains intoxiqués par une exposition à de très fortes doses. On possède suffisamment de données pour déterminer la dose journalière tolérable par l'Homme, données notamment fournies par des études de toxicité chronique ainsi qu'une étude de toxicité génésique portant sur deux générations. Les études menées sur des volontaires pendant des périodes allant jusqu'à 12 semaines n'ont pas permis de mettre en évidence le moindre effet hématologique, même à la dose la plus forte utilisée, à savoir 36 µg/kg p.c. j^{-1}. Ces études n'ayant pas permis de déterminer la dose à partir duquel se manifestent des effets toxiques, on ne peut rien en tirer quant à l'ordre de grandeur de la marge de sécurité.

Une étude portant sur deux générations de rats a permis de fixer la NOAEL à 2,9 mg/kg p.c. j^{-1}, les critères retenus étant la diminution de l'amplitude du tressaillement auditif, la réduction du poids du cerveau dans les générations F_1 et F_2 et la modification du poids du foie dans les deux générations. En estimant que la marge d'incertitude correspond à un facteur 100 (un facteur de 10 à chaque fois pour tenir compte des variations intra- et interspécifiques), on en a déduit que la dose journalière tolérable était de 30 µg/kg p.c. Les études effectuées sur des volontaires confirment cette valeur.

10) Chlorates

Comme dans le cas des chlorites, le principal problème d'ordre toxicologique tient aux lésions oxydatives qui se produisent au niveau des érythrocytes. De même que pour l'ion chlorite, on a constaté qu'une dose quotidienne de chlorates de 0,036 mg/kg p.c. pendant 12 semaines ne provoquait aucun effet indésirable chez des volontaires. La base de données relative aux chlorates est moins riche que pour les chlorites mais on dispose cependant des résultats d'une récente étude de 90 jours sur le rat, qui a permis de déterminer la NOAEL en prenant comme critère une déplétion des colloïdes dans la glande thyroïde. La valeur obtenue est de 30 mg/kg p.c. j^{-1}. On est dans l'attente des résultats d'une autre étude à long terme, aussi n'a t-on pas cherché à fixer la valeur de la dose journalière tolérable car cette étude devrait fournir des données plus complètes sur l'exposition chronique aux chlorates.

11) Bromates

Les bromates se comportent comme des oxydants actifs vis-à-vis des systèmes biologiques et on a montré qu'ils provoquaient une augmentation du nombre de tumeurs rénales, de mésothéliomes péritonéaux et de tumeurs folliculaires de la thyroïde chez le rat et, dans une moindre mesure, chez le hamster. Chez la souris en revanche, on ne constate qu'une légère augmentation des tumeurs du rein. La dose la plus faible à laquelle on ait observé une augmentation de l'incidence des tumeurs rénales chez le rat est égale à 6 mg/kg p.c. j^{-1}.

Il a également été montré que les bromates provoquaient des aberrations chromosomiques dans des cellules mammaliennes *in vitro* et *in vivo*, mais on n'a pas constaté de mutations ponctuelles lors d'épreuves sur bactéries. Un ensemble de plus en plus important de données, confirmées par des tests de génotoxicité, incitent à penser que l'ion bromate agit en donnant naissance à des radicaux oxygénés à l'intérieur de la cellule.

Dans les *Directives de qualité pour l'eau de boisson* (avant-dernière édition), on a utilisé un modèle linéaire multistade pour étudier l'incidence des tumeurs rénales lors d'une étude de 2 ans sur des rats, mais il avait été cependant noté que si le mécanisme de cancérogenèse repose un stress oxydatif des cellules rénales, il n'était peut-être pas approprié d'utiliser un modèle de cancérisation faisant intervenir de faibles doses. La limite supérieure de l'intervalle de confiance à 95 % pour un risque de 10^{-5}, a été estimée à 0,1 µg/kg p.c. j^{-1}.

Chez le rat, la dose quotidienne sans effet est de 1,3 mg/kg p.c., si l'effet retenu est la formation de tumeurs rénales. Si l'on considère qu'à partir de cette valeur la relation dose-réponse n'est plus linéaire et en prenant une marge de sécurité correspondant à un facteur 1000 (un facteur de 10 à chaque fois pour tenir compte des variations intra-interspécifiques plus un facteur 10 pour prendre en compte la cancéro-génicité possible du composé), on peut fixer à 1 µg/kg p.c. la dose journalière tolérable. Cette valeur est à rapprocher de la valeur de 0,1 µg/kg j^{-1} obtenue dans le cas d'un risque de cancer de 10^{-5} sur toute la durée de l'existence.

Pour l'instant, on ne possède pas suffisamment de données pour savoir si les tumeurs dues aux bromates s'expliquent par un phénomène de cytotoxicité, par une hyperplasie réparatrice ou par un effet génotoxique.

Le CIRC a placé le bromate de potassium dans le groupe 2B (composés peut-être cancérogènes pour l'Homme).

5.1.2 *Etudes épidémiologiques*

Il faut procéder à une évaluation minutieuse des études épidémi-ologiques afin de s'assurer qu'elles ne comportent aucun biais et qu'elles sont effectivement conçues pour mettre en évidence une relation causale éventuelle. On peut procéder à l'évaluation de cette relation causale lorsqu'on dispose d'éléments d'appréciation suffisants fournis par plusieurs études bien conçues menées dans différentes régions. Il importe également de disposer de données toxicologiques et pharmacologiques à l'appui de l'hypothèse que l'on cherche à vérifier. Les données épidémiologiques fournies par les études écol-ogiques relatives à la désinfection de l'eau sont d'une interprétation particulièrement difficile et on les utilise essentiellement pour la formulation d'hypothèses à examiner plus avant.

Les résultats des études épidémiologiques analytiques ne permettent pas, à eux seuls, d'établir une relation de cause à effet dans le cas de telle ou telle association observée. Les résultats des études analytiques qui sont actuellement publiées sont particulièrement difficiles à interpréter car ils ne donnent pas assez de renseignements sur l'exposition aux à certains contaminants présents dans l'eau, qui pourraient constituer des facteurs de confusion ou tout au moins modifier le risque. Etant donné que l'on ne s'est pas suffisamment préoccupé d'évaluer l'exposition à ces contaminants, il n'est pas possible d'estimer correctement l'excès de risque relatif observé. Il n'est en effet pas exclu que ce risque soit dû à d'autres contaminants présents dans l'eau ou à d'autres facteurs dont l'action serait attribuée à tort à l'eau chlorée et aux THM qu'elle peut contenir.

5.2   Caractérisation de l'exposition

5.2.1   Fréquence des désinfectants et des sous-produits de chloration

On utilise le plus souvent des doses de désinfectants de plusieurs milligrammes par litre, qui sont nécessaires pour inactiver les germes présents dans l'eau (désinfection primaire) ou maintenir une concentration résiduelle dans le réseau d'adduction (désinfection secondaire).

Pour évaluer l'exposition, il faut savoir quels sont les SPC présents et à quelle concentration. Il n'existe malheureusement guère d'études publiées au niveau international qui aillent au-delà de la simple étude cas-témoins ou dont la portée ne soit pas limitée à une région.

L'étude des données disponibles indique, qu'en moyenne, il y a 35 à 50 µg/litre de THM totaux dans l'eau de boisson traitée par le chlore et que les espèces chimiques prédominantes sont, dans l'ordre, le chloroforme et le bromodichlorométhane. En ce qui concerne l'exposition aux HAA, on peut dire qu'elle est approximativement égale à la somme de cinq espèces chimiques appartenant à ce groupe, dont la concentration totale serait à peu près la moitié de celle des THM (cette proportion peut toutefois varier assez sensiblement); les composés prédominants sont, dans l'ordre, l'acide dichloracétique et l'acide trichloracétique. Dans les eaux où le rapport des bromates aux composés organiques totaux est élevé ou encore où les bromures prédominent par rapport aux chlorures, il y a vraisemblablement formation plus importante de THM et de HAA bromés. Si on utilise une solution d'hypochlorite de préférence à du chlore à l'état gazeux, le processus de chloration peut entraîner la formation de chlorates.

L'exposition aux SPC qui se forment lorsqu'on traite l'eau par la chloramine est fonction de la méthode employée pour générer la chloramine; par exemple, si on commence par injecter du chlore puis de l'ammoniac, il se forme moins de SPC (THM et HAA) pendant la période où le chlore est à l'état libre; toutefois, à la diminution de la formation de chloroforme et d'acide trichloracétique ne correspond pas une diminution proportionnelle de la formation d'acide dichlor-acétique.

Toutes choses égales par ailleurs, la concentration des bromures et la dose d'ozone sont les paramètres qui permettent le mieux de prévoir la formation de bromates au cours de l'ozonisation, le taux de conversion des bromures en bromates étant d'environ 50 %. Une étude portant sur diverses compagnies européennes de distribution d'eau a montré que la concentration des bromates dans l'eau quittant les installations de traitement allait de valeurs inférieures à la limite de détection (2 µg/litre) à 16 µg/litre. Les sous-produits bromés qui se forment au cours du processus d'ozonisation sont généralement présents à faible concentration. Si on utilise du dioxyde de chlore, il est possible d'estimer la quantité de chlorites formés par une simple proportion (50-70 %) de la dose utilisée.

5.2.2   *Incertitudes des données relatives à la qualité de l'eau*

Dans une étude toxicologique, on s'efforce de d'extrapoler à l'Homme une réaction (contrôlée) observée sur un animal de laboratoire. On peut par exemple en tirer une estimation du risque de cancer. Dans une étude épidémiologique, on tente de relier des effets sur la santé humaine (par exemple, la formation de cancers) à l'action d'un ou de plusieurs agents (par exemple des SPC) et il faut pour cela évaluer l'exposition à ces agents.

Il peut y avoir plusieurs modes d'exposition aux risques que présente la consommation d'eau chlorée : i) l'ingestion de SPC avec l'eau qui les contient; ii) l'ingestion de désinfectants chimiques contenus dans l'eau de boisson et la formation intragastrique de SPC; iii) l'inhalation de SPC volatils en prenant une douche. La formation de SPC *in vivo* ou leur inhalation pendant une douche peut poser problème sur le plan sanitaire, mais la discussion qui suit repose sur l'hypothèse que l'ingestion des SPC présents dans l'eau de boisson constitue le mode d'exposition le plus important.

L'exposition humaine aux SPC dépend à la fois de leur concentration et de la durée de contact. Plus précisément, les effets que ces composés peuvent exercer sur la santé humaine sont fonction de l'exposition à des mélanges complexes de SPC (par exemple THM plutôt que HAA, dérivés bromés plutôt que chlorés) dont la composition peut varier au cours du temps, avec la saison (par ex. selon la température, la nature et la concentration des matières organiques naturelles) ou encore en différents points (à l'intérieur du réseau d'adduction par exemple). Chaque désinfectant utilisé pour traiter l'eau peut donner naissance à un mélange de SPC et un traitement associant plusieurs désinfectants va conduire à la formation de mélanges encore plus complexes. Lorsqu'ils se forment, la plupart de ces SPC sont stables mais certains d'entre eux peuvent subir des transformations, notamment par hydrolyse. Si l'on ne possède pas de données sur les SPC, il est possible d'obtenir une évaluation indirecte de l'exposition en utilisant à la place la dose de chlore (ou la demande de chlore), la teneur en carbone organique total (ou l'absorbance dans l'ultraviolet à 254 nm [UVA_{254}]) ou encore la teneur en bromures. Si on ne connaît pas la concentration en précurseurs organiques des SPC, on peut lui substituer la teneur en carbone organique total, mais l'absorbance à 254 nm donne une meilleure idée des caractéristiques des matières organiques naturelles, qui peuvent être soumises à des variations géographiques. Deux variables très importantes qui affectent la qualité de l'eau, à savoir la teneur en bromures et le pH, ont un effet sensible sur la nature et la concentration des SPC formés.

Lorsqu'on cherche à évaluer l'exposition, il faut tout d'abord s'efforcer de déterminer quels sont les SPC susceptibles de se former et de coexister simultanément. Il faut ensuite connaître l'évolution de leur concentration au cours du temps, qui va dépendre de leur stabilité et de leur transport à travers le réseau de distribution. En ce qui concerne les études épidémiologiques, il existe des bases de données historiques sur la concentration des désinfectants (par exemple le chlore) et éventuellement des précurseurs de SPC (par exemple le carbone organique total) ou encore des THM totaux (parfois sur certains THM bien déterminés). Contrairement aux THM qui sont depuis longtemps sous surveillance pour des raisons réglementaires, les données de surveillance concernant les HAA en général ou certains membres de ce groupe, les bromates et les chlorites sont beaucoup plus récentes et par conséquent peu abondantes. On peut toutefois faire appel à la modélisation pour simuler des données manquantes ou anciennes. La documentation relative à l'évolution des méthodes de traitement de l'eau est également un élément important à prendre en considération.

5.2.3   *Incertitudes des données épidémiologiques*

Même dans les études bien conçues et bien menées, on s'aperçoit que l'évaluation de l'exposition laisse à désirer. Dans la plupart des cas, on a pris en considération la durée de l'exposition et la source d'eau. L'exposition a été déterminée en étudiant la situation générale des habitations ainsi que les dossiers des compagnies de distribution ou des services publics. Il n'existe que très peu d'études dans lesquelles on ait tenté d'estimer la consommation d'eau des participants et leur exposition à divers THM ou mélanges de THM. Il n'y en a qu'une où l'on se soit efforcé de déterminer l'exposition aux autres SPC. Lorsqu'on cherche à évaluer certains risques, par exemple un risque d'issue défavorable pour une grossesse qui pourrait être lié à une exposition relativement brève à des sous-produits volatils, il n'est pas inutile de prendre en considération la voie respiratoire aussi bien que la voie digestive. Dans un certain nombre d'études, on a tenté d'estimer la teneur en SPC pendant la période étiologiquement significative ainsi que l'exposition cumulée. Il existe des modèles appropriés ou des analyses de simulation comme la méthode de Monte Carlo qui permettent d'estimer l'exposition au cours des périodes voulues.

L'incertitude est très importante en ce qui concerne l'interprétation des associations observées, car on n'a pris en considération que l'exposition à un nombre relativement restreint de contaminants présents dans l'eau. Il est difficile, à la lumière des données actuelles, de déterminer dans quelle mesure les SPC ou autres contaminants qui n'ont pas été dosés ont pu influer sur l'estimation du risque relatif.

Il y a eu davantage d'études consacrées au cancer de la vessie qu'à tout autre cancer. Les auteurs des études les plus récemment publiées au sujet du risque de cancer vésical mettent en garde contre toute interprétation simpliste des associations observées. Les éléments d'appréciation dont on dispose à l'appui d'un risque accru de cancer de la vessie ne sont pas concordants - on trouve un risque différent pour les fumeurs et les non fumeurs, pour les hommes et les femmes et selon que la consommation d'eau est forte ou faible. Le risque peut différer selon la région car les mélanges de SPC ne sont pas forcément identiques ou parce que l'eau peut contenir d'autres contaminants. Il faut rassembler des données beaucoup plus complètes sur la qualité de l'eau - ou les obtenir le cas échéant par simulation - pour permettre une meilleure évaluation de l'exposition en vue des études épidémiologiques.

RESUMEN Y EVALUACION

El cloro (Cl_2) se ha utilizado ampliamente en todo el mundo como desinfectante químico, siendo la principal barrera contra los contaminantes microbianos del agua de bebida. Las notables propiedades biocidas del cloro se han visto neutralizadas en parte por la formación, durante el proceso de cloración, de subproductos de los desinfectantes (SPD) que son motivo de preocupación para la salud pública. En consecuencia, se están utilizando cada vez más desinfectantes químicos alternativos, como el ozono (O_3), el dióxido de cloro (ClO_2) y las cloraminas (NH_2Cl, monocloramina); sin embargo, se ha demostrado que cada uno de ellos forma su propia serie de SPD. Aunque no se puede comprometer la calidad microbiológica del agua de bebida, es necesario conocer mejor la química, la toxicología y la epidemiología de los desinfectantes químicos y de sus SPD asociados, a fin de tener un mayor conocimiento de los riesgos para la salud (microbianos y químicos) asociados con el agua de bebida y buscar un equilibrio entre ambos riesgos. Es posible reducir el riesgo químico que representan los SPD sin comprometer la calidad microbiológica.

1. Química de los desinfectantes y de los subproductos de los desinfectantes

Los desinfectantes químicos más utilizados son el cloro, el ozono, el dióxido de cloro y la cloramina. Las propiedades físicas y químicas de los desinfectantes y los SPD pueden influir en su comportamiento en el agua de bebida, así como en su toxicología y su epidemiología. Todos los desinfectantes químicos que se examinan en el presente documento son oxidantes solubles en agua, que se producen *in situ* (por ejemplo, el ozono) o *ex situ* (por ejemplo, el cloro). Se administran en forma de gas (por ejemplo, el ozono) o de líquido (por ejemplo, el hipoclorito) a dosis normales de varios miligramos por litro, solos o bien mezclados. Los SPD que se examinan aquí se pueden medir por cromatografía de gases o líquida y clasificarse como orgánicos o inorgánicos, halogenados (clorados o bromados) o no halogenados y volátiles o no volátiles. Al formarse, los SPD pueden ser estables o inestables (por ejemplo, descomposición por hidrólisis).

Los SPD se forman en la reacción de desinfectantes químicos con precursores de los SPD. La materia orgánica natural, que normalmente se mide por el carbono orgánico total, actúa como precursor orgánico, mientras que el ión bromuro (Br⁻) es el precursor inorgánico. En la formación de los SPD influyen la calidad del agua (por ejemplo, el carbono orgánico total, el bromuro, el pH, la temperatura, el amoníaco y la alcalinidad por carbonatos) y las condiciones del tratamiento (por ejemplo, la dosis de desinfectante, el tiempo de contacto, la eliminación de la materia orgánica natural antes de la aplicación del desinfectante, la adición previa del desinfectante).

El cloro en forma de ácido hipocloroso/ión hipoclorito (ClOH/ClO⁻) reacciona con el ión bromuro, oxidándolo a ácido hipobromoso/ión hipobromito (BrOH/BrO⁻). El ácido hipocloroso (oxidante más potente) y el ácido hipobromoso (agente halogenante más eficaz) reaccionan conjuntamente con la materia orgánica natural para formar SPD del cloro, entre ellos trihalometanos (THM), ácidos haloacéticos (AHA), haloacetonitrilos (HAN), halocetonas, hidrato de cloral y cloropicrina. El predominio de los grupos de SPD del cloro suele disminuir en el orden siguiente: THM, AHA y HAN. Las cantidades relativas de carbono orgánico total, bromuro y cloruro influyen en la distribución por especies de THM (cuatro especies: cloroformo, bromoformo, bromodiclorometano y dibromoclorometano), de los AHA (hasta nueve especies cloradas/bromadas) y de los HAN (varias especies cloradas/bromadas). En general predominan las especies de THM, AHA y HAN cloradas sobre las bromadas, aunque se puede dar el caso contrario en aguas con un alto contenido de bromuro. Si bien se han identificado numerosos SPD específicos del cloro, hay un porcentaje considerable de halógenos orgánicos totales que siguen sin conocerse. Otra de las reacciones del cloro es la que da lugar a la formación de clorato (ClO_3^-) en soluciones concentradas de hipocloritos.

El ozono puede reaccionar directa o indirectamente con el bromuro para formar SPD de ozono bromados, incluido el ión bromato (BrO_3^-). En presencia de materia orgánica natural, durante la ozonación se producen SPD orgánicos no halogenados, como aldehídos, cetoácidos y ácidos carboxílicos, predominando los aldehídos (por ejemplo, el formaldehído). En presencia de materia orgánica natural y de bromuro, la ozonación forma ácido hipobromoso, que a su vez da lugar a la formación de compuestos organohalogenados bromados (por ejemplo, el bromoformo).

Los principales SPD del dióxido de cloro son los iones clorito (ClO_2^-) y clorato, sin formación directa de SPD organohalogenados. A diferencia de otros desinfectantes, los SPD más importantes del dióxido de cloro proceden de la descomposición del desinfectante, y no de la reacción con los precursores.

El uso de la cloramina como desinfectante secundario suele dar lugar a la formación de cloruro de cianógeno (ClCN), un compuesto de nitrógeno, y concentraciones significativamente reducidas de SPD del cloro. Un problema conexo es la presencia de nitrito (NO_2^-) en sistemas de distribución cloraminados.

Teniendo en cuenta el conocimiento actual acerca de la presencia y los efectos en la salud, los SPD de mayor interés son los THM, los AHA, el bromato y el clorito.

Se ha comprobado que el grupo predominante de SPD del cloro son los THM, siendo el cloroformo y el bromodiclorometano la primera y la segunda especies. El segundo grupo más importante lo forman los AHA, siendo el ácido dicloroacético y el ácido tricloro-acético la primera y la segunda especies.

La conversión de bromuro en bromato durante la ozonación depende de la materia orgánica natural, el pH y la temperatura, entre otros factores. Los niveles pueden oscilar entre valores inferiores al nivel de detección (2 μg/litro) y varias decenas de miligramos por litro. Las concentraciones de cloruro suelen ser muy previsibles, variando entre el 50% y el 70% aproximadamente de la dosis de dióxido de cloro administrada.

Los SPD están presentes en mezclas complejas que dependen del desinfectante químico utilizado, de la calidad del agua y de las condiciones del tratamiento; otros factores son la combinación/uso secuencial de desinfectantes/oxidantes múltiples. Además, la composición de estas mezclas puede cambiar con las estaciones. Es evidente que los efectos químicos potenciales relacionados con la salud serán función de la exposición a las mezclas de SPD.

Aparte de los SPD del cloro (en particular los THM), hay muy pocos datos sobre la presencia de SPD en el agua tratada y los sistemas de distribución. A partir de las bases de datos de laboratorio, se han elaborado modelos empíricos para pronosticar las concentraciones de THM (THM totales y sus especies), de AHA (AHA totales y sus especies) y de bromato. Estos modelos se pueden utilizar en la evaluación del rendimiento para predecir el efecto de los cambios de tratamiento y en la evaluación de la exposición para simular datos que falten o pasados (por ejemplo, para pronosticar las concentraciones de AHA a partir de los datos relativos a los THM).

Los SPD se pueden controlar mediante la inspección y eliminación de sus precursores o con prácticas de desinfección modificadas. La materia orgánica natural se puede eliminar mediante coagulación, carbono granular activado, filtración por membrana y biofiltración de ozono. Si se exceptúa la utilización de membranas, hay pocas posibilidades de eliminar el bromuro con eficacia. Si se desea evitar el tratamiento del agua habrá que proteger y controlar las fuentes. No es posible eliminar los SPD tras su formación en el caso de los SPD orgánicos, mientras que el bromato y el clorito se pueden eliminar con carbono activado o agentes reductores. Cabe prever que el uso óptimo de combinaciones de desinfectantes, utilizados como desinfectantes primarios y secundarios, permitirá controlar ulteriormente los SPD. Hay una tendencia a la utilización simultánea o sucesiva de diversos desinfectantes; el ozono se utiliza exclusivamente como desinfectante primario, las cloraminas sólo como secundario, y tanto el cloro como el dióxido de cloro en ambos casos.

2. Cinética y metabolismo en animales de laboratorio y en el ser humano

2.1 Desinfectantes

Los desinfectantes residuales son productos químicos reactivos que reaccionan con compuestos orgánicos presentes en la saliva y en el contenido del estómago para formar subproductos. Hay diferencias significativas en la farmacocinética del ^{36}Cl según se obtenga a partir del cloro, de la cloramina o del dióxido de cloro.

2.2   Trihalometanos

Tras la exposición oral o por inhalación, los mamíferos absorben, metabolizan y eliminan con rapidez los THM. Después de la absorción, las concentraciones tisulares más elevadas se producen en la grasa, el hígado y los riñones. La semivida suele oscilar entre 0,5 y tres horas y la vía primaria de eliminación es la metabolización en anhídrido carbónico. La toxicidad de los THM sólo se manifiesta previa activación metabólica a intermediarios reactivos, y las tres especies bromadas se metabolizan con mayor rapidez y en mayor medida que el cloroformo. La ruta metabólica más importante para todos los THM es la oxidación a través del citocromo P450 (CYP)2E1, que da lugar a la formación de dihalocarbonilos (es decir, fosgeno y compuestos análogos bromados), que se pueden hidrolizar para formar anhídrido carbónico o unirse a macromoléculas de los tejidos. Las vías metabólicas secundarias son la deshalogenación por reducción a través del citocromo CYP2B1/2/2E1 (que da lugar a la formación de radicales libres) y la conjugación del glutatión mediante la glutatión-*S*-transferasa T1-1, que forma intermediarios mutágenos. Los THM bromados tienen muchas más probabilidades que el cloroformo de seguir las vías secundarias, y la conjugación del cloroformo con el glutatión mediante la glutatión-*S*-transferasa se puede producir solamente a concentraciones o dosis extraordinariamente elevadas de cloroformo.

2.3   Ácidos haloacéticos

La cinética y el metabolismo de los ácidos dihaloacéticos y trihaloacéticos difieren considerablemente. En la medida en que se metabolizan, las principales reacciones de los ácidos trihaloacéticos se producen en la fracción microsomal, mientras que más del 90% del metabolismo de los ácidos dihaloacéticos, fundamentalmente por intervención de las glutatión-transferasas, tiene lugar en el citosol. El ácido tricloroacético tiene una semivida biológica de 50 horas en el ser humano. La semivida de los otros ácidos trihaloacéticos disminuye considerablemente con la sustitución del bromo, y con ácidos trihaloacéticos bromados se pueden detectar cantidades mensurables de ácidos dihaloacéticos como productos. La semivida de los ácidos dihaloacéticos a dosis bajas es muy breve, pero se puede elevar radicalmente con el aumento de las dosis.

2.4   Haloaldehídos y halocetonas

Se dispone de datos limitados sobre la cinética del hidrato de cloral. Sus dos metabolitos principales son el tricloroetanol y el ácido tricloroacético. El tricloroetanol sufre una glucuronidación rápida, con circulación enterohepática, hidrólisis y oxidación para dar ácido tricloroacético. La decloración del tricloroetanol o del hidrato de cloral daría lugar a la formación de ácido dicloroacético. Luego, éste se puede transformar de nuevo en monocloroacetato, glioxalato, glicolato y oxalato, probablemente a través de un intermediario reactivo. No se encontró información sobre los demás haloaldehídos y halocetonas.

2.5   Haloacetonitrilos

No se han estudiado el metabolismo y la cinética de los haloacetonitrilos. Los datos cualitativos indican que entre los productos del metabolismo figuran el cianuro, el formaldehído, el cianuro de formilo y los haluros de formilo.

2.6   Derivados halogenados de las hidroxifuranonas

El miembro del grupo de las hidroxifuranonas que se ha estudiado más a fondo es la 3-cloro-4-(diclorometil)-5-hidroxi-2 (5H)-furanona (MX). De los estudios en animales parece deducirse que la MX marcada con ^{14}C se absorbe con rapidez en el tracto gastrointestinal y pasa a la circulación sistémica. No se ha determinado la concentración de la propia MX en la sangre. La MX marcada se excreta fundamentalmente en la orina y en las heces, siendo la orina la vía principal de excreción. Es muy pequeña la concentración del producto inicial radiomarcado que se retiene en el organismo después de cinco días.

2.7   Clorito

El ^{36}Cl del clorito se absorbe con rapidez. Menos de la mitad de la dosis pasa a la orina como cloruro y una pequeña proporción lo hace en forma de clorito. Probablemente un porcentaje importante entra a formar parte de la reserva de cloruros del organismo, pero no hay información detallada debido a la falta de métodos analíticos para valorar el clorito en muestras biológicas.

2.8 Clorato

El clorato se comporta de manera semejante al clorito. Existen los mismos problemas analíticos.

2.9 Bromato

El bromato se absorbe y excreta con rapidez, fundamentalmente en la orina, en forma de bromuro. Se detecta bromato en la orina a dosis de 5 mg/kg de peso corporal o superiores. Las concentraciones de bromato en la orina alcanzan un máximo cuando ha transcurrido alrededor de una hora, y después de dos horas no es posible detectarlo en el plasma.

3. Toxicología de los desinfectantes y de los subproductos de los desinfectantes

3.1 Desinfectantes

El gas cloro, la cloramina y el dióxido de cloro son irritantes respiratorios potentes. El hipoclorito de sodio (ClONa) se utiliza también como blanqueante y con frecuencia produce intoxicación en el ser humano. Sin embargo, estas exposiciones no guardan relación con la exposición en el agua de bebida. Se han realizado relativamente pocas evaluaciones de los efectos tóxicos de estos desinfectantes, cuando están presentes en el agua, para los animales de experimentación o el ser humano. Los estudios realizados al respecto parecen indicar que el cloro, las soluciones de hipoclorito, la cloramina y el dióxido de cloro probablemente no contribuyan como tales a la aparición de cáncer o de cualquier efecto tóxico. La atención se ha concentrado en la amplia variedad de subproductos que se originan en las reacciones del cloro y de otros desinfectantes con la materia orgánica natural, que se encuentra prácticamente en todas las fuentes de agua.

3.2 Trihalometanos

Los THM inducen citotoxicidad hepática y renal en roedores expuestos a dosis de unos 0,5 mmoles/kg de peso corporal. El vehículo de administración influye notablemente en la toxicidad de los THM.

Éstos tienen escasa toxicidad en la reproducción o el desarrollo, pero se ha demostrado que el bromodiclorometano reduce la motilidad de los espermatozoides en ratas que consumen 39 mg/kg de peso corporal al día en el agua. Al igual que el cloroformo, cuando el bromodiclorometano se administra en aceite de maíz induce la formación de cáncer de hígado y de riñón tras la exposición a lo largo de toda la vida a dosis altas. A diferencia del cloroformo y del dibromoclorometano, el bromodiclorometano y el bromoformo inducen la formación de tumores en el intestino grueso de ratas expuestas al aceite de maíz mediante sonda. El bromodiclorometano induce la formación de tumores en los tres lugares a los que llega y a dosis más bajas que los demás THM. Desde la publicación en 1994 de los criterios de salud ambiental de la OMS sobre el cloroformo, se han añadido a la suma de datos acumulados nuevos estudios que indican que el cloroformo no es un carcinógeno mutágeno capaz de reaccionar de forma directa con el ADN. En cambio, los THM bromados parecen tener una débil acción mutágena, probablemente debido a la conjugación con el glutatión.

3.3   Ácidos haloacéticos

Los AHA tienen efectos toxicológicos diversos en los animales de laboratorio. Los que suscitan mayor preocupación son los que tienen efectos carcinógenos o en la reproducción y el desarrollo. Los efectos neurotóxicos son importantes a las elevadas dosis de ácido dicloroacético que se utilizan con fines terapéuticos. Los efectos carcinógenos parecen limitarse al hígado y a las dosis altas. La mayor parte de los datos pruebas indican que los efectos tumorígenos del ácido dicloroacético y del ácido tricloroacético dependen de la modificación de los procesos de división y muerte celular más que de su actividad mutágena, que es muy débil. El choque oxidativo es también una característica de la toxicidad de los análogos bromados comprendidos en esta categoría. Tanto el ácido dicloroacético como el tricloroacético provocan a dosis altas malformaciones cardíacas en ratas.

3.4   Haloaldehídos y halocetonas

El hidrato de cloral induce necrosis hepática en ratas a dosis iguales o superiores a 120 mg/kg de peso corporal al día. Su efecto depresor del sistema nervioso central en el ser humano probablemente esté relacionado con su metabolito tricloroetanol. Hay pocos datos de toxicidad para los otros aldehídos y cetonas halogenados. La exposición al cloroacetaldehído provoca en las ratas efectos hematológicos. La exposición de los ratones a la 1,1-dicloropropanona, pero no a la 1,3-dicloropropanona, produce toxicidad hepática.

El hidrato de cloral dio resultados negativos en la mayor parte de las pruebas bacterianas de mutaciones puntuales, pero no en todas, y en estudios *in vivo* sobre daños cromosómicos. Sin embargo, se ha demostrado que puede inducir aberraciones cromosómicas estructurales *in vitro* e *in vivo*. Se ha notificado que el hidrato de cloral provoca tumores hepáticos en ratones. No está claro si es el compuesto original o sus metabolitos los que inducen el efecto carcinógeno. Los dos metabolitos del hidrato de cloral, el ácido tricloroacético y el ácido dicloroacético, han provocado la inducción de tumores hepáticos en ratones.

Algunos aldehídos y cetonas halogenados son potentes inductores de mutaciones en bacterias. Se han notificado efectos clastógenos para las propanonas cloradas. En un estudio con exposición de animales durante toda su vida al cloroacetaldehído, agregado al agua de bebida, se observó la formación de tumores hepáticos. Se han identificado otros aldehídos halogenados, por ejemplo el 2-cloropropenal, como inductores de la formación de tumores cutáneos en ratones. No se han sometido a prueba las halocetonas para investigar la carcinogenicidad en el agua de bebida. Sin embargo, en un estudio de carcinogenicidad cutánea en ratones la 1,3-dicloropropanona actuó como inductora de tumores.

3.5   **Haloacetonitrilos**

Se han realizado hasta ahora pocas pruebas con estos compuestos para investigar los efectos toxicológicos. Algunos de los grupos son mutágenos, pero no hay una relación clara de esos efectos con la actividad de los productos químicos como inductores de tumores cutáneos. Son muy pocos los estudios que se han realizado sobre la carcinogenicidad de este tipo de sustancias. Parece que los indicios precoces de toxicidad de los miembros de este grupo en el desarrollo se deben fundamentalmente al vehículo utilizado para su administración.

3.6 *Derivados halogenados de la hidroxifuranona*

Los estudios experimentales parecen indicar que los efectos de mayor importancia de la MX son su mutagenicidad y su carcinogenicidad. En varios estudios *in vitro* se ha comprobado que la MX es mutágena en sistemas de prueba con bacterias y mamíferos. La MX provocó aberraciones cromosómicas e indujo lesiones en el ADN de células hepáticas y testiculares aisladas, así como el intercambio de cromátidas hermanas en linfocitos periféricos de ratas expuestas *in vivo*. Una evaluación general de los datos de mutagenicidad pone de manifiesto que la MX es mutágena *in vitro* e *in vivo*. En un estudio de carcinogenicidad en ratas se observó un aumento de la frecuencia de tumores en varios órganos.

3.7 *Clorito*

La acción tóxica del clorito se produce fundamentalmente en forma de daño oxidativo en los glóbulos rojos a dosis de apenas 10 mg/kg de peso corporal. Hay indicios de efectos leves en el neurocomportamiento de crías de rata con 5,6 mg/kg de peso corporal al día. Los datos sobre la genotoxicidad del clorito son contradictorios. En estudios de exposición crónicos, el clorito no produjo un aumento de tumores en animales de laboratorio.

3.8 *Clorato*

La toxicidad del clorato es semejante a la del clorito, pero como oxidante este compuesto causa menos lesiones. No parece ser teratógeno o genotóxico *in vivo*. No hay datos de estudios de carcinogenicidad prolongados.

3.9 *Bromato*

A dosis elevadas el bromato provoca lesiones en los túbulos renales de las ratas expuestas. En estudios crónicos induce tumores en el riñón, el peritoneo y el tiroides de las ratas sometidas a dosis de 6 mg/kg de peso corporal y superiores. Los hámsteres son menos sensibles y los ratones considerablemente menos. El bromato a dosis elevadas es también genotóxico *in vivo* en ratas . La carcinogenicidad parece ser un efecto secundario del choque oxidativo en la célula.

4. Estudios epidemiológicos

4.1 *Enfermedades cardiovasculares*

En los estudios epidemiológicos no se ha identificado un riesgo mayor de enfermedad cardiovascular asociado con el agua de bebida que contiene cloro o cloramina. No se han realizado estudios de otros desinfectantes.

4.2 *Cáncer*

Las pruebas epidemiológicas no son suficientes para confirmar la existencia de una relación causal entre el cáncer de vejiga y la exposición prolongada al agua de bebida clorada, a los THM, al cloroformo u a otras especies de THM. Los datos epidemiológicos son poco concluyentes y equívocos con respecto a una asociación entre el cáncer de colon y la exposición prolongada al agua clorada, a los THM, al cloroformo u a otras especies de THM. La información no es suficiente para permitir una evaluación de los riesgos observados de cáncer de recto y los riesgos de otros tipos de cáncer detectados en estudios analíticos aislados.

En varios tipos de estudios epidemiológicos se ha intentado evaluar los riesgos de cáncer que pueden estar asociados con la exposición al agua clorada. En dos estudios se examinó el agua con cloramina. En varios estudios se ha intentado estimar la exposición a la totalidad de los THM o al cloroformo y a las otras especies de THM, pero en los estudios no se examinaron las exposiciones a otros SPD o a otros contaminantes del agua, que pueden ser diferentes para las fuentes de agua superficial y freática. En un estudio se examinó la mutagenicidad del agua medida mediante la valoración de *Salmonella typhimurium*. No se han realizado evaluaciones de los posibles riesgos de cáncer que pueden estar asociados con el agua desinfectada con ozono o dióxido de cloro.

Diversos estudios de casos y testigos basados en datos ecológicos o en certificados de defunción han permitido formular hipótesis que deberán evaluarse más detenidamente en estudios analíticos que tomen en consideración el consumo individual de agua de bebida y los posibles factores de confusión.

En los estudios analíticos se ha notificado un aumento de escaso a moderado del riesgo relativo de cáncer de vejiga, colon, recto, páncreas, mama, cerebro o pulmón asociado con la exposición prolongada al agua clorada. En estudios individuales se notificaron asociaciones entre la exposición al agua clorada y el cáncer de páncreas, de mama o de cerebro; sin embargo, para determinar si esas asociaciones epidemiológicas corresponden efectivamente a una relación causal se necesitará más de un estudio. En un estudio se asoció un ligero aumento del riesgo relativo de cáncer de pulmón con el consumo de aguas superficiales, pero la magnitud del riesgo era demasiado pequeña para descartar la presencia de un factor de confusión residual.

En un estudio de casos y testigos se notificó una asociación moderadamente elevada entre el cáncer de recto y la exposición prolongada al agua clorada o la exposición acumulativa a los THM, pero en estudios de cohortes se ha comprobado que no aumenta el riesgo o es demasiado pequeño para que se pueda descartar la presencia de un factor de confusión residual.

La disminución del riesgo de cáncer de vejiga se asoció con la mayor duración de la exposición al agua de bebida con cloramina, pero no hay base biológica para suponer un efecto protector de este tipo de agua.

Aunque en varios estudios se observó un aumento del riesgo de cáncer de vejiga asociado con la exposición prolongada al agua clorada y la exposición acumulativa a los THM, se notificaron resultados contradictorios de los estudios sobre el riesgo de cáncer de vejiga entre fumadores y no fumadores y entre hombres y mujeres. En tres de estos estudios se examinó la exposición estimada a los THM. En uno de ellos no se encontró ninguna relación con la exposición acumulativa estimada a los THM; en otro estudio se asoció un aumento moderadamente alto del riesgo relativo con una mayor exposición acumulativa a los THM en los hombres, pero no en las mujeres. En el tercer estudio se notificó un ligero aumento del riesgo relativo asociado con una exposición acumulativa estimada de 1957-6425 µg de THM por litro al año; se notificaron asimismo asociaciones de ligeras a moderadas para la exposición a concentraciones de THM superiores a 24 µg/litro, superiores a 49 µg/litro y superiores a 74 µg/litro. En una cohorte de mujeres no se asoció un aumento del riesgo relativo de cáncer de vejiga con la exposición al consumo de aguas superficiales municipales cloradas, al cloroformo o a otras especies de THM, pero el período de verificación de ocho años fue muy corto, por lo que se pudieron estudiar pocos casos.

Habida cuenta de que en los estudios epidemiológicos no se ha prestado la debida atención a la evaluación de la exposición a los contaminantes del agua, no es posible valorar de manera adecuada el aumento de los riesgos relativos que se notificaron. Los riesgos específicos pueden deberse a otros SPD, a mezclas de subproductos u a otros contaminantes del agua, o bien a otros factores cuyos efectos se atribuirían al agua clorada o a los THM.

4.3   Resultados adversos en la gestación

En algunos estudios se ha examinado la posible correlación entre el consumo de agua clorada o la exposición a los THM o especies de THM y diversos resultados adversos del embarazo. Un grupo científico especial convocado recientemente por la Agencia para la Protección del Medio Ambiente de los Estados Unidos examinó los estudios epidemiológicos y llegó a la conclusión de que los resultados de los estudios publicados actualmente no prueban de manera convincente de que el agua clorada o los THM provoquen resultados adversos en el embarazo.

Los resultados de los primeros estudios son difíciles de interpretar debido a las limitaciones metodológicas o a un probable sesgo.

En un estudio de casos y testigos concluido recientemente pero que todavía no se ha publicado se notifica un aumento moderado del riesgo relativo de defectos del tubo neural en niños cuyas madres residieron al comienzo del embarazo en una zona donde los niveles de THM eran superiores a 40 µg/litro. Para evaluar de manera adecuada esta asociación habría que confirmar los resultados en otra zona. En un estudio realizado anteriormente en la misma zona geográfica se notificó una asociación semejante, pero el estudio presentaba limitaciones metodológicas.

En un reciente estudio de cohortes se encontró un riesgo mayor de aborto asociado con un consumo elevado de agua (cinco o más vasos de agua de grifo fría al día) con niveles altos (≥75 µg/litro) de THM. Cuando se examinaron THM concretos, sólo se asoció con el riesgo de aborto un consumo elevado de agua con bromodiclorometano (≥18 µg/litro). Teniendo en cuenta que éste es el primer estudio que parece indicar un efecto reproductivo adverso asociado con un subproducto bromado, un grupo científico especial recomendó que se realizase otro estudio en una zona geográfica diferente para tratar de reproducir esos resultados y que se hicieran nuevos esfuerzos para evaluar las exposiciones de la cohorte a otros contaminantes del agua.

5.   Caracterización del riesgo

Hay que señalar que el uso de desinfectantes químicos en el tratamiento del agua suele dar lugar a la formación de subproductos químicos, algunos de los cuales son potencialmente peligrosos. Sin embargo, los riesgos para la salud de estos subproductos en las concentraciones en las cuales se encuentran en el agua de bebida son muy pequeños en comparación con los riesgos asociados con una desinfección inadecuada. Así pues, es importante que al intentar controlar dichos subproductos no se comprometa la desinfección.

5.1   Caracterización del peligro y de la relación dosis-respuesta

5.1.1   Estudios toxicológicos

1)   Cloro

Un Grupo de Trabajo de la OMS reunido en 1993 para preparar las *Guías para la calidad del agua de bebida* examinó el problema del cloro. Fijó una ingesta diaria tolerable (IDT) de 150 µg/kg de peso corporal para el cloro libre basada en una concentración sin efectos adversos observados (NOAEL) de unos 15 mg/kg de peso corporal al día en estudios de dos años en ratas y ratones y aplicando un factor de incertidumbre de 100 (10 por la variación intraespecífica y 10 por la interespecífica). No hay nuevos datos que indiquen la necesidad de cambiar esta IDT.

2) Monocloramina

El mencionado Grupo de Trabajo de la OMS sobre las *Guías para la calidad del agua de bebida* examinó el caso de la monocloramina. Fijó una ingesta diaria tolerable (IDT) de 94 µg/kg de peso corporal basada en una concentración sin efectos adversos observados (NOAEL) de alrededor de 9,4 mg/kg de peso corporal al día, la dosis más alta sometida a prueba, en una biovaloración de dos años en ratas y aplicando un factor de incertidumbre de 100 (10 por la variación intraespecífica y 10 por la interespecífica). No hay nuevos datos que indiquen la necesidad de cambiar esta IDT.

3) Dióxido de cloro

La química del dióxido de cloro en el agua es compleja, pero el principal producto de su degradación es el clorito. Al establecer una IDT específica para el dióxido de cloro, se pueden considerar los datos relativos al dióxido de cloro y al clorito, dada la rápida hidrólisis a clorito. Por consiguiente, la IDT por vía oral para el dióxido de cloro es de 30 µg/kg de peso corporal, basada en una NOAEL de 2,9 mg/kg de peso corporal al día para los efectos del clorito en el desarrollo neural de las ratas.

4) Trihalometanos

El riesgo de cáncer tras la exposición crónica es el principal motivo de preocupación en relación con esta clase de subproductos. Debido a que los datos relativos al cloroformo indican que puede inducir cáncer en animales sólo tras la exposición crónica a dosis citotóxicas, es evidente que la exposición a concentraciones bajas de este compuesto en el agua de bebida no representa un riesgo carcinógeno. La NOAEL para la citoletalidad y la hiperplasia degenerativa en ratones fue de 10 mg/kg de peso corporal al día tras la administración de cloroformo en aceite de maíz durante tres semanas. Tomando como base los datos relativos al mecanismo de acción para la carcinogenicidad del cloroformo, se obtuvo una IDT de 10 μg/kg de peso corporal utilizando la NOAEL para la citotoxicidad en ratones y aplicando un factor de incertidumbre de 1000 (10 por la variación interespecífica, 10 por la intraespecífica y 10 por la brevedad del estudio). Respaldan este enfoque varios estudios adicionales. Esta IDT es semejante a la que se determinó en la edición de 1998 de las *Guías para la calidad del agua de bebida* de la OMS, basada en un estudio de 1979 en el cual se expusieron perros durante 7,5 años al cloroformo.

Entre los THM bromados, reviste particular interés el bromodiclorometano porque induce la formación de tumores en ratas y ratones y en varios lugares (hígado, riñones, intestino grueso) tras el suministro con sonda de aceite de maíz. La inducción de tumores de colon en ratas por el bromodiclorometano (y por el bromoformo) es también interesante debido a las asociaciones epidemiológicas con el cáncer de colon y recto. El bromodiclorometano y los otros THM bromados son también débilmente mutágenos. En general, se supone que los carcinógenos mutágenos a dosis bajas producirán relaciones dosis-respuesta lineales, puesto que se suele considerar que la mutagénesis es un efecto irreversible y acumulativo.

En una biovaloración de dos años, el bromodiclorometano administrado con aceite de maíz mediante sonda indujo la formación de tumores (junto con citotoxicidad y un aumento de la proliferación) en los riñones de ratones y ratas a dosis de 50 y 100 mg/kg de peso corporal al día, respectivamente. Se observaron tumores en el intestino grueso de ratas tras la exposición tanto a 50 como a 100 mg/kg de peso corporal al día. Utilizando la incidencia de tumores de riñón en ratones macho observada en este estudio, se han calculado estimaciones del riesgo cuantitativo, obteniéndose un factor CSF (*cancer slope factor*) de $4,8 \times 10^{-3}$ [mg/kg de peso corporal al día]$^{-1}$ y una dosis calculada de 2,1 μg/kg de peso corporal al día para un nivel de riesgo de 10^{-5}. Se estableció un CSF de $4,2 \times 10^{-3}$ [mg/kg de peso corporal al día]$^{-1}$ (2,4 μg/kg de peso corporal al día para un riesgo de 10^{-5}) sobre la base de la incidencia de carcinoma en el intestino grueso de ratas macho. El Centro Internacional de Investigaciones sobre el Cáncer (CIIC) ha clasificado el bromodiclorometano en el grupo 2B (posiblemente carcinógeno para el ser humano).

El dibromoclorometano y el bromoformo se estudiaron en biovaloraciones prolongadas. En un estudio de dos años con aceite de maíz administrado mediante sonda, el dibromoclorometano indujo la formación de tumores hepáticos en ratones hembra, pero no en ratas, a una dosis de 100 mg/kg de peso corporal al día. En evaluaciones anteriores se había indicado que el aceite de maíz como vehículo podía desempeñar una función en la inducción de tumores en ratones hembra. En el estudio del bromoformo a dosis de 200 mg/kg de peso corporal al día se observó un pequeño aumento del número de tumores del intestino grueso de ratas. Los CSF basados en estos tumores son $6,5 \times 10^{-3}$ [mg/kg de peso corporal al día]$^{-1}$ para el dibromoclorometano, o de 1,5 µg/kg de peso corporal al día para un riesgo de 10^{-5}, y de $1,3 \times 10^{-3}$ [mg/kg de peso corporal al día]$^{-1}$, ó 7,7 µg/kg de peso corporal al día para un riesgo de 10^{-5} en el caso del bromoformo.

Estos dos trihalometanos bromados se comportaron como mutágenos débiles en algunas valoraciones y fueron con diferencia los subproductos más mutágenos del grupo en el sistema de evaluación basado en la glutatión-S-transferasa. Puesto que éstos son los THM más lipófilos, se deberían examinar aspectos adicionales para determinar si en los estudios prolongados el aceite de maíz puede haber influido en su biodisponibilidad. Se ha establecido una NOAEL para el dibromoclorometano de 30 mg/kg de peso corporal al día basada en la ausencia de efectos histopatológicos en el hígado de ratas después de 13 semanas de exposición con aceite de maíz administrado por sonda. El CIIC ha clasificado el dibromoclorometano en el grupo 3 (no clasificable en cuanto a su carcinogenicidad para el ser humano). Se determinó una IDT para este producto de 30 µg/kg de peso corporal basada en una NOAEL para la toxicidad hepática de 30 mg/kg de peso corporal al día y un factor de incertidumbre de 1000 (10 por la variación interespecífica, 10 por la intraespecífica y 10 por la brevedad del estudio y la posible carcinogenicidad).

De igual forma, se puede determinar para el bromoformo una NOAEL de 25 mg/kg de peso corporal al día sobre la base de la ausencia de lesiones hepáticas en ratas después de 13 semanas de administración mediante sonda con aceite de maíz. Se estableció para el bromoformo una IDT de 25 µg/kg de peso corporal sobre la base de esta NOAEL para la toxicidad hepática y un factor de incertidumbre de 1000 (10 por la variación interespecífica, 10 por la intraespecífica y 10 por la brevedad del estudio y la posible carcinogenicidad). El CIIC ha clasificado el bromoformo en el grupo 3 (no clasificable en cuanto a su carcinogenicidad para el ser humano).

5) Ácidos haloacéticos

Es muy poco probable que el ácido dicloroacético induzca mutaciones a dosis tan bajas como las que se encontrarían en el agua clorada. Los datos disponibles indican que el ácido dicloroacético influye de distinta manera en la velocidad de replicación de los hepatocitos normales y de los hepatocitos en los que ha habido iniciación. Las relaciones dosis-respuesta son complejas, estimulando inicialmente el ácido dicloroacético la división de los hepatocitos normales. Sin embargo, a las dosis crónicas más bajas utilizadas en los estudios con animales (pero todavía muy altas en relación con las que se encontrarían en el agua), la velocidad de replicación de los hepatocitos normales se inhibe de forma radical con el tiempo. Esto indica que a larga los hepatocitos normales regulan a la baja esas vías que son sensibles al efecto estimulante del ácido dicloroacético. Sin embargo, los efectos en células alteradas, particularmente en las que sintetizan grandes cantidades de una proteína que es inmunorreactiva frente a un anticuerpo c-Jun, no parecen capaces de regular a la baja esta respuesta. Así pues, la velocidad de replicación en las lesiones preneoplásicas con este fenotipo es muy elevada a las dosis de ácido dicloroacético que provocan la aparición de tumores, siendo el período de latencia muy bajo. Los datos preliminares parecen indicar que esta alteración continuada en la velocidad de formación y muerte celular es también necesaria en la evolución de los tumores hacia la malignidad. Respaldan esta interpretación estudios en los que se utilizan también modelos de iniciación de la alteración/estímulo.

Teniendo en cuenta lo expuesto, se propone la modificación de las estimaciones de riesgo de cáncer establecidas actualmente para el ácido dicloroacético con la incorporación de la nueva información que se está obteniendo sobre su metabolismo comparativo y los mecanismos de acción para formular un modelo de dosis-respuesta con una base biológica. En este momento no se dispone de esos datos, pero se podrán obtener en el plazo de los próximos 2-3 años.

Los efectos del ácido dicloroacético parecen hallarse en estrecha correlación con las dosis que inducen hepatomegalia y acumulación de glucógeno en ratones. La concentración más baja con efectos adversos observados (LOAEL) para estos efectos en un estudio de ocho semanas en ratones fue de 0,5 g/litro, equivalentes a unos 100 mg/kg de peso corporal al día, y la NOAEL fue de 0,2 g/litro, es decir, unos 40 mg/kg de peso corporal al día. Se ha calculado una IDT de 40 µg/kg de peso corporal, aplicando a esta NOAEL un factor de incertidumbre de 1000 (10 por la variación interespecífica, 10 por la intraespecífica y 10 por la brevedad del estudio y la posible carcinogenicidad). El CIIC ha clasificado el ácido dicloroacético en el grupo 3 (no clasificable en cuanto a su carcinogenicidad para el ser humano).

El ácido tricloroacético es uno de los activadores más débiles conocidos de los receptores PPAR (*peroxisome proliferator-activated receptors*). Parece tener una actividad solamente marginal como proliferador de los perixosomas, incluso en ratas. Además, el tratamiento de ratas con concentraciones altas de ácido tricloroacético en el agua de bebida no induce la formación de tumores hepáticos. Estos datos indican claramente que el ácido tricloroacético presenta poco peligro carcinógeno para el ser humano en las bajas concentraciones que se encuentran en el agua.

Desde una perspectiva toxicológica más amplia, los efectos finales más preocupantes del ácido tricloroacético son las consecuencias en el desarrollo. Los animales parecen tolerar concentraciones de ácido tricloroacético en el agua de bebida de 0 ,5 g/litro (unos 50 mg/kg de peso corporal al día) con poco o ningún signo de efectos adversos. Con 2 g/litro, el único signo de efectos adversos parece ser la hepatomegalia. Ésta no se observa en ratones a una dosis de 0,35 g de ácido tricloroacético por litro de agua, que se estima que es equivalente a 40 mg/kg de peso corporal al día.

En otro estudio se observaron anomalías en los tejidos blandos con un índice aproximadamente tres veces superior a los testigos a la dosis más baja administrada, 330 mg/kg de peso corporal al día. A esta dosis las anomalías fueron leves, y la dosis es claramente de la misma magnitud que la que provocaría hepatomegalia (y efectos carcinógenos). Teniendo en cuenta el hecho de que el PPAR interacciona con los mecanismos de señalización celular que pueden afectar a los procesos de desarrollo normales, se debe considerar la posibilidad de que exista un mecanismo común a la hepatomegalia, a los efectos carcinógenos y a los efectos en el desarrollo provocados por este compuesto.

La IDT para el ácido tricloroacético se basa en una NOAEL estimada de 40 mg/kg de peso corporal al día para la toxicidad hepática en un estudio prolongado en ratones. La aplicación de un factor de incertidumbre de 1000 (10 por la variación interespecífica, 10 por la intraespecífica y 10 por la posible carcinogenicidad) a la NOAEL estimada proporciona una IDT de 40 µg/kg de peso corporal. El CIIC ha clasificado el ácido tricloroacético en el grupo 3 (no clasificable en cuanto a su carcinogenicidad para el ser humano).

Los datos sobre la carcinogenicidad de los ácidos acéticos bromados son demasiado preliminares para ser útiles en la caracterización del riesgo. Los datos obtenibles de los resúmenes analíticos parecen indicar, sin embargo, que las dosis necesarias para inducir respuestas hepatocarcinógenas en ratones no son muy diferentes de las de los ácidos acéticos clorados. Además de los mecanismos que intervienen en la inducción de cáncer por los ácidos dicloroacético y tricloroacético, es posible que contribuya a sus efectos un aumento del choque oxidativo resultante de su metabolismo.

Hay datos abundantes sobre los efectos del ácido dibromoacético en la función reproductiva masculina. No se observaron efectos en ratas a una dosis de 2 mg/kg de peso corporal al día durante 79 días, mientras que con 10 mg/kg de peso corporal al día se detectó una mayor retención de espermátidas en la fase 19. A dosis más elevadas los efectos fueron progresivamente más graves, en particular una atrofia acentuada de los túbulos seminíferos con 250 mg/kg de peso corporal al día, sin que se hubiera producido una reversión seis meses después de la suspensión del tratamiento. Se estableció una IDT de 20 µg/kg de peso corporal mediante la asignación de un factor de incertidumbre de 100 (10 por la variación intraespecífica y 10 por la interespecífica) a la NOAEL de 2 mg/kg de peso corporal al día.

6) Hidrato de cloral

Con concentraciones de hidrato de cloral de 1 g/litro de agua (166 mg/kg de peso corporal al día) se indujo la formación de tumores hepáticos en ratones expuestos durante 104 semanas. No se han evaluado dosis inferiores. Se ha demostrado que el hidrato de cloral ha inducido anomalías cromosómicas en varias pruebas *in vitro*, pero dio resultados en gran parte negativos cuando se evaluó *in vivo*. Es probable que en la inducción de tumores hepáticos por el hidrato de cloral intervenga la formación de ácido tricloroacético y/o ácido dicloroacético en su metabolismo. Como se ha señalado más arriba, se considera que estos compuestos actúan como estimulantes de la formación de tumores. El CIIC ha clasificado el hidrato de cloral en el grupo 3 (no clasificable en cuanto a su carcinogenicidad para el ser humano).

La administración de hidrato de cloral en el agua a ratas durante 90 días indujo necrosis hepatocelular con concentraciones de 1200 mg/litro y superiores, sin que se observasen efectos con 600 mg/litro (unos 60 mg/kg de peso corporal al día). Se detectó hepatomegalia en ratones que recibieron dosis de 144 mg/kg de peso corporal al día mediante sonda durante 14 días. No se observaron efectos con 14,4 mg/kg de peso corporal al día en un estudio de 14 días, pero se detectó una ligera hepatomegalia cuando se administró hidrato de cloral en el agua en una concentración de 70 mg/litro (16 mg/kg de peso corporal al día) en un estudio complementario de 90 días. La aplicación de un factor de incertidumbre de 1000 (10 por la variación interespecífica, 10 por la intraespecífica y 10 por utilizar una LOAEL en lugar de la NOAEL) a este valor permite establecer una IDT de 16 µg/kg de peso corporal.

7) Haloacetonitrilos

Sin datos adecuados para el ser humano o un estudio en animales de experimentación que comprenda una gran parte de su vida, no existe una base unánimemente aceptada para la estimación del riesgo carcinógeno de los haloacetonitrilos.

Los datos obtenidos en estudios subcrónicos proporcionan algunos indicios de las NOAEL para la toxicidad general del dicloroacetonitrilo y del dibromoacetonitrilo. Se identificaron unas NOAEL de 8 y 23 mg/kg de peso corporal al día en estudios de 90 días en ratas para el dicloroacetonitrilo y el dibromoacetonitrilo, respectivamente, basadas en la disminución del peso corporal a las siguientes dosis más altas de 33 y 45 mg/kg de peso corporal al día, respectivamente.

Un Grupo de Trabajo de la OMS reunido en 1993 para preparar las *Guías para la calidad del agua de bebida* examinó el dicloroacetonitrilo y el dibromoacetonitrilo. Fijó una IDT de 15 µg/kg de peso corporal para el primero sobre la base de una NOAEL de 15 mg/kg de peso corporal al día obtenida en un estudio de toxicidad reproductiva en ratas y aplicando un factor de incertidumbre de 1000 (10 por la variación intraespecífica, 10 por la interespecífica y 10 por la intensidad de los efectos). Solamente se observaron efectos reproductivos y en el desarrollo para el dibromoacetonitrilo a dosis que superaban las establecidas para la toxicidad general (unos 45 mg/kg de peso corporal al día). Se calculó una IDT de 23 µg/kg de peso corporal para el dibromoacetonitrilo basada en una NOAEL de 23 mg/kg de peso corporal al día obtenida en un estudio de 90 días en ratas y aplicando un factor de incertidumbre de 1000 (10 por la variación intraespecífica, 10 por la interespecífica y 10 por la brevedad el estudio). No hay datos nuevos que indiquen que deban cambiarse estas IDT.

Se identificó una LOAEL para el tricloroacetonitrilo de 7,5 mg/kg de peso corporal al día para la embriotoxicidad y de 15 mg/kg de peso corporal al día para los efectos en el desarrollo. Sin embargo, estudios posteriores parecen indicar que estas respuestas fueron función del vehículo utilizado. No se puede establecer una IDT para el tricloroacetonitrilo.

No hay datos útiles para la caracterización del riesgo imputable a otros miembros del grupo de los haloacetonitrilos.

8) MX

Recientemente se ha estudiado el mutágeno MX en un estudio prolongado en ratas en el cual se observaron algunas respuestas carcinógenas. Estos datos indican que el MX induce la formación de tumores de tiroides y de los conductos biliares. Se observó un aumento de la incidencia de tumores de tiroides a la dosis más baja de MX administrada (0,4 mg/kg de peso corporal al día). La inducción de tumores de tiroides a dosis elevadas de productos químicos se ha relacionado desde hace tiempo con los compuestos halogenados. En la inducción de tumores foliculares tiroideos podrían intervenir modificaciones en la función del tiroides o un mecanismo de acción mutágeno. Se observó asimismo un aumento de la incidencia de colangiomas y colangiocarcinomas relacionado con la dosis, comenzando con la dosis baja en ratas hembra, con una respuesta menor en ratas macho. Se utilizó el aumento de los colangiomas y colangiocarcinomas en ratas hembra para obtener un factor CSF para el cáncer. Se calculó un límite de confianza superior al 95% para un riesgo a lo largo de toda la vida de 10^{-5} basado en un modelo línealizado en fases múltiples de 0,06 μg/kg de peso corporal al día.

9)   Clorito

El efecto principal y más constante derivado de la exposición al clorito es el choque oxidativo que provoca cambios en los glóbulos rojos. Este efecto final se observa en animales de laboratorio y, por analogía con el clorato, en personas expuestas a dosis elevadas en casos de intoxicación. Hay datos suficientes para estimar una IDT en las personas expuestas al clorito, en particular estudios de toxicidad crónica y un estudio de toxicidad reproductiva de dos generaciones. En estudios de hasta 12 semanas con voluntarios no se identificó efecto alguno en los parámetros sanguíneos a la dosis más alta utilizada, a saber, 36 μg/kg de peso corporal al día. Debido a que en estos estudios no se identifica una concentración con efectos, no se pueden utilizar para el establecimiento de un margen de inocuidad.

En un estudio de dos generaciones en ratas se identificó una NOAEL de 2,9 mg/kg de peso corporal al día basada en una disminución de la reacción de sobresalto auditivo, la disminución del peso absoluto del cerebro en las generaciones F_1 y F_2 y la alteración del peso del hígado en dos generaciones. La aplicación a esta NOAEL de un factor de incertidumbre de 100 (10 por la variación interespecífica y 10 por la intraespecífica) permite establecer una IDT de 30 μg/kg de peso corporal. Los estudios con voluntarios confirman esta IDT.

10) Clorato

Al igual que en el caso del clorito, el principal motivo de preocupación con el clorato es el daño oxidativo de los glóbulos rojos. Al igual que con el clorito, 0,036 mg de clorato por kg de peso corporal al día durante 12 semanas no provocaron efectos adversos en voluntarios. Aunque la base de datos para el clorato es menos amplia que para el clorito, en un estudio reciente de 90 días en ratas bien realizado se identificó una NOAEL de 30 mg/kg de peso corporal al día basada en la reducción de los coloides de la glándula tiroidea a la dosis siguiente más alta de 100 mg/kg de peso corporal al día. No se determina una IDT porque está en curso un estudio prolongado que debe proporcionar más información sobre la exposición crónica al clorato.

11) Bromato

El bromato es un oxidante activo de los sistemas biológicos y se ha demostrado que provoca un aumento de la aparición de tumores renales, mesoteliomas peritoneales y tumores de las células foliculares tiroideas en ratas, y en menor medida en hámsteres, y sólo un pequeño aumento de los tumores de riñón en ratones. La dosis más baja a la cual se observó un aumento de la incidencia de tumores renales en ratas fue de 6 mg/kg de peso corporal al día.

Se ha demostrado asimismo que el bromato da resultados positivos para las aberraciones cromosómicas en células de mamíferos *in vitro* e *in vivo*, pero no en valoraciones bacterianas para las mutaciones puntuales. Hay cada vez más pruebas, respaldadas por los datos de genotoxicidad, que parecen indicar que la acción del bromato consiste en generar radicales de oxígeno en la célula.

En las *Guías para la calidad del agua de bebida* de 1993 de la OMS se aplicó el modelo linealizado en fases múltiples a la incidencia de tumores renales en un estudio de carcinogenicidad de dos años en ratas, aunque se observó que, si el mecanismo de inducción de tumores es el daño oxidativo en el riñón, podría no ser adecuada la aplicación del modelo de cáncer a dosis bajas. El intervalo de confianza superior del 95% calculado para un riesgo de 10^{-5} fue de 0,1 µg/kg de peso corporal al día.

La concentración sin efectos para la formación de tumores en las células renales de ratas es de 1,3 mg/kg de peso corporal al día. Si se considera que a partir de este valor la relación dosis-respuesta ya no es lineal y se aplica un factor de incertidumbre de 1000 (10 por la variación interespecífica, 10 por la intraespecífica y 10 por la posible carcinogenicidad), se puede calcular una IDT de 1 μg/kg de peso corporal, frente a un valor de 0,1 μg/kg de peso corporal al día asociado con un exceso de riesgo de cáncer de 10^{-5} a lo largo de toda la vida.

De momento no hay datos suficientes para saber si los tumores inducidos por el bromato se deben a la citotoxicidad y la hiperplasia reparativa o son un efecto genotóxico.

El CIIC ha incluido el bromato de potasio en el grupo 2B (posible carcinógeno para el ser humano).

5.1.2 Estudios epidemiológicos

Los estudios epidemiológicos se deben evaluar con cuidado para garantizar que las asociaciones observadas no se deban a un sesgo y que el diseño sea adecuado para evaluar una posible relación causal. La causalidad se puede evaluar cuando hay datos suficientes de diversos estudios bien definidos y realizados en distintas zonas geográficas. También es importante el respaldo de datos toxicológicos y farmacológicos. Es especialmente difícil interpretar los datos epidemiológicos de los estudios ecológicos del agua desinfectada, y esos resultados se utilizan fundamentalmente como ayuda en la formulación de hipótesis para un ulterior estudio.

Los resultados de los estudios epidemiológicos analíticos son insuficientes para respaldar una relación causal en el caso de cualquiera de las asociaciones observadas. Es especialmente difícil interpretar los resultados de los estudios analíticos publicados actualmente a causa de la información incompleta acerca de la exposición a contaminantes específicos del agua que podrían constituir un factor de confusión o modificar el riesgo. Debido a que en los estudios epidemiológicos no se ha prestado suficiente atención a la evaluación de la exposición a los contaminantes del agua, no es posible evaluar de manera adecuada el aumento de los riesgos relativos notificados. Los riesgos se pueden deber a otros contaminantes del agua o a otros factores cuya acción se atribuiría sin razón al agua clorada o a los THM.

5.2 *Caracterización de la exposición*

5.2.1 *Presencia de desinfectantes y de subproductos de los desinfectantes*

Se suelen utilizar dosis de desinfectantes de varios miligramos por litro, que son las dosis necesarias para inactivar los microorganismos (desinfección primaria) o las dosis necesarias para mantener una concentración residual en el sistema de distribución (desinfección secundaria).

Para la evaluación de la exposición se necesita saber cuáles son los SPD presentes en el agua y en qué concentración. Desafortunadamente, hay pocos estudios internacionales publicados que vayan más allá del estudio de casos o de los datos regionales.

Los datos disponibles parecen indicar la presencia, como promedio, de alrededor de 35-50 μg de THM totales por litro en el agua clorada, siendo el cloroformo y el bromodiclorometano la primera y segunda especies predominantes. La exposición a los AHA se puede calcular de manera aproximada mediante la concentración total de los AHA (suma de cinco especies) correspondiente a alrededor de la mitad de la concentración total de THM (aunque esta proporción puede variar significativamente); los ácidos dicloroacético y tricloroacético son la primera y la segunda especies más importantes. En el agua con una proporción bromuro/carbono orgánico total elevada o con una proporción bromuro/cloro elevada, cabe prever una mayor formación de THM y AHA bromados. Cuando se utiliza una solución de hipoclorito (con preferencia al cloro gaseoso), también se puede producir clorato durante la cloración.

La exposición a los SPD en el agua cloraminada depende del sistema de cloraminación, con la secuencia de cloro seguido de amoníaco para dar lugar a la formación de (niveles más bajos de) SPD del cloro (es decir, THM y AHA) durante el periodo de cloro libre; sin embargo, la supresión de la formación de cloroformo y ácido tricloroacético no se corresponde con una reducción proporcional de la formación de ácido dicloroacético.

En igualdad de condiciones, la concentración de bromuro y la dosis de ozono son los mejores indicadores de la formación de bromato durante la ozonación, con una conversión de bromuro a bromato de alrededor del 50%. En un estudio de diferentes servicios europeos de abastecimiento de agua se puso de manifiesto que los niveles de bromato en el agua al salir de las instalaciones de tratamiento oscilaba entre una concentración inferior al límite de detección (2 µg/litro) y 16 µg/litro. Los SPD orgánicos bromados que se forman durante la ozonación se suelen encontrar en concentraciones bajas. La formación de clorito se puede calcular como un simple porcentaje (50%-70%) de la dosis de dióxido de cloro aplicada.

5.2.2   *Incertidumbre de los datos sobre la calidad del agua*

En un estudio toxicológico se intenta extrapolar una respuesta (controlada) de animales de laboratorio a una respuesta humana potencial; un posible resultado es la estimación de los factores de riesgo de cáncer. En un estudio epidemiológico se intenta relacionar los efectos en la salud humana (por ejemplo, cáncer) con uno o varios agentes causales (por ejemplo, un SPD), para lo cual se necesita una evaluación de la exposición.

Los riesgos químicos asociados con el agua de bebida desinfectada se basan potencialmente en varias vías de exposición: i) ingestión de SPD en el agua de bebida; ii) ingestión de desinfectantes químicos en el agua de bebida y formación concomitante de SPD en el estómago; y iii) inhalación de SPD volátiles durante la ducha. Aunque la formación *in vivo* de SPD y la inhalación de estos SPD volátiles puede ser un motivo potencial de preocupación para la salud, el examen que se expone a continuación se basa en la premisa de que la ingestión de los SPD presentes en el agua de bebida es la vía de exposición más importante.

La exposición humana depende tanto de la concentración de SPD como del tiempo de exposición. Más en concreto, los efectos en la salud humana dependen de la exposición a mezclas complejas de SPD (por ejemplo, THM más bien que AHA, especies cloradas más bien que bromadas) que pueden sufrir cambios estacionales/temporales (por ejemplo, en función de la temperatura, las características y la concentración de la materia orgánica natural) y espaciales (es decir, en la totalidad de un sistema de distribución). Cada desinfectante químico concreto puede formar una mezcla de SPD; las combinaciones de desinfectantes químicos pueden formar incluso mezclas más complejas. Al formarse, la mayoría de los SPD son estables, pero algunos se pueden transformar, por ejemplo, mediante hidrólisis. En ausencia de datos sobre los SPD, se pueden utilizar en su lugar la dosis de cloro (o la demanda de cloro), el carbono orgánico total (o la absorción ultravioleta a 254 nm [UVA_{254}]) o el bromuro para estimar indirectamente la exposición. Aunque el carbono orgánico total es un buen sustitutivo de los precursores orgánicos de los SPD, la UVA_{254} proporciona información adicional sobre las características de la materia orgánica natural, que pueden variar en función de la zona geográfica. Se han identificado dos variables fundamentales de la calidad del agua, el pH y la concentración de bromuro, como factores que influyen de manera considerable en el tipo y las concentraciones de SPD que se forman.

En una evaluación de la exposición se debe intentar definir en primer lugar los tipos específicos de SPD y las mezclas resultantes que probablemente se formarán, así como sus concentraciones a lo largo del tiempo, en las que influyen su estabilidad y el transporte a través del sistema de distribución. Para los estudios epidemiológicos existen algunas bases de datos históricos sobre la concentración de desinfectantes (por ejemplo, de cloro) y posiblemente de los precursores de los SPD (por ejemplo, el carbono orgánico total) o de los THM totales (y, en algunos casos, especies de THM). En contraste con los THM, que se han vigilado durante periodos de tiempo más largos por razones reglamentarias, los datos de vigilancia de los AHA (y sus especies), el bromato y el clorito, son mucho más recientes y, por consiguiente, poco abundantes. Sin embargo, se pueden utilizar modelos de SPD para simular los datos que faltan o datos pasados. Otro aspecto importante es la documentación relativa a la evolución de las prácticas de tratamiento de agua.

5.2.3 Incertidumbres de los datos epidemiológicos

Incluso en estudios analíticos bien diseñados y realizados, se llevaron a cabo evaluaciones relativamente deficientes de la exposición. En la mayor parte de los estudios se examinó la duración de la exposición al agua de bebida desinfectada y a la fuente de agua. Estas exposiciones se estimaron a partir de los historiales de los residentes y de los registros de los servicios de agua de bebida o de los gobiernos. Sólo en un pequeño número de estudios se intentó estimar el consumo de agua de los participantes en un estudio y la exposición a los THM totales o a especies aisladas de THM. Sólo en un estudio se intentó estimar la exposición a otros SPD. Al evaluar algunos riesgos potenciales, es decir, los resultados adversos en el embarazo, que pueden estar asociados con exposiciones relativamente breves a subproductos volátiles, puede ser importante examinar la inhalación además de la vía de exposición por ingestión de agua de bebida. En algunos estudios se intentó estimar tanto las concentraciones de subproductos en el agua de bebida durante períodos de tiempo importantes desde el punto de vista etiológico como la exposición acumulativa. Se pueden utilizar modelos adecuados y análisis de sensibilidad, como la simulación de Monte Carlo, para estimar estas exposiciones durante los períodos que interese estudiar.

La incertidumbre es grande en lo que se refiere a la interpretación de las asociaciones observadas, puesto que se han examinado exposiciones a un número relativamente pequeño de contaminantes del agua. Con los datos actuales, es difícil evaluar cómo pueden haber influido las concentraciones de SPD o de otros contaminantes sin dosificar en las estimaciones de los riesgos relativos observados.

Se han dedicado más estudios al cáncer de vejiga que a cualquier otro tipo de cáncer. Los autores de los resultados notificados más recientemente para los riesgos de cáncer de vejiga advierten contra una interpretación simplista de las asociaciones observadas. Los indicios epidemiológicos de un aumento del riesgo relativo de cáncer de vejiga no son concordantes: se notifican riesgos diferentes para fumadores y no fumadores, para hombres y mujeres y para un consumo alto y bajo de agua. Los riesgos pueden variar entre diversas zonas geográficas debido a que las mezclas de SPD pueden ser distintas o porque el agua puede contener también otros contaminantes. Hay que recopilar, u obtener mediante simulación, datos más exhaustivos sobre la calidad del agua a fin de mejorar la evaluación de la exposición con miras a los estudios epidemiológicos.

Food additives and contaminants in food, principles for the safety assessment of (No. 70, 1987)
Formaldehyde (No. 89, 1989)
Genetic effects in human populations, guidelines for the study of (No. 46, 1985)
Glyphosate (No. 159, 1994)
Guidance values for human exposure limits (No. 170, 1994)
Heptachlor (No. 38, 1984)
Hexachlorobenzene (No. 195, 1997)
Hexachlorobutadiene (No. 156, 1994)
Alpha- and beta-hexachlorocyclohexanes (No. 123, 1992)
Hexachlorocyclopentadiene (No. 120, 1991)
n-Hexane (No. 122, 1991)
Human exposure assessment (No. 214, 1999)
Hydrazine (No. 68, 1987)
Hydrogen sulfide (No. 19, 1981)
Hydroquinone (No. 157, 1994)
Immunotoxicity associated with exposure to chemicals, principles and methods for assessment (No. 180, 1996)
Infancy and early childhood, principles for evaluating health risks from chemicals during (No. 59, 1986)
Isobenzan (No. 129, 1991)
Isophorone (No. 174, 1995)
Kelevan (No. 66, 1986)
Lasers and optical radiation (No. 23, 1982)
Lead (No. 3, 1977)[a]
Lead, inorganic (No. 165, 1995)
Lead – environmental aspects (No. 85, 1989)
Lindane (No. 124, 1991)
Linear alkylbenzene sulfonates and related compounds (No. 169, 1996)
Magnetic fields (No. 69, 1987)
Man-made mineral fibres (No. 77, 1988)
Manganese (No. 17, 1981)
Mercury (No. 1, 1976)[a]
Mercury – environmental aspects (No. 86, 1989)
Mercury, inorganic (No. 118, 1991)
Methanol (No. 196, 1997)
Methomyl (No. 178, 1996)
2-Methoxyethanol, 2-ethoxyethanol, and their acetates (No. 115, 1990)
Methyl bromide (No. 166, 1995)
Methylene chloride
(No. 32, 1984, 1st edition)
(No. 164, 1996, 2nd edition)
Methyl ethyl ketone (No. 143, 1992)
Methyl isobutyl ketone (No. 117, 1990)
Methylmercury (No. 101, 1990)
Methyl parathion (No. 145, 1992)
Methyl tertiary-butyl ether (No. 206, 1998)
Mirex (No. 44, 1984)
Morpholine (No. 179, 1996)
Mutagenic and carcinogenic chemicals, guide to short-term tests for detecting (No. 51, 1985)
Mycotoxins (No. 11, 1979)

Mycotoxins, selected: ochratoxins, trichothecenes, ergot (No. 105, 1990)
Nephrotoxicity associated with exposure to chemicals, principles and methods for the assessment of (No. 119, 1991)
Neurotoxicity associated with exposure to chemicals, principles and methods for the assessment of (No. 60, 1986)
Nickel (No. 108, 1991)
Nitrates, nitrites, and N-nitroso compounds (No. 5, 1978)[a]
Nitrogen oxides
(No. 4, 1977, 1st edition)[a]
(No. 188, 1997, 2nd edition)
2-Nitropropane (No. 138, 1992)
Noise (No. 12, 1980)[a]
Organophosphorus insecticides: a general introduction (No. 63, 1986)
Paraquat and diquat (No. 39, 1984)
Pentachlorophenol (No. 71, 1987)
Permethrin (No. 94, 1990)
Pesticide residues in food, principles for the toxicological assessment of (No. 104, 1990)
Petroleum products, selected (No. 20, 1982)
Phenol (No. 161, 1994)
d-Phenothrin (No. 96, 1990)
Phosgene (No. 193, 1997)
Phosphine and selected metal phosphides (No. 73, 1988)
Photochemical oxidants (No. 7, 1978)
Platinum (No. 125, 1991)
Polybrominated biphenyls (No. 152, 1994)
Polybrominated dibenzo-p-dioxins and dibenzofurans (No. 205, 1998)
Polychlorinated biphenyls and terphenyls
(No. 2, 1976, 1st edition)[a]
(No. 140, 1992, 2nd edition)
Polychlorinated dibenzo-p-dioxins and dibenzofurans (No. 88, 1989)
Polycyclic aromatic hydrocarbons, selected non-heterocyclic (No. 202, 1998)
Progeny, principles for evaluating health risks associated with exposure to chemicals during pregnancy (No. 30, 1984)
1-Propanol (No. 102, 1990)
2-Propanol (No. 103, 1990)
Propachlor (No. 147, 1993)
Propylene oxide (No. 56, 1985)
Pyrrolizidine alkaloids (No. 80, 1988)
Quintozene (No. 41, 1984)
Quality management for chemical safety testing (No. 141, 1992)
Radiofrequency and microwaves (No. 16, 1981)
Radionuclides, selected (No. 25, 1983)
Resmethrins (No. 92, 1989)
Synthetic organic fibres, selected (No. 151, 1993)
Selenium (No. 58, 1986)
Styrene (No. 26, 1983)
Sulfur oxides and suspended particulate matter (No. 8, 1979)
Tecnazene (No. 42, 1984)

---

[a]   Out of print